Handbook of Poisoning

Handbook of Poisoning:

Prevention, Diagnosis & Treatment

TWELFTH EDITION

ROBERT H. DREISBACH, MD, PhD

Clinical Professor of Environmental Health,
School of Public Health and Community Medicine,
University of Washington, Seattle,
and
Professor (Emeritus) of Pharmacology,
Stanford University School of Medicine,
Stanford, California

WILLIAM O. ROBERTSON, MD

Professor of Pediatrics,
School of Medicine,
University of Washington, Seattle,
and
Medical Director,
Seattle Poison Center,
Washington Poison Network

Appleton & Lange
Norwalk, Connecticut/Los Altos, California

Copyright © 1987 by Appleton & Lange
A Publishing Division of Prentice-Hall
Copyright © 1983 by Lange Medical Publications

87 88 89 90 / 5 4 3 2 1

Prentice-Hall of Australia, Pty. Ltd., Sydney
Prentice-Hall Canada, Inc.
Prentice-Hall Hispanoamericana, S.A., Mexico
Prentice-Hall of India Private Limited, New Delhi
Prentice-Hall International (UK) Limited, London
Prentice-Hall of Japan, Inc., Tokyo
Prentice-Hall of Southeast Asia (Pte.) Ltd., Singapore
Whitehall Books Ltd., Wellington, New Zealand
Editora Prentice-Hall do Brasil Ltda., Rio de Janeiro

Spanish Edition: Editorial El Manual Moderno, S.A. de C.V., Av. Sonora 206, Col. Hipodromo, 06100-Mexico, D.F.
Portuguese Edition: Atheneu Editora São Paulo Ltda., Rua Marconi, 131–2.o andar, 01047 São Paulo, Brazil
Polish Edition: Panstwowy Zaklad Wydawnictw Lekarskich, P.O. Box 379, 00-950 Warsaw 1, Poland
Japanese Edition: Hirokawa Publishing Company, 27-14, Hongo 3, Bunkyo-ku, Tokyo 113, Japan
Serbo-Croatian Edition: Savremena Administracija, Crnotravska 7-9. 11100 Belgrade, Yugoslavia

ISBN: 0-8385-3643-3

PRINTED IN THE UNITED STATES OF AMERICA

Table of Contents

Index to Tables

Preface

Handbook of Poisoning provides a concise summary of the diagnosis and treatment of poisoning for medical students, house officers, and practicing physicians. It is not intended to be encyclopedic; rather, it is designed as a guide and ready reference. The handbook contains listings of more extensive sources of information about poisons, as well as selected references for specific poisons.

Organization of the Book

Chapters 1–4 provide a grounding in the prevention, diagnosis, and treatment of poisoning. Chapter 5 considers the important medicolegal aspects of poisoning. Specific poisons are discussed in the remainder of the book and are organized into agricultural, industrial, household, medicinal, and natural hazards, since this method allows correlation of poisons with types of exposure. In some cases, chemically similar agents with varied uses appear in more than one section. Insofar as is possible, chemically and, in some cases, pharmacologically related agents have been grouped together.

To enable the physician to identify the toxic principle in a given proprietary preparation, brand-named products likely to be encountered clinically or whose composition is not obvious are listed in the index. This group includes many insecticides and medicinal agents.

New Features

The twelfth edition of *Handbook of Poisoning* has been substantially revised and includes the following new features:

- Sections on diagnosis and treatment revised and updated to reflect the latest procedures in use in emergency rooms and poison centers.

- Sections on water and electrolyte balance and acidosis simplified for easier use in emergencies.

- Significant reorganization of the section on agricultural poisons, with the addition of many new compounds.

- Addition of an index to tables following the Table of Contents.

- Reference lists restricted to useful recent articles plus essential older ones.

This book has been used by thousands of students and physicians all over the world since its first edition more than 30 years ago. It is now available in Spanish, Portuguese, Polish, Japanese, and Serbo-Croatian translations.

With the twelfth edition, Dr William O. Robertson joins Dr Robert H. Dreisbach as an author of this book. Both authors wish to thank all of those who have taken the time to offer helpful criticisms and suggestions for improvement of *Handbook of Poisoning*. Correspondence is always welcome and may be addressed to Dr Dreisbach at

University of Washington, SC-34
Seattle, WA 98195

Robert H. Dreisbach
William O. Robertson

Seattle
December, 1986

I. General Considerations

Prevention of Poisoning | 1

More than 12,000 deaths due to poisoning occur in the USA each year. Many of these deaths are avoidable regardless of whether the poisoning is purposeful or accidental, occupational or environmental, or carcinogenic or mutagenic. Prevention of poisoning requires adequate knowledge of the hazardous properties of substances by users.

When prescribing drugs, always be alert to their toxic potentialities so that the first signs will be recognized and proper action taken. Drugs should not be used during pregnancy unless maternal need overrides the risk to the fetus.

HOUSEHOLD POISONING

Safe Storage & Use
(1) All containers should have safety closures. Medicines, insecticides, and rodenticides should be stored in locked cabinets. If a locked cabinet is not available, a suitcase with a lock is satisfactory.

(2) Lye, polishes, kerosene, and other household chemicals should never be left on a low shelf or on the floor. Again, locked storage is best. Do not leave these materials exposed in the kitchen or bathroom.

(3) Dangerous solutions should never be left in drinking glasses or in beverage bottles. Store them only in their original containers.

(4) Combustion devices should be adequately vented.

(5) Inhalation of spray or fumes must be prevented during painting and application of insecticides.

(6) Unnecessary toxic substances, such as boric acid and unused medicines, should be discarded by being flushed down a drain.

(7) Carefully check the label of any medicine before taking. Do not put different tablets or capsules in the same bottle, and avoid transferring them to envelopes or purses for convenience.

Education
(1) Parents should be educated to the dangers present in medicines and household chemicals. All adults should be familiar with the concept of risk versus benefit in using chemicals at home, in the workplace, or in the environment. A poison label should appear on all dangerous

3

Table 1—1. Checklist of household poisons.

House

    Insecticides—All ant, roach, and moth poisons. Animal flea collars.

    Inflammables and extinguishers—

        Kerosene and gasoline

        Fire lighter—Methanol, petroleum hydrocarbons, denatured alcohol

        Fire starting tablets—Metaldehyde, methenamine

        Fire extinguishers—Carbon dioxide

    Cleaning supplies—

        Chlorinated hydrocarbons

        Solvent distillate

        Lye (sodium hydroxide)

        Ammonia

        Bleach—Sodium hypochlorite, oxalic acid

        Drain cleaner—Lye, sodium acid sulfate

        Rug cleaner—Chlorinated hydrocarbons

        Wallpaper cleaner—Kerosene

        Laundry ink—Aniline

    Medicines—

        Salicylates—Aspirin, methyl salicylate

        Acetaminophen

        Sedatives—Barbiturates, bromides, benzodiazepines, ethanol

        Antidepressants—Imipramine, amitriptyline, doxepin

        Antiepileptic agents—Barbiturates, hydantoins

        Antihistamines—"Cold" tablets and seasickness pills

        Cathartic pills—Strychnine, atropine, drastic cathartics

        Cough mixtures—Codeine, methadone, other opiates

        Nose drops—Ephedrine, Privine, Neo-Synephrine, etc

        Reducing or slimming tablets—Amphetamines, thyroid, digitalis

        Cardiac drugs—Digitalis, quinidine, etc

        Antiseptics—Boric acid, mercuric chloride, iodine, phenol

        Hematinics—Ferrous sulfate

        Liniment—Methyl salicylate, alcohols

        Drugs of abuse—Amphetamines, PCP, methadone, LSD, etc

    Cosmetics—

        Hair—Silver salts, anilines, potassium bromate, selenium sulfide

    Hobby—Toluene (cement), methanol (stencils), photography chemicals

Storeroom

    Paints and painting supplies—

        Paint—Thinner, lead, arsenic, chlorinated hydrocarbons

        Paint remover—Chlorinated hydrocarbons, acids, alkalies

        Lacquer—Ethyl acetate, amyl acetate, methanol

        Shellac—Methanol

        Wood bleach—Oxalic acid

    Pesticides—Moth balls (naphthalene, paradichlorophenol)

Yard or Storage (Garage)

    Insecticides—(Organic solvents used in some of these are also poisonous.)

        Chlordane and lindane

        Toxaphene

        Arsenic and lead

        Malathion, Diazinon

        Fumigants

        Nicotine

Table 1–1 (cont'd). Checklist of household poisons.

Yard or Storage (Garage) (cont'd)
  Rodenticides—
    Sodium fluoroacetate, phosphorus, thallium, barium
    Strychnine
    Methyl bromide
    Cyanides
  Plants (See also Tables 36–1 and 36–2.)—
    Foxglove—Digitalis
    Cherry—Cyanide
    Thorn apple—Atropine
    Mushrooms
    Oleander
    Poison ivy

medicines, including aspirin, soluble iron salts, and sedatives. Combinations of different drugs with or without alcohol may increase the hazard. A checklist of dangerous household chemicals and medicines (Table 1–1) should be given to parents when their children become mobile. The relative hazards of the various substances and the means of seeking emergency treatment should be explained.

(2) Parents must begin to teach their children at an early age the danger of touching, eating, or playing with medicines, pesticides, household chemicals, or plants. They should never refer to flavored drugs as candy, nor should they make the giving of a medication a game.

Benson BE et al: Warning labels: A source of toxicity information for parents. *Clin Pediatr* 1984;**23**:441.

Craft AW et al: Accidental childhood poisoning with household products. *Br Med J* 1984;**288**:682.

Dershewitz RA et al: Effectiveness of a health education program in a lower socioeconomic population: Replication of an ipecac guidance study. *Clin Pediatr* 1984;**23**:686.

Dine MS, McGovern ME: Intentional poisoning of children: An overlooked category of child abuse. *Pediatrics* 1982;**70**:32.

Fischler RS: Poisoning: A syndrome of child abuse. *Am Fam Physician* (Dec) 1983;**28**:103.

Kleoppel JW: Potential holiday poisonings. *Vet Hum Toxicol* 1985;**27**:113.

McIntire MS et al: Trends in childhood poisoning: A collaborative study 1970, 1975, 1980. *J Toxicol Clin Toxicol* 1983;**21**:321.

Pearn J et al: Accidental poisoning in childhood: Five-year urban population study with 15-year analysis of fatality. *Br Med J* 1984;**288**:44.

Poisoning among children—United States. *MMWR* 1983;**33**:129.

Vernberg K et al: The deterrent effect of poison-warning labels. *Am J Dis Child* 1984;**138**:1018.

AGRICULTURAL POISONS
(Insecticides, Rodenticides, Fungicides, Etc)

Persons exposed to agricultural poisons are divided into 2 groups: those who work with agricultural poisons during manufacture, preparation for use, storage, or application; and those who come in contact with these chemicals accidentally, either through improper storage, by entering sprayed areas, or by eating sprayed foods from which spray residues have not been removed. Poisoning can be prevented by giving attention to the cautionary measures listed below.

Storage of Poisons

(1) Poisons must be stored in well-marked containers with safety closures, preferably under lock and key.

(2) Mixtures of poisons with flour or cereals must not be stored near food. Sweet mixtures are the most dangerous. Warning labels on such mixtures should be obvious even to illiterate persons.

(3) Emptied containers must be burned immediately to destroy residual poisons. Cans should be opened before burning.

(4) Storage in food containers such as beverage bottles is extremely dangerous.

Protective Clothing & Equipment

(1) Use masks and exhaust ventilation during dry mixing.

(2) Wear protective clothing, goggles, and oil-resistant neoprene gloves when prolonged handling of poisons in petroleum oils or other organic solvents is necessary. Protective clothing should be removed and exposed skin washed thoroughly before eating.

(3) Wear respirators, goggles, protective clothing, and gloves during preparation and use of sprays, mists, or aerosols when skin contamination or inhalation may occur. Protective equipment made of rubber should be used in the handling of chlorinated hydrocarbons, and equipment made of neoprene or other oil-resistant materials should be employed for handling poisons in organic solvents. The indane derivatives and cholinesterase inhibitors are especially dangerous. Mix pesticides only in totally enclosed systems.

Other Protective Measures

(1) Always spray downwind. If wind velocity is insufficient, spraying should be discontinued to avoid contact with the mist.

(2) Avoid exposure for more than 8 hours per day in a closed area where an insecticide vaporizer is being operated. Such vaporizers *must* be adjusted to release not more than 1 g of lindane per 425 m^3 per 24 hours at a rate constant within 25%. No other insecticides are safe for

use in vaporizers. Vaporizers should never be used in living quarters or where food is stored, prepared, or served.

(3) Do not apply chlorinated or phosphate ester insecticides where body contact with residues is likely to occur.

(4) Food and forage plants should not be sprayed with insecticides unless the procedure used has been clearly shown not to leave a residue above tolerance limits.

(5) For protection of the consumer, specific tolerances have been established by the Food and Drug Administration, US Department of Health and Human Services, and represent levels above which foods are not allowed to be sold. These tolerances are maintained partly by field inspection and control of pesticide use and partly by analysis of selected portions of foods reaching the market.

Hayes WJ: *Pesticides Studied in Man*. Williams & Wilkins, 1982.
Rogan WJ: Persistent pesticides and polychlorinated biphenyls. *Annu Rev Public Health* 1983;**4**:381.

INDUSTRIAL CHEMICALS: RESPIRATORY & SKIN HAZARDS

In many states, the department of health or industrial safety has field inspectors who assist in establishing proper safeguards for workers and analyzing air in working areas.

Environmental Controls

(1) Dust-forming operations must be conducted in closed systems with local exhaust ventilation. Ordinary room ventilation is never sufficient to control air contamination.

(2) Hoods for local exhaust ventilation should enclose the process as completely as possible to prevent dispersion of contaminants.

(3) Materials should be transported by enclosed mechanical conveyors whenever possible.

(4) Areas where hazardous materials are used should have impervious floors and work tables to allow adequate cleaning and to prevent accumulations of hazardous dusts or liquids. Drains should be provided to allow frequent and thorough flushing.

(5) Spilled dusts should be removed by vacuum cleaning.

(6) Sweeping should be done only with wet or oiled sweeping compounds.

(7) Spilled liquids should be removed by flushing.

(8) Room ventilation should be provided by fresh air.

(9) Less toxic substances should be substituted wherever possible.

For example, toluene or xylene can be substituted for benzene in many operations.

(10) Control of temperature should be provided where decomposition to dangerous by-products is possible.

(11) Exposure limit values for work or ambient atmospheres have been established as permissible exposure limits by the Occupational Safety and Health Administration (OSHA) and the National Institute of Occupational Safety and Health (NIOSH) and as threshold limit values (TLVs) by the American Conference of Governmental Industrial Hygienists (ACGIH). The exposure limit given in this book is the lowest value published by any of these sources. Such established concentrations are ordinarily safe for an exposure time of 8 hours per day for 5 days per week. If the time of exposure is increased, then the safe exposure level is less. For gases, these concentrations are ordinarily given in parts per million parts (ppm) or in milligrams per cubic meter (mg/m³) of air. For particulates, concentrations are given only in mg/m³. Since the volume occupied by a given weight of a gas is dependent on the molecular weight, the following formula must be used to convert from ppm to mg/m³ (formula correct at 25 °C):

$$\text{mg/m}^3 = \frac{\text{ppm} \times \text{Molecular weight}}{24.5}$$

For example, the exposure limit of carbon tetrachloride, 5 ppm, represents a concentration of 32 mg/m³ (1 m³ = 35.3 cu ft).

Safe concentrations of substances in air can only be established by analysis, since in many instances the odor threshold is well above the exposure limit value (Table 1–2).

Table 1–2. Odor thresholds (ppm) for substances with odor thresholds greater than exposure limit.

Allyl chloride	25	Epichlorohydrin	10
Arsine	1	Ethanolamine	4
Benzene	100	Ethylene oxide	300
Bromine	3.5	Isopropyl amine	10
Carbon dioxide	None	Methanol	2000
Carbon monoxide	None	Methyl chloroform	500
Carbon tetrachloride	79	Methylene chloride	300
Chlorine	5	Nickel carbonyl	1
Chlorobromomethane	400	Nitromethane	200
Chloroform	200	Propylene oxide	200
Chloropicrin	1.1	n-Propyl nitrate	50
Diglycidyl ether	5	Tolylene-2,4-diisocyanate	0.4
1,1-Dimethyl hydrazine	6	Turpentine	200
Dioxane	200	Vinyl chloride	4100

Instructions for & Provision of Safety Equipment

Simple instructions for the use of safety equipment and of procedures for emergencies should be posted in areas in which hazardous chemicals are in use. Many institutions have special departments that are prepared to monitor hazardous operations and give instructions in the use of equipment and in maintaining safe working conditions.

(1) Workers should be trained to understand the hazards involved and to avoid exposure by proper use of safety equipment. They should be instructed to evacuate rooms in which spills of hazardous chemicals have occurred. If possible, electrical equipment should be disconnected if volatile explosive substances are involved. Decontamination of spills should be undertaken only by personnel with adequate safety equipment.

(2) Gloves, goggles, aprons, and protective clothing should be used wherever necessary.

(3) Eye fountains and showers must be provided for rapid removal of corrosive materials.

(4) Protective clothing should be laundered daily.

(5) For operations where local control of contaminants is impractical, supplied-air masks, gas masks, or self-contained oxygen helmets should be provided.

(6) Supplied-air masks or gas masks should be available for emergency use wherever dangerous substances are being used. A safety harness and lifeline are necessary to evacuate personnel from areas that may become dangerously contaminated.

(7) Workers handling poisonous substances should be required to wash properly before eating or smoking. A change of clothing after work also should be required.

(8) Workers should be instructed to report for examination at the first evidence of illness or injury.

Adequate Medical Program

(1) Workers in hazardous occupations must be examined every 6 months to 1 year as a check against failures in control measures. Examinations should be made more often during periods of high risk of exposure to cumulative poisons. Examinations should include complete blood count and urinalysis and, if possible, analysis of blood and urine for the particular hazardous agent in use. Workers in dusty trades should have chest x-rays yearly.

(2) Facilities should be inspected weekly or monthly in order to detect failures or inadequacies in control methods. Adequate inspection may require continuous or intermittent sampling of air.

(3) Preplacement physical examinations should be used to detect chronic respiratory, kidney, liver, or other systemic disease. Individu-

als with any disease should not be exposed to toxic fumes. A preemployment urinalysis for drug abuse is also useful.

Analysis of trace metals for occupationally exposed workers. *MMWR* 1984;**33**:664.

Biological Abstracts. Biosciences Information Services. Serial publication. Abstracts on health effects of environmental pollutants.

Burgess WA: *Recognition of Health Hazards in Industry*. Wiley, 1981.

Cherry N et al: The acute behavioural effects of solvent exposure. *J Soc Occup Med* 1983;**33**:13.

Clayton GD, Clayton FE (editors): *Patty's Industrial Hygiene and Toxicology*, 3rd ed. 4 vols. Wiley, 1981, 1982.

Dangerous Properties of Industrial Materials Report. Van Nostrand Reinhold. Bimonthly serial.

Gregersen P et al: Neurotoxic effects of organic solvents in exposed workers. *Am J Ind Med* 1984;**5**:201.

Guengerich FP et al: Enzymatic activation of chemicals to toxic metabolites. *CRC Crit Rev Toxicol* 1985;**14**:259.

Himmelstein JS et al: The right to know about toxic exposures: Implications for physicians. *N Engl J Med* 1984;**312**:687.

Hunter D (editor): *The Diseases of Occupations*, 6th ed. Little, Brown, 1979.

LaDou J: Potential occupational health hazards in the microelectronics industry. *Scand J Work Environ Health* 1983;**9**:42.

Last JM: *Preventive Medicine and Public Health*, 11th ed. Appleton-Century-Crofts, 1980.

Leading work-related diseases and injuries—United States. *MMWR* 1983;**32**:24.

Lotti M et al: Occupational peripheral neuropathies. *West J Med* 1982;**137**:493.

National Institute for Occupational Safety and Health: *The Industrial Environment: Its Evaluation and Control*. US Department of Health, Education, and Welfare, 1973.

National Institute for Occupational Safety and Health: *Occupational Health Guidelines for Chemical Hazards*. DHHS Publication No. (NIOSH) 81–123. US Department of Health and Human Services, 1981.

National Institute for Occupational Safety and Health: *Pocket Guide to Chemical Hazards*. DHEW Publication No. (NIOSH) 78–210. US Department of Health, Education, and Welfare, 1978.

Omenn GS, Morris SL: Occupational hazards to health care workers. *Am J Ind Med* 1984;**6**:129.

Pond SM: Effects on the liver of chemicals encountered in the workplace. *West J Med* 1982;**137**:506.

Sax NI: *Dangerous Properties of Industrial Materials*, 6th ed. Van Nostrand Reinhold, 1984.

Schrag SD, Dixon RL: Occupational exposures associated with male reproductive dysfunction. *Annu Rev Pharmacol Toxicol* 1985;**25**:567.

Sewer collapse and toxic illness in sewer repairmen—Ohio. *MMWR* 1981;**30**:89.

Sheppard D: Occupational asthma. *West J Med* 1982;**137**:480.

Sittig M: *Handbook of Toxic and Hazardous Chemicals and Carcinogens*. Noyes, 1985.

Threshold Limit Values for Chemical Substances and Physical Agents in the Workroom Environment, With Intended Changes. American Conference of

Governmental Industrial Hygienists, PO Box 1937, Cincinnati, OH 45201. Annual publication.

Whorton MD: Male occupational reproductive hazards. *West J Med* 1982;**137**:521.

CANCER

A sizable part of the present incidence of cancer appears to be the result of chemical carcinogenesis; estimates range from 4 to 60% or more. The Occupational Safety and Health Administration (OSHA) has established zero tolerance levels for working atmospheres for the following substances suspected of being carcinogens in humans: 2-acetyl-aminofluorene, 4-aminodiphenyl, benzidine (and its salts), 3,3'-di-chlorobenzidine (and its salts), 4-dimethylaminoazobenzene, alpha-naphthylamine, beta-naphthylamine, 4-nitrobiphenyl, N-nitro-sodimethylamine, beta-propiolactone, bis-chloromethyl ether, methyl-chloromethyl ether, 4,4'-methylene(bis)-2-chloroaniline, ethylene-imine (see NIOSH: *Registry of Toxic Effects of Chemical Substances*). Table 1–3 lists a number of suspected or confirmed environmental carcinogens. A number of substances can be considered possible carcinogens on the basis of their structural similarity to vinyl chloride: bromoprene, epibromohydrin, epichlorohydrin, perbromoethylene, perchloroethylene, tribromoethylene, styrene (vinyl benzene), vinyl bromide, vinylidene bromide, vinylidene chloride.

Becker CE, Coye MJ: Recent advances in occupational cancer. *J Toxicol Clin Toxicol* 1984;**22**:195.

CIP Bulletin. Carcinogen Information Program, PO Box 6057, St. Louis, MO 63139.

Coombs MM: Chemical carcinogenesis: A view at the end of the first half century. *J Pathol* 1980;**130**:117.

Crump KS, Guess HA: Drinking water and cancer: Review of recent epidemiological findings and assessment of risks. *Annu Rev Public Health* 1982;**3**:339.

Dubrow R, Wegman DH: Cancer and occupation in Massachusetts: A death certificate study. *Am J Ind Med* 1984;**6**:207.

Ernst P: Known occupational carcinogens and their significance. *Can Med Assoc J* 1984;**130**:863.

Hooper K: Epigenetic carcinogens: Problems with identification and risk estimation. *J Toxicol Clin Toxicol* 1984;**22**:283.

IARC Monographs on the Evaluation of Carcinogenic Risks of Chemicals in Human Beings. Serial publication.

Landrigan PJ, Rinsky RA: The application of epidemiology to the prevention of occupational cancer. *J Toxicol Clin Toxicol* 1984;**22**:209.

Leading work-related diseases and injuries—United States. *MMWR* 1983;**33**:125.

National Institute of Occupational Safety and Health: *Registry of Toxic Effects of Chemical Substances.* US Government Printing Office. Annual publication.

Table 1–3. Environmental substances carcinogenic for humans.*

Target Organ	Confirmed	Suspected
Bone		Beryllium.
Brain	Vinyl chloride.	
Endometrium	Estrogens.	
Esophagus	Alcohol, lye, tobacco smoking.	
Gastrointestinal tract	Asbestos.	Smoked meats.
Hematopoietic tissue (leukemia)	Alkylating agents: cyclophospha-mide, melphalan, busulfan; ben-zene; styrene butadiene, other syn-thetic rubbers.	
Kidney	Coke oven emissions, phenacetin.	Lead.
Larynx	Alcohol, asbestos, chromium, mus-tard gas, tobacco smoking.	
Liver	Aflatoxin, alcohol, anabolic ste-roids, contraceptive steroids, vinyl chloride.	Aldrin, dieldrin, hep-tachlor, chlordecone, mirex, DDT, carbon tetrachloride, chloro-form, PCBs, trichlor-ethylene.
Lung	Arsenic, asbestos, bis(chloromethyl) ether, chloromethyl methyl ether, chromium, coke oven emissions, mustard gas, nickel, polycyclic hy-drocarbons, soots and tars, tobacco smoking, uranium, vinyl chloride.	Beryllium, cadmium, chloroprene, lead.
Lymphatic tissue		Arsenic, benzene.
Mouth	Alcohol, betel, limes, tobacco.	
Nasal mucosa	Chromium, formaldehyde, isopro-pyl alcohol, leather manufacture, nickel, wood dust.	
Pancreas		Benzidine, PCBs.
Peritoneum	Asbestos.	
Pharynx	Alcohol, tobacco smoking.	
Pleural cavity	Asbestos.	
Prostate	Cadmium.	
Reticuloendothelium	Immunosuppressive drugs.	
Scrotum	Polycyclic hydrocarbons, soots and tars.	Chloroprene.
Skin	Arsenic, cutting oils, coke oven emissions, polycyclic hydrocarbons, soots and tars.	
Urinary bladder	Alkylating agents: cyclophospha-mide, melphalan; 4-aminobiphenyl; benzidine; chlornaphazine; β-naphthylamine; tobacco smoking.	Auramine, magenta, 4-nitrodiphenyl.
Vagina	Estrogens.	

*Modified from Key MM et al (editors): *Occupational Diseases, A Guide to Their Recognition.* DHEW Publication No. (NIOSH) 77–181. US Department of Health, Education, and Welfare, 1977.

Peters JM et al: Occupational epidemiology: Detection of cancer in the work-place. *West J Med* 1982;**137**:555.

Robbins A et al: Conference on the role of metals in carcinogenesis. *Environ Health Perspect* 1981;**40**:1.

Rosenstock L: Occupational cancer: Clinical interpretation and application of scientific evidence. *J Toxicol Clin Toxicol* 1984;**22**:261.

Sax NI: *Cancer Causing Chemicals*. Van Nostrand Reinhold, 1981.

Wegman DH: Approaches to surveillance of occupational cancer. *J Toxicol Clin Toxicol* 1984;**22**:239.

AIR POLLUTION
& ENVIRONMENTAL CONTAMINATION

No clear-cut relationship has been found between air pollution and acute, self-limited disease. However, not only do fatal illnesses increase in air pollution disasters such as occurred in Donora, Pennsylvania, in 1948 and in London in 1952, but an increase in the incidence of fatalities can also be shown in relation to the intensity of community air pollution. For example, in New York City, during a period of stable inversion with increase in sulfur dioxide concentration and particulate density, deaths increased about 10% for a total of 300 excess deaths in the 7-day period from November 23 to 29, 1966.

Air pollution may aggravate preexisting respiratory and cardiac conditions and is responsible for some of the present incidence of cancer. Those conditions most likely to be affected by air pollution episodes are chronic bronchitis, chronic obstructive pulmonary disease, pulmonary emphysema, bronchial asthma, and coronary vascular disease. The physician is faced with the problem of determining whether to take steps to ameliorate the possible effects of air pollution on patients with the above conditions.

Lead, carcinogens, halogenated hydrocarbons, and pesticides are the chief environmental contaminants under discussion at present. These and other individual air pollutants and environmental contaminants are discussed elsewhere in this book (see Index):

Carbon monoxide	Organic compounds
Hydrogen sulfide	Oxidants
Lead	Particulates
Nitrogen oxides	Sulfur oxides

Berger BB: Water and wastewater quality control and the public health. *Annu Rev Public Health* 1982;**3**:359.

Brown SL: Quantitative risk assessment of environmental hazards. *Annu Rev Public Health* 1985;**6**:247.

Goyer RA: Health effects of toxic chemical waste dumps. *Environ Health Perspect* 1983;**48:**1.

Harris RH et al: Hazardous waste disposal: Emerging technologies and public policies to reduce public health risks. *Annu Rev Public Health* 1985;**6:**269.

Holmberg B et al: Mutagenicity and carcinogenicity of air pollutants. *Environ Health Perspect* 1983;**47:**1.

Honicky RE et al: Symptoms of respiratory illness in young children and the use of wood-burning stoves for indoor heating. *Pediatrics* 1985;**75:**587.

Kirsch LS: The problem of indoor pollutants. *Environment* (March) 1983;**25:**16.

Landrigan PJ: Occupational and community exposure to toxic metals: Lead, cadmium, mercury, and arsenic. *West J Med* 1982:**137:**531.

Lebowitz MD: Health effects of indoor pollutants. *Annu Rev Public Health* 1983;**4:**203.

Rom WN: *Environmental and Occupational Medicine.* Little, Brown, 1983.

Samuel HD: Chronic disease in the workplace and the environment. *Arch Environ Health* 1984;**39:**133.

Stark AD et al: Hazardous waste sites: Will the community call on you to assess their effect? (Editorial.) *Postgrad Med* (March) 1985;**77:**13.

Zervos C et al: Exposure assessment: Problems and perspectives. *J Toxicol Clin Toxicol* 1983;**21:**1.

SUICIDAL POISONING

Recognition of Suicidal Tendencies

A. Symptoms and Signs of Depression:

1. Insomnia–True insomnia may be an early symptom of depression. The patient is unable to go to sleep at night or may awaken during the night or early in the morning and be unable to go back to sleep.

2. Anorexia–The patient may have a striking history of weight loss and may complain that food no longer "tastes good" or that it "tastes like straw."

3. Lack of interest in surroundings–The patient shows no interest in occupation, friends, or hobbies. This person may quit a job and at the same time profess an interest in continuing the same type of work.

B. Medical Evaluation: An evaluation should be made of every patient who mentions or attempts suicide or is depressed. Hospitalization may be necessary for proper evaluation.

Prevention

(1) The physician should avoid prescribing sedatives, hypnotics, or tranquilizers for depressed or possibly suicidal persons, since they are responsible for more than 20% of suicidal deaths. Relatives should be informed of possible suicidal tendencies in a patient.

(2) Persons who have made unsuccessful attempts at suicide should have adequate follow-up psychiatric therapy.

Deykin EY et al: Nonfatal suicidal and life-threatening behavior among 13–17-year-old adolescents seeking emergency medical care. *Am J Public Health* 1985;**85**:90.
Kessel N: Patients who take overdoses. *Br Med J* 1985;**290**:1297.
Prescott LF et al: Drugs prescribed for self poisoners. *Br Med J* 1985;**290**:1633.
Stern TA et al: Life-threatening drug overdose. *JAMA* 1984;**251**:1983.

TERATOGENS: DRUG & CHEMICAL INJURY TO THE FETUS

Evidence for the safety of drugs must be established before they are used during pregnancy. Self-administration of drugs and chemicals should be discouraged during the childbearing years, since pregnancy may not be recognized during the important first trimester, when fetal injury commonly occurs.

Drugs Especially to Be Avoided During First Trimester

All drugs, including prescription drugs, over-the-counter drugs, caffeine, alcohol, and tobacco and other drugs of abuse, should be avoided in the first trimester of pregnancy unless maternal need overrides the hazard to the fetus. The following are known to be hazardous:

A. Antineoplastic Agents: (Anomalies and abortion.) Aminopterin, chlorambucil, melphalan, methotrexate, radioiodine, cyclophosphamide, DON, 6-azauridine, fluorouracil.

B. Antihistamines and Antinauseants: (Anomalies.) Chlorcyclizine, cyclizine, meclizine.

C. New or Incompletely Studied Drugs: (Check package literature before prescribing.) Carbamazepine, cholestyramine, furosemide, pargyline, phenylbutazone, propranolol, metronidazole.

D. Antibiotics: (Anomalies.) Amphotericin B, mitomycin.

Drugs to Be Avoided Throughout Pregnancy & Neonatal Period

A. Sex Hormones: (Masculinization and advanced bone age.) Androgens, estrogens, progestogens, anabolic steroids.

B. Acne Medication: (Microcephalus, hydrocephalus, heart defects, other major abnormalities.) Retinoids, Accutane.

C. Antithyroid Drugs: (Goiter, mental retardation.) Potassium iodide, propylthiouracil, methimazole.

D. Corticosteroids: Cleft palate.

E. Antidiabetic Agents: (Anomalies.) Excess insulin (from hypoglycemia), acetohexamide, chlorpropamide, phenformin, tolbutamide.

F. Anticonvulsants: Phenytoin (mental retardation, heart defects, cleft palate, midfacial defects, finger abnormalities—the "phenytoin syndrome"), valproic acid (multiple malformations including neural tube defects).

G. Chemotherapeutic Agents: Streptomycin (deafness), sulfonamides (kernicterus), chloramphenicol (death), novobiocin (hyperbilirubinemia), erythromycin (liver damage?), nitrofurantoin (hemolysis), tetracyclines (inhibition of bone growth, discoloration of teeth), chloroquine (retinal damage), quinine (thrombocytopenia).

H. Anticoagulants: (Fetal death or hemorrhage.) Dicumarol, ethyl biscoumacetate, warfarin.

I. Vitamin K: Hyperbilirubinemia.

J. Central Nervous System Drugs: Morphine and heroin (death, convulsions, tremors), meprobamate (retarded development), phenobarbital (bleeding), phenothiazines (hyperbilirubinemia).

K. Cardiovascular Drugs: Ammonium chloride (acidosis), hexamethonium (neonatal ileus), reserpine (nasal congestion, depression), thiazides (thrombocytopenia).

L. Analgesics: Salicylates (neonatal bleeding), acetaminophen (liver injury).

M. Nicotine and Alcohol: Effects on growth and mental development.

N. Drugs and Chemicals Dangerous to Nursing Infants: All drugs and chemicals absorbed by the mother appear in the breast milk to some extent. Most of these have little effect on the nursing infant because they appear in relatively small amounts in the milk. Heroin addiction in the mother is associated with withdrawal in the infant whether or not the infant nurses.

Barlow SM, Sullivan FM: *Reproductive Hazards of Industrial Chemicals.* Academic Press, 1982.

Briggs GG et al: *Drugs in Pregnancy and Lactation.* Williams & Wilkins, 1983.

Clarkson TW et al: Reproductive and developmental toxicity of metals. *Scand J Work Environ Health* 1985;**11**:145.

Rao KS, Schwetz BA: Reproductive toxicity of environmental agents. *Annu Rev Public Health* 1982;**3**:1.

Savitz DA et al: Survey of reproductive hazards among oil, chemical, and atomic workers exposed to halogenated hydrocarbons. *Am J Ind Med* 1984;**6**:253.

Schilling S, Lalich NR: Maternal occupation and industry and the pregnancy outcome of US married women, 1980. *Public Health Rep* 1984;**99**:152.

Shepard TS: *Catalog of Teratogenic Agents,* 5th ed. Johns Hopkins Univ Press, 1986.

DRUG-INDUCED REACTIONS & FATALITIES

Drug-induced reactions can occur with drug abuse or with medical or dental treatment. Prevention of drug reactions due to therapeutic use of drugs is discussed below; drug abuse is considered in Chapter 3.

Prevention of drug fatalities should be one of the physician's paramount concerns. Dosage errors due to mistakes in reading or writing decimal places can have devastating effects. The physician should continually evaluate the need for and appropriateness of any drug therapy and should be alert to recognize the early signs of drug reaction. Laboratory procedures for monitoring a drug or the effects of a drug must be used for maximum safety.

Fatalities are uncommon (3.6% of hospital deaths in one series), and potentially dangerous therapy seldom results in a medical catastrophe. Thus, the physician can be lulled into a false sense of security when using dangerous drugs. The potentially most lethal drugs are intravenous medications of all sorts, depressants, penicillins, anticoagulants, cardiac drugs, potassium chloride and other potassium salts, diuretics, and insulin.

Dahiya U, Noronha P: Drug-induced acute dystonic reactions in children. *Postgrad Med* (Apr) 1984;**75**:286.

Davies DM: *Textbook of Adverse Drug Reactions.* Oxford Univ Press, 1981.

Dukes MNG (editor): *Meyler's Side Effects of Drugs,* 10th ed. Excerpta Medica, 1984.

Dukes MNG: *Side Effects of Drugs.* Excerpta Medica. Annual publication.

Garriott JC et al: Death in the dental chair: Three drug fatalities in dental patients. *J Toxicol Clin Toxicol* 1982;**19**:987.

Kramer MS et al: Adverse drug reactions in general pediatric outpatients. *J Pediatr* 1985;**106**:305.

Pentel P: Toxicity of over-the-counter stimulants. *JAMA* 1984;**252**:1898.

Podrid PJ: Aggravation of ventricular arrhythmia: A drug-induced complication. *Drugs* 1985;**29(Suppl 4)**:33.

Rawlins MD: Postmarketing surveillance of adverse reactions to drugs. *Br Med J* 1984;**288**:879.

Ruskin JN et al: Antiarrhythmic drugs: A possible cause of out-of-hospital cardiac arrest. *N Engl J Med* 1983;**309**:1302.

Ryan AJ: Causes and remedies for drug misuse and abuse by athletes. *JAMA* 1984;**252**:517.

Stephan P et al: Drug-induced Parkinsonism in the elderly. *Lancet* 1984;**2**:1082.

Vaino H: Inhalation anesthetics, anticancer drugs and sterilants as chemical hazards in hospitals. *Scand J Work Environ Health* 1982;**8**:94.

DRUG & CHEMICAL INTERACTIONS

Chronic exposure to many drugs and chemicals induces greater production of hepatic microsomal drug-metabolizing enzymes, with the result that drugs and other substances metabolized in the liver are processed more rapidly. Some drugs are metabolized to less active or inactive metabolites and hence are less active in the presence of a liver enzyme inducer: barbiturates, coumarin anticoagulants, phenytoin, digitoxin, desipramine, antipyrine, aminopyrine, phenylbutazone, amphetamine, adrenocorticosteroids, estrogens, and progestogens. If the dosage of a drug is increased to compensate for the concurrent administration of an inducer and the inducer is later withdrawn, drug toxicity may occur. Pregnancy has occurred in women taking estrogen-progestogens who have been given rifampin. Other drugs and chemicals are metabolized to more active or toxic substances; hence, in the presence of a liver enzyme inducer, the toxicity of these substances is increased. The pesticide Guthion is not active as a cholinesterase inhibitor as such but must be metabolized in the body to the active substance. In the presence of induced liver enzymes, Guthion is more toxic. The hepatic toxicity of acetaminophen depends on metabolism to toxic products, and in the presence of induced liver enzymes, toxicity can occur at lower doses of acetaminophen. The toxicity of phenacetin for the hematopoietic system is the result of its metabolism to toxic products, and this toxicity is increased in the presence of induced liver enzymes. Since most environmental carcinogens enter the body as procarcinogens, the possibility exists that in the presence of induced metabolizing enzymes, a greater fraction of such procarcinogens will be converted, increasing the carcinogenicity.

Several drugs, including methylphenidate, oxyphenbutazone, methandrostenolone, phenyramidol, nortriptyline, allopurinol, and disulfiram, depress drug metabolism in general.

Pharmacologic interactions of other drugs and chemicals will be considered in each chapter and are ordinarily included only once, either as inducer or as recipient.

Hansten PD: *Drug Interactions*, 5th ed. Lea & Febiger, 1984.

Emergency Management of Poisoning | 2

With a case of known or suspected poisoning, the physician must first activate routine life-support measures—airway, cardiac support, etc—if necessary and then direct attention to other aspects of the case. Any available historical information should be obtained; further inquiries may be necessary later. The patient and any materials accompanying the patient should be examined for evidence that may clarify the problem. If, for example, an overdose is suspected and tablets or capsules have been found, the drugs can be identified from the manufacturer's drug imprint on them.

In order to treat poisoning properly when called upon in an emergency, the physician must possess some special knowledge and equipment. First of all, a knowledge of adequate emergency treatment is essential. If called by telephone, the physician must decide quickly if first-aid treatment is necessary and be able to give instructions for appropriate measures (see Inside Front Cover). After the type of exposure (inhalation, skin contact, etc) has been determined and procedures to minimize further absorption instituted, an attempt must be made to identify the poison. If the label does not give the ingredients or if the container is not available, then all known information (physical state [eg, liquid], odor, type of container, trade name, manufacturer's drug imprint [on tablets or capsules], use, presence of poison label) must be obtained in an effort to determine the toxic nature of the poison (Table 3–1). If available, the container with its contents should be brought with the patient for further attempts at identification. Vomitus should be brought for the same reason.

After first-aid measures (see Table 2–1) have been instituted, definitive or supportive treatment must be planned. This usually involves bringing the patient by car or ambulance to an emergency room or to the doctor's office. The physician or the staff may need to arrange transportation by either ambulance or taxi (list phone number on Inside Back Cover) if transportation is not already available. The emergency room should be alerted when transportation has been arranged.

While awaiting the arrival of the patient, the physician should try to identify the poison from the information given. For this purpose, thorough familiarity with the index of this book and other information sources is helpful (see p 32). The telephone number of a functioning

Table 2—1. Summary of emergency management of poisoning.

I. When notified that poisoning has occurred—
1. Give first-aid advice (see Inside Front and Back Covers).
2. Give instructions to save suspected poison in original container and place vomitus in a clean jar or plastic bag. Bring specimens with patient for possible identification (see p 31).
3. Provide for transportation to emergency treatment center and alert the center.

II. Maintain respiration and control shock (see pp 56 and 66).

III. Identify poison if possible (Table 3—1), but do not delay adequate control of respiration and blood pressure.

IV. Remove poison to minimize further absorption and injury—
1. Ingested poisons—
   a. Give emetics (see p 21) or perform gastric lavage (see p 24).
   b. Give activated charcoal (see p 25).
   c. Give milk or liquid detergent if syrup of ipecac or activated charcoal is not available.
2. Injected poisons—Immobilize patient. Give antidote.
3. Snakebite (see Chapter 33)—
   a. Immobilize patient immediately. Do not use any form of cooling.
   b. Give specific antiserum as soon as possible.
   c. To move patient, carry on a stretcher as gently as possible.
4. Skin or eye contamination—Flood with running water for 15 minutes.
5. Inhaled poisons—Remove from exposure and give O_2 or artificial respiration as necessary.
6. Poison by rectum—Give enema.

V. Give specific antidote, if available, while proceeding with the removal of the poison. Toxic antidotes should not be used unless positive identification of the poison has been made.

VI. Give supportive treatment (see p 46).

---

poison information center should also be available (list telephone number on Inside Back Cover). The local or regional poison center can supply information about ingredients of the poison, specific toxic consequences, and details of management.

Before sending a patient to an emergency room, the physician must check the facilities to be sure they are adequate for the treatment of poisoning. A suitable list of equipment and supplies is given in Tables 2–2 and 2–3. These or adequate substitutes should be available in any emergency station or hospital. No delay can be tolerated in obtaining necessary equipment or drugs. The physician must also know how to use the equipment properly and must be certain that the personnel in the emergency room are adequately trained.

The emergency management of poisoning is aimed at maintaining life and preventing absorption of the poison beyond that amount which the body can safely detoxify or which can be effectively antagonized by antidotes. This can be accomplished by delaying absorption and removing the poison from the body.

INGESTED POISONS

The comparative efficacy of gastric lavage versus emesis for the removal of ingested poisons is controversial. The prompt use of syrup of ipecac, 15–30 mL orally, is safe and effective.

Emergency Medical Measures

(1) Maintain respiration and circulation (see pp 57 and 66). If patient is drowsy or in shock, administration of oral fluids is hazardous.

(2) Induce emesis by giving 15–30 mL (1–2 tablespoons) of syrup of ipecac orally followed by $\frac{1}{2}$ glass of water. Repeat in 20 minutes if not effective initially. If syrup of ipecac is not available, liquid detergent can be used as an emetic.

(3) Give activated charcoal (see p 25).

(4) In patients with depressed respiration or if emesis is not produced, perform gastric lavage cautiously—or not at all after poisoning with corrosives or kerosene (see p 24).

Treatment

The treatment of acute poisoning consists of the application of the following general procedures as rapidly as possible: (1) maintain vital functions (see pp 57 and 66), (2) remove poison, and (3) delay absorption.

A. Emesis:

1. Indications–Induction of emesis by syrup of ipecac is possibly more effective than gastric lavage in removing swallowed poisons. If emesis occurs within 1 hour after ingestion of a poison, 30–60% of the poison may be returned; emesis after 1 hour may yield less than 20% of the poison. Vomiting may be associated with aspiration of gastric contents, and aspiration of hydrocarbons is dangerous. However, this occurs so infrequently that emesis is advised if the patient is conscious and a significantly toxic hydrocarbon, eg, parathion, is involved.

2. Contraindications–Do not induce emesis if the patient is drowsy or unconscious; in such cases, if a swallowed poison must be removed, gastric lavage should be performed following insertion of a cuffed endotracheal tube. Do not induce emesis if the patient has ingested any of the following:

a. Acids or alkalies–Emesis increases the likelihood of gastric perforation.

b. Convulsants–Vomiting may induce convulsions.

3. Materials–Syrup of ipecac is considered sufficiently safe that it can be kept in the home for administration to children when emesis is indicated. Liquid detergent is also an effective emetic. Syrup of ipecac is supplied in 30-mL (1-oz) containers. It is not effective after activated charcoal has been used. *Do not use* fluidextract of ipecac. Apomorphine is too hazardous for routine use.

Table 2–2. List of drugs useful in treatment of poisoning.

Drug	Use
N-Acetylcysteine (Mucomyst), 20%*	Acetaminophen
Aminophylline, 250 mg*	Propranolol
Ammonium chloride, 30 mL, 120 meq*	Phencyclidine, amphetamine
Ammonium chloride, 0.9%, 500 mL	Phencyclidine, amphetamine
Amyl nitrite, 0.3 mL, breakable*†	Cyanide
Antihistamine, in tablet form, 10 tabs	Bee sting
Anti-snakebite serum, polyvalent, 10 mL*	North American snakes
Atropine sulfate, 2 mg† (ampules)	Phosphate ester insecticides
Botulism antitoxin, 20,000 units*	Botulism
Bretylium, 500 mg*	Cardiac arrest
Calcium disodium edetate, 5 mL, 1 g*	Lead
Calcium gluconate, 10 mL, 1 g*	Fluoride, black widow spider
Charcoal, activated, 25–50 g (See p 25.)	Adsorbent
Dantrolene, 20 mg*	Hyperthermia
Deferoxamine, 500 mg*	Iron
Dextrose, 50%*	Cerebral edema
Dextrose, 5%, 1L*	Fluid replacement
Dextrose, 5% in normal saline, 1L*	Fluid replacement
Diazepam (Valium), 5 mg/mL in 2 mL	Anticonvulsant
Dimercaprol (BAL), 5 mL, 10% in oil*	Arsenic, mercury
Diphenhydramine (Benadryl), 10 mL, 100 mg*†	Bee sting, anaphylaxis
Distilled water, 10 mL*	Diluent
Epinephrine, 1 mL, 1 mg*	Sensitivity reactions
Ethanol, 95%	Methanol
Ethanol, 5% in normal saline, 1L*	Methanol
Fluorescein solution, 2% (sterile)	Eye contamination
Furosemide, 20 mg*	Diuretic
Glucagon, 1 mg*	Propranolol
Ipecac, syrup of, 60 mL	Emetic
Isoproterenol, 0.2 mg*	Propranolol
Lidocaine, 1 g*	Cardiac arrest
Mannitol, 20% in 500 mL*	Cerebral edema
Methylene blue, 50 mL, 0.5 g*	Methemoglobinemia
Milk, evaporated, 1 can, and opener†	Acids
Milk of magnesia, 1 L	Acids
Morphine sulfate, 10 mg*	Pain
Naloxone (Narcan), 0.4 mg in 1 mL* and 0.04 mg in 2 mL*	Narcotic antagonist
Norepinephrine bitartrate, 4 mL, 8 mg*†	Cardiac arrest
Paraldehyde	Acute alcoholic mania
Penicillamine, 250-mg capsules	Lead, copper
Pentobarbital sodium, 0.5 g, 5-mL ampule and 30-mL vial*‡	Anticonvulsant
Phenobarbital sodium, 2 mL, 0.3 g*‡	Anticonvulsant

*In ampules; at least 6 should be available.
†Must be available for immediate use.
‡One of these anticonvulsants must be available at all times.

Table 2–2 (cont'd). List of drugs useful in treatment of poisoning.

Drug	Use
Phenytoin (Dilantin), 100 mg*	Arrhythmias
Physostigmine, 2 mg in 2 mL*	Atropine, anticholinergics
Potassium chloride, 20 meq in 10 mL	Electrolyte replacement
Pralidoxime, 1 g	Phosphate ester insecticides
Prednisolone, 20 mg/mL* and 100 mg/mL*	Cerebral edema
Procainamide, 1 g*	Cardiac arrest
Propranolol, 1 mg*	Arrhythmias
Pyridoxine, 1 g in 10 mL*	Mushrooms, sulfides, isoniazid
Sodium bicarbonate, 7.5%, 50 mL*	Acidosis
Sodium chloride solution, isotonic, 1 L*	Fluid replacement
Sodium nitrite, 10 mL, 3%*†	Cyanide
Sodium sulfate, 1 lb†	Barium, cathartic
Sodium thiosulfate, 25%, 50 mL*†	Cyanide, bleaching solution
Starch, 1 lb†	Iodine
Succinylcholine chloride, 2%, 10 mL*	Anticonvulsant
Thiopental sodium, 500 mg*‡	Anticonvulsant
Urea, 50%*	Sulfides
Vitamin K$_1$ emulsion, 1 mL, 50 mg*	Dicumarol, warfarin

*In ampules; at least 6 should be available.

†Must be available for immediate use.

‡One of these anticonvulsants must be available at all times.

Table 2–3. Emergency equipment for treatment of poisoning.

Gastric lavage: Mouth gag; gastric tubes No. 22 and No. 32; and Asepto syringe to fit (see p 25). Levin tube to fit Asepto syringe.

Hypodermic syringes, 2-, 10-, and 20-mL, with needles sizes 20, 22, and 24.

Oxygen inhaler: Oronasal masks (large, medium, small), rebreathing bag, tubing, regulator, humidifier, and oxygen tank.

Oropharyngeal airways (sizes 1, 3, 5) and endotracheal tubes (see p 58).

Urethral catheters (sizes 12F, 16F, and 20F) and suction apparatus.

Resuscitation apparatus.

Tracheostomy set (see p 59).

Rubber-band tourniquet, 1 X 60 cm (½ X 24 inch).

Intravenous infusion set (including polyethylene tubing in various sizes).

Transfusion equipment.

Sterile cutdown set to expose veins for emergency intravenous injection.

Lumbar puncture kit.

Cardiac resuscitation supplies and equipment.

Restraints, sheets, blankets.

Chemically clean specimen bottles with screw-top plastic-lined lids for vomitus and excreta.

Can opener.

Laryngoscope.

4. Technique–

a. Give 15–30 mL (1–2 tablespoons) of syrup of ipecac followed by $\frac{1}{2}$ glass of water. If emesis does not occur within 30 minutes after a 15-mL dose, repeat with the same dose of syrup of ipecac. For children under age 1 year, the dose should be 10–15 mL (2–3 teaspoons) of syrup of ipecac.

b. If indicated, save specimens of emesis for analysis.

B. Gastric Lavage:

1. Indications–

a. Gastric lavage is most effective when ingestion is discovered within 4 hours. After ingestion of salicylate, glutethimide, ethchlorvynol, or tricyclic antidepressants, or when the patient is in coma or shock with inaudible bowel sounds, substantial amounts of drug may be recovered even later. In such instances, intestinal lavage is useful (see p 27).

b. Lavage is indicated for removal of poisons in hysterical, comatose, or otherwise uncooperative patients. In such patients, the airway must be protected with a cuffed endotracheal tube.

2. Contraindications, precautions, and complications–

a. In acid or alkali ingestion, do not perform gastric lavage more than 30 minutes after ingestion. By this time, tissue destruction may have progressed to the point where perforation may occur. A small flexible Levin tube may be passed cautiously and left in place without danger of perforation.

b. Passing a gastric tube is likely to induce severe retching and vomiting, and this may be dangerous in hydrocarbon poisoning because hydrocarbons apparently pass readily into the trachea. Aspiration can be prevented by intubating the trachea with a tube having an inflatable cuff (see p 58). Endotracheal tubes generally fit tightly enough in children under age 2 that no additional cuff is advised.

c. If convulsions are present, any attempt to pass a stomach tube may increase the frequency and severity of convulsions. If there is reason to believe that unabsorbed poison remains in the gastrointestinal tract, a stomach tube can be passed after convulsions are controlled. Place a cuffed endotracheal tube to facilitate control of respiration and prevent aspiration (see p 58).

d. Because excess fluid tends to increase the absorption of poisons by forcing gastric emptying, quantities of fluid introduced at one time should be small and removal should be as complete as possible.

e. Complications include aspiration pneumonitis, perforation, bleeding, gagging, psychic trauma, and cardiac arrest.

3. Materials–The following supplies and equipment for gastric lavage should be available in hospital emergency rooms, in other emergency treatment centers, and in doctors' offices:

a. Stomach tubes, No. 22 (0.7 cm) and No. 32 (1.1 cm), rubber with removable funnel, with at least 2 through-and-through perforations at the end. The larger size facilitates removal of tablet fragments.

b. Asepto irrigating syringe, 4-oz, to fit the stomach tubes.

c. Levin tube, No. 12, with syringe to fit.

d. Endotracheal tubes with inflatable cuffs, in sizes for children and adults (see p 58).

e. Mouth gag.

f. Suction machine, syringe, or aspirating bulb, with tubing and soft rubber catheters, sizes 12F, 16F, and 20F, for removing mucus from the pharynx and trachea.

g. Canned milk (for treatment of poisoning with corrosives and to delay absorption) and can opener.

h. Activated charcoal is the most effective adsorbent and is available at pharmacies in 25- to 40-g containers. It is now available in a sorbitol suspension. Although activated charcoal is sufficiently safe that use in the home has been recommended, since prompt use can prevent symptoms from lethal amounts of poisons, it may not be palatable enough for routine home use; in emergency rooms, charcoal must still be administered by tube in many cases because patients refuse to swallow it. Do not use "universal antidote" or burned toast as a substitute. To 50 g of activated charcoal in a 500-mL polyethylene bottle, add 400 mL of distilled water and shake. Make certain that all of the charcoal has been wetted; the consistency should be that of slightly thickened soup or heavy cream. Of this mixture, give portions equivalent to about 5 mL for each kilogram of body weight, orally or by gastric lavage. Remove by suction or emesis, and repeat the procedure until a total of 100 g of charcoal has been introduced and recovered. Each gram of activated charcoal will adsorb 100–1000 mg of poison. Charcoal is ineffective against boric acid, ferrous sulfate, DDT, cyanide, ethanol, methanol, water-insoluble substances, mineral acids, alkalies, and many metallic compounds.

i. Saline solution, sodium bicarbonate, and milk of magnesia should also be on hand.

j. Chemically clean containers for specimens.

4. Technique–*Speed is essential*.

a. Give the patient a glass of water to drink before passing the stomach tube.

b. Lay the patient on one side, with the head lower than the waist to prevent fluid from entering the trachea. A struggling patient should be immobilized in a sheet or a blanket.

c. Measure the distance on the tube from the mouth to the epigastrium, and mark the tube with an indelible marking pencil or a piece of adhesive tape.

d. Remove dentures and other foreign objects from the patient's mouth.

e. Open the patient's mouth, using a gag if necessary. Extend the head by lifting the chin.

f. Pass the tube over the tongue and toward the back of the throat without extending the head or the neck. The tube will curve down the back wall of the pharynx and enter the esophagus. If an obstruction is met before the mark on the tube reaches the level of the teeth, do not use force but simply remove the tube and repeat the procedure until the tube passes readily to the mark indicated. The end of the tube may then be placed in a glass of water. If the tube meets an obstruction when introduced about halfway to the mark, it has probably entered the trachea. Sudden aphonia also indicates tracheal intubation. Bubbling on expiration indicates placement in the trachea.

g. After the tube has entered the stomach, always aspirate first to remove stomach contents by using an irrigating syringe.

h. After the stomach contents have been removed and saved for later toxicologic examination, repeat the introduction and withdrawal of aliquots of 100–300 mL of warm (37°C) water or 0.5 N (0.45%) saline solution until at least 3 L of clear return is obtained. If available, activated charcoal may be used at the beginning of lavage to aid in inactivating the poison. At the end of lavage, leave 50 g of charcoal suspended in water in the stomach. If the introduction and removal of lavage fluid by gravity alone requires more than 5 minutes, assist the process gently with the use of an Asepto syringe. Prevent possible aspiration by placing a cuffed endotracheal tube (see p 58). Avoid giving large quantities of water; this might force the stomach contents through the pylorus. In children, gastric lavage solutions should contain 0.45–0.9% sodium chloride to avoid the danger of water intoxication.

i. If the patient is comatose, intubate the trachea with a cuffed endotracheal tube (see p 58) in order to prevent aspiration of gastric contents. Succinylcholine can be given by experienced personnel (anesthesiologist) to ease the insertion of the tracheal catheter prior to the passage of the stomach tube.

C. Gastrotomy (Surgical Removal):

1. Indications–

a. Capsules or tablets ingested in large quantities sometimes form a mass of drug in the stomach that cannot be removed by gastric lavage or emesis. Such a mass of drug can contribute to late deterioration of the patient.

b. Medications containing iron or bromine can be seen on x-ray, and masses of drug capsules or tablets can be observed after giving barium sulfate contrast media. Some drugs include a contrast medium as part of the formulation.

2. Contraindications and precautions–Gastrotomy can only be done if the condition of the patient is satisfactory from the standpoint of circulation and respiration. Thus, the procedure should be considered before deterioration is advanced.

D. Catharsis and Intestinal Lavage:

1. Indications–Catharsis or intestinal lavage can be used to remove unabsorbed poisons or poisons that have been excreted into the intestine.

2. Contraindications–

a. When a corrosive has been ingested, administration of a cathartic may increase the extent of the intestinal injury.

b. Do not use catharsis in a patient already showing disturbed electrolyte balance.

c. Irritant cathartics such as the vegetable cathartics (aloes, cascara) should not be used in any type of poisoning.

d. Hypertonic cathartics and enemas are hazardous in the presence of impaired renal function (see p 72).

e. Do not give cathartics containing magnesium to patients with renal disease or those exposed to nephrotoxins, or to any patient in whom myoglobinuria or hemoglobinuria is present or threatened.

3. Materials–

a. Sodium sulfate–This substance is less toxic than magnesium sulfate, but it can cause hypernatremia.

b. Sodium phosphate–Fleet's Phospho-Soda is a palatable form.

c. Castor oil–Castor oil is bland until it is hydrolyzed to an irritant in the intestine. It has been recommended in phenol poisoning, since phenols are highly soluble in castor oil, but data on its effectiveness are not available. Removal of the castor oil by use of a saline cathartic is advisable. Castor oil is contraindicated in poisoning by chlorinated insecticides, since it may increase intestinal absorption.

d. Sorbitol or mannitol–These poorly absorbed carbohydrates can be used as lavage agents to remove excreted poisons from the small intestine.

4. Technique–

a. Give 30 g of sodium sulfate dissolved in a glass of water or 15–60 mL Fleet's Phospho-Soda diluted 1:4. The cathartic effect should follow within 30–60 minutes.

b. For intestinal lavage, instill 100- to 250-mL portions of 20–40% sorbitol or mannitol into the small intestine by means of an intestinal suction tube and remove by gentle continuous suction.

E. Adsorption and Delay of Gastric Emptying:

1. Indications–Ingestion of poisons of all types.

2. Contraindications and precautions–The quantity of liquid given should not exceed 50 mL/10 kg body weight; otherwise, gastric contents could be forced past the pylorus and absorption speeded.

3. Materials and technique–Give activated charcoal (see p 25) or evaporated milk within the first few minutes after ingestion. Milk effectively delays gastric emptying time and therefore reduces absorption in the intestine; little absorption takes place in the stomach.

SNAKEBITE

Tourniquet

Apply a 1×60 cm ($\frac{1}{2} \times 24$ inch) rubber-band tourniquet proximal to the injection site. The pulse in vessels distal to the tourniquet should not disappear, nor should the tourniquet produce a throbbing sensation. Slight venous engorgement should occur. A tourniquet should not be applied to fingers or toes. The tourniquet should be left in place until an antidote can be given.

Cold

Application of cold is too hazardous for emergency use.

Incision

Incision and suction removes up to 20% of subcutaneously injected snake venom in the first 10 minutes after bites of some snakes (see p 473). Damage to underlying structures is common.

Specific Antidote

If a specific antidote is available (eg, snake venom antiserum), give according to the directions included with the package.

SKIN CONTAMINATION

Flood the contaminated area with copious amounts of water from a hose or shower or poured from a bucket to dilute and remove the poison. Remove the clothing while a continuous stream of water is played on the skin. Protect emergency personnel against contamination by use of rubber gloves and aprons if necessary. The rapidity and volume of washing are extremely important in reducing the extent of injury from corrosives or other agents that injure the skin.

Do not use chemical antidotes. The heat liberated by a chemical reaction may increase the extent of injury.

Further treatment to involved areas should be the same as for burns of similar severity.

EYE INJURY DUE TO CHEMICAL IRRITANTS

In industries where eye contamination is liable to occur, foot-operated eyewash fountains with rubber eye pieces should be available for immediate use. If an eyewash fountain is not available, the victim should be taken to a hose or sink where the eye can be flooded with water under low pressure while the lids are held apart. Washing is continued for a full 15 minutes and the patient is then taken to a first-aid station. Washing must begin immediately, since a delay of a few seconds can greatly increase the extent of injury.

Do not use chemical antidotes. These may actually increase the extent of the injury by liberating heat.

At the first-aid station, place the patient in a reclining chair and irrigate the eyes for 15 more minutes with sterile normal saline solution or sterile water. Then instill a few drops of 2% fluorescein solution *(must be sterile)* into the eye. (Sterile fluorescein papers or single-dose containers may also be used.) If the fluorescein produces a yellow or green stain, irrigate the eye for another 5 minutes and then send the patient to an ophthalmologist for further examination and treatment. If possible, the patient should be seen by an ophthalmologist within 2 hours after the injury.

INHALED POISONS

Remove from exposure, establish an adequate airway, and give O_2 and artificial respiration as indicated. Determine blood pressure frequently during the use of positive-pressure resuscitation equipment. A prolonged inspiratory cycle will impair venous return and lower blood pressure. Maintain body temperature.

Use a specific antidote when available (eg, amyl nitrite for cyanide poisoning).

RECTALLY ADMINISTERED POISONS

Dilute the poison with tap water by enema and allow its expulsion. Catharsis may also be necessary.

References

Curtis RA et al: Efficacy of ipecac and activated charcoal/cathartic. *Arch Intern Med* 1984;**144**:48.

Kulig K: Management of acutely poisoned patients with gastric emptying. *Ann Emerg Med* 1985;**14**:562.

Oderda GM, Klein-Schwartz W: General management of the poisoned patient. *Critical Care Quarterly* 1982;**4(4):**1.

Picchioni AL et al: Evaluation of activated charcoal-sorbitol suspension as an antidote. *J Toxicol Clin Toxicol* 1982;**19:**433.

Pond SM et al: Randomized study of the treatment of phenobarbital overdose with repeated doses of activated charcoal. *JAMA* 1984;**251:**3104.

Diagnosis & Evaluation of Poisoning | 3

PRINCIPLES OF DIAGNOSIS

The first responsibility of a physician called upon to treat a case of poisoning is to decide whether any treatment is necessary and, if so, to retard absorption or otherwise limit the effect of the poison. A decision must then be made about whether the poisoning is sufficiently serious to require further treatment. Cases of poisoning generally fall into 3 categories: (1) exposure to a known poison, (2) exposure to an unknown substance that may be a poison, and (3) disease of undetermined cause in which poisoning must be considered as part of the differential diagnosis.

EXPOSURE TO KNOWN POISONS

In many cases of poisoning, the agent responsible is known, and the physician's only problem is to determine whether the degree of exposure is sufficient to require more than emergency treatment. However, in many instances the history is inaccurate. The exact quantity of poison absorbed by the patient will probably be unknown, but the physician may be able to estimate the greatest amount the patient could have absorbed by examining the container from which the poison was obtained and by questioning relatives or coworkers to determine the amount present in the container previously. The missing quantity can then be compared with the known fatal dose.

Reported minimum lethal doses may be useful indications of the relative hazards of poisonous substances, but the fatal dose may vary greatly. If the estimated amount of poison is known to have caused serious or potentially fatal poisoning, treatment must be vigorous.

Lethal Dose (LD) & Lethal Concentration (LC)

In order to facilitate estimation of the severity of poisoning after exposure to substances for which clinical experience does not provide an indication of dangerous doses for humans, lethal doses for experimental animals are given in the tables of toxic substances in this book. Unless otherwise indicated, these constitute the smallest median lethal dose (LD50) that has been reported in any experimental animal by either oral administration or skin application. The LD50 is the amount of chemical that will kill approximately 50% of a group of animals. For some substances, the lethal concentration (LC) is given. This is the lowest concentration, in parts per million parts of air (ppm) or parts per billion parts of air (ppb), that is lethal to any animal species after short or long exposure. When known, the dose that has been fatal to humans is included in the text. Depending on the steepness of the dose-response curve—ie, the relationship between the smallest dose that will kill any animals and the largest dose that some of the animals will survive—the dangerous dose for humans may be 1–10% or less of the indicated lethal dose. The sources for the lethal doses in the tables are the references listed below. **For emphasis:** Because there are enormous intraspecies differences in susceptibility to poisons, LD50s can be misleading and must be used with caution.

American Conference of Governmental Industrial Hygienists: *Documentation of the Threshold Limit Values,* 4th ed. American Conference of Governmental Industrial Hygienists, 1980. Supplemented in 1981.

Berg GL (editor): *Farm Chemicals Handbook.* Meister. Annual publication.

National Institute of Occupational Safety and Health: *Registry of Toxic Effects of Chemical Substances.* US Government Printing Office. Annual publication.

Negherbon WO: *Insecticides.* Vol 3 of: *Handbook of Toxicology.* Saunders, 1959.

Spector WS (editor): *Acute Toxicities of Solids, Liquids, and Gases to Laboratory Animals.* Vol 1 of: *Handbook of Toxicology.* Saunders, 1956.

EXPOSURE TO SUBSTANCES THAT MAY BE POISONOUS

If a patient has been exposed to a substance whose ingredients are not known, the physician must identify the contents without delay. This problem is complicated by the great numbers of trade-named mixtures and the rapidity with which the formulas for such mixtures change. Since some trade-named chemical mixtures do not list the ingredients on the label, it may not be possible to evaluate the significance of contact with such materials without further information. In the 1980s, most labels contain a list of ingredients. The sources given below are suggested for evaluating trade-named mixtures. **For emphasis:** Physicians should be cautious in incriminating a chemical as the cause of symptoms *unless* a clear association is obvious or laboratory confirmation has been made, particularly when the symptoms are chronic.

Index of This Book
The index of this book lists the main toxic ingredient of some of the

most poisonous trade-named mixtures or indicates the poison that most closely represents the overall effects of the mixture. Many other commercial products are listed according to the nature or use of the product, since it would be impractical to list all trade names. For these general listings, the one ingredient that best represents the toxic potentialities of the product is indicated. Unless further information concerning the toxic ingredients can be obtained, the patient exposed to such a mixture should be treated as if this toxic substance were present. For example, some poster paints contain gamboge. A child who has eaten "poster paint" should be observed for the possibility of gamboge poisoning unless the physician knows that the paint eaten did not contain this substance. Toxic antidotes should not be given without definite evidence that poisoning has occurred.

Poison Information Center

Obtain the telephone number of the nearest poison information center from the local medical society or health officer. Make certain that 24-hour service is available. Poison information centers are in most cases able to identify the ingredients of trade-named mixtures, give some estimate of their toxicity, and suggest the necessary treatment. Most have access to Poisindex (see reference 10, below)

Manufacturer or Local Representative

One of the quickest and most reliable ways to find out the contents of a questionably poisonous substance is to telephone the manufacturer or one of its local or regional representatives. These individuals may also have information concerning the type of toxic hazard to be expected from the material in question and methods of treatment.

References Useful in Determining the Contents of Proprietary Mixtures

Since available proprietary mixtures number in the hundreds of thousands, it is impractical to include all of these names in a reference work. A number of sources, among them this one (see Index), are useful in determining the contents of mixtures and should be available to every physician.

(1) *Pesticide Handbook.* Entoma Society. Annual publication; lists 9000 pesticide mixtures.

(2) *Farm Chemicals Handbook.* Berg GL (editor). Meister. Annual publication.

(3) *Clinical Toxicology of Commercial Products,* 5th ed. Gosselin RE et al. Williams & Wilkins, 1984.

(4) *The Merck Index,* 10th ed. Merck & Co, 1983.

(5) *Trade Names Index.* American Conference of Governmental Industrial Hygienists, 1965 (and annual supplements).

(6) *American Drug Index*. Billups NF, Billups SM (editors). Lippincott. Annual publication.

(7) *Physicians' Desk Reference*. Medical Economics, Inc. Annual publication. Lists about 7000 proprietary medicinal agents and contains product identification section.

(8) *Hospital Formulary*. American Society of Hospital Pharmacists, 4630 Montgomery Ave, Washington, DC 20014. Annual publication.

(9) *Handbook of Nonprescription Drugs*, 7th ed. American Pharmaceutical Association, 1982.

(10) *Poisindex*. Rumack BH (editor). Micromedex, Inc., Denver. A computerized microfiche system containing information on more than 300,000 commercial compounds. Revised quarterly.

(11) *Toxifile*. Likes KE (editor). Chicago Micro Corporation, Chicago 60625. A microfiche information system.

DIFFERENTIAL DIAGNOSIS OF DISEASE THAT MAY BE THE RESULT OF POISONING

In any disease state of unknown origin, poisoning must be considered as part of the differential diagnosis. For example, the high number

Table 3–1. Summary of diagnosis and evaluation of poisoning.

I. **Acute Poisoning:** *Speed is essential.* Acute poisoning should be considered if—
   1. Patient has symptoms that began shortly after exposure to a known poison.
   2. Patient has been exposed to a poison known to have caused fatalities.
   3. Patient has been exposed to a substance whose ingredients are not known.
      Proceed as follows:
      a. Search index of this book to find trade name or type of use.
      b. Check available references (see p 33).
      c. Call poison information center (list telephone number on Inside Back Cover).
      d. Call manufacturer or local representative.

II. **Chronic Poisoning:** This should be considered in—
   1. Patient with symptoms—
      a. After known exposure—Proceed as follows:
         (1) Determine severity of exposure (history; concentration in excreta).
         (2) Determine magnitude of organ involvement (see specific poison).
      b. Without history of exposure—Proceed as follows:
         (1) Careful history and physical examination with attention to poisons listed in Table 3–2.
         (2) Search for exposure to common poisons (Table 3–2).
         (3) Conduct laboratory tests for common poisons (see p 43).
   2. Patient without symptoms after known exposure—
      a. Determine severity of exposure (history; concentration in excreta).
      b. Investigate possibility that asymptomatic impairment of function has occurred in certain organs (see specific poison).

Table 3–2. Diagnosis of unrecognized poisoning.

Agent	History	Physical Examination	Clinical and Laboratory Evidence
Arsenic (paint, weed-killer, pesticides)	Gastrointestinal disturbances, dizziness, restlessness, muscular cramps, polyneuritis (anesthesias, paresthesias).	Skin: bronzing, hyperkeratosis, waxiness. Low blood pressure, jaundice, weight loss, enlarged or cirrhotic liver.	Oliguria, anuria, proteinuria, hematuria, anemia, liver function impairment, bilirubinemia, arsenic in hair, nails, urine.
Carbon monoxide (exhaust gas from any combustion device, artificial gas)	Headache, irritability, shortness of breath, nausea, fainting, peripheral sensory loss, mental deterioration.	Cyanosis, positive Romberg sign.	Leukocytosis, proteinuria, increased carboxyhemoglobin concentration in blood.
Chlorinated compounds: insecticides (DDT, chlordane, etc) and solvents (carbon tetrachloride, etc)	Fatigue, weakness, loss of appetite, blurred vision, memory loss, drowsiness, paresthesias, tremor, coma, jaundice, convulsions.	Weight loss, low blood pressure, cardiac irregularities, enlarged or cirrhotic liver, convulsions, skin eruptions.	Anemia, leukocytosis, oliguria, hematuria, proteinuria, impaired liver function, organic chlorine compound in urine or body fat.
Fluoride (insecticides, phosphates)	General ill health, weakness.	Weight loss.	Anemia, increased density of bones radiographically, fluoride in urine.
Hypnotics and sedatives (barbiturates, narcotics, etc)	Mental confusion, emotional instability, poor judgment, neglect of appearance.	Ataxia, pinpoint pupils (narcotics), coma.	Barbiturates or other hypnotics in urine or blood, alkaloids in urine.
Lead (paint, toys, gasoline, bootleg alcohol)	Vomiting, constipation, irritability, convulsions, metallic taste, dizziness, weakness, abdominal pain.	Weight loss, lethargy, nerve paralysis, pallor, bluish lead line on gums, jaundice.	Anemia, reticulocytosis, hematuria, proteinuria, coproporphyrinuria, elevated CSF pressure and protein, subepiphyseal increase in bone density.
Mercury (paint, medicinals, antiseptics, pesticides)	Stomatitis, salivation, diarrhea, photophobia, extreme restlessness, muscular pains, mental deterioration, amnesia.	Palmar erythema, loosening of teeth, black lead line on gums.	Oliguria, anuria, proteinuria, hematuria, urine mercury excretion over 0.1 mg/d, increase in urine mercury after dimercaprol.
Phosphate ester insecticides	Weakness, anxiety, tremors, vomiting, salivation, and pulmonary secretions.	Dyspnea, miosis, cyanosis, slow pulse.	Cholinesterase levels of red blood cells markedly reduced.
Salicylates	Vomiting, abdominal pain, irritability, tinnitus, convulsions.	Fever, hyperpnea, restlessness, ecchymoses, blood in stool.	Blood CO_2 below 20 meq/L. Salicylate in urine. Blood salicylate over 30 mg/dL.
Silica	Dyspnea, cough.	Decreased vital capacity.	Granular or linear increase in lung density.
Thallium (insecticide or rodenticide)	Pain in extremities, ataxia, lethargy, coryza, gastrointestinal disturbances, salivation.	Ptosis, conjunctivitis, loss of hair, fever, tremors, convulsions, atrophy of skin, peripheral sensory loss.	Hematuria, proteinuria, eosinophilia, leukocytosis, thallium in urine.

Table 3—3. History and physical examination in diagnosis of coma from poisoning.

History and Physical Findings	Most Likely Poison
Children	Aspirin, antihistamines, iron tablets.
Alcohol ingestion	Alcohols.
Suicide	Barbiturates, antidepressants.
Dry cleaning	Chlorinated compounds, petroleum hydrocarbons.
Spray painting	Chlorinated compounds, petroleum hydrocarbons.
Lacquering	Chlorinated hydrocarbons, organic solvents.
Insecticide use	Chlorinated or cholinesterase inhibitor pesticides.
Epilepsy	Anticonvulsants.
Odor of breath:	
Alcohol	Phenols, cyanide, chloral hydrate, alcohols.
Acetone	Lacquer, alcohol.
Coal gas	Carbon monoxide.
Acrid	Paraldehyde.
Color of skin and mucous membranes:	
Hyperemia	Cyanide, alcohol.
Cyanosis	Aniline, nitrobenzene, nitrates, marking ink.
Pallor	Benzene, carbon monoxide.
Jaundice	Mushrooms, quinacrine, nitro compounds, phosphorus, carbon tetrachloride.
Temperature:	
Increased	Dinitrophenol.
Decreased	Chloral hydrate, morphine, barbiturates.
Pulse:	
Rapid	Theophylline, amphetamines.
Irregular	Insecticides, tricyclic antidepressants.
Slow	Morphine.
Respiration:	
Kussmaul	Salicylates, acetanilid, cinchophen.
Increased	Dinitrophenol, carbon monoxide, cyanide.
Wheezing	Cholinesterase inhibitor pesticides.
Convulsions	Alcohol, insecticides, strychnine, isoniazid.
Vomiting	Any poison.
Neck stiffness	Strychnine, cocaine.
Distention and spasticity of the abdomen	Corrosives.
Muscular twitchings	Cholinesterase inhibitor pesticides.

of cases of lead poisoning which have been discovered in a few medical centers indicates that many cases must go unrecognized. Some of these patients had had symptoms for more than a year and had been seen by several different physicians. Admittedly, the diagnosis of lead poisoning is difficult, but the possibility of this disorder must be considered before the necessary steps to confirm the diagnosis can be taken.

On the basis of exposure possibilities and clinical reports, a small group of poisons appears to be responsible for most disabilities resulting from unrecognized poisoning. The symptoms, physical changes, and laboratory findings for these poisons are summarized in Table 3–2. In any patient with a disease of undetermined cause, these poisons should be considered if symptoms are suggestive.

The diagnostic workup of a patient who may be a victim of unrecognized poisoning consists of (1) a complete history, (2) complete physical examination, and (3) appropriate laboratory tests.

History

The history may be obtained from parents, friends, or neighbors. For example, in cases of poisoning in children, the parents may not be helpful, whereas a neighbor might have seen the child eating a plant or other poisonous substance. The various individuals should be questioned separately to avoid overlooking important items.

The history should be taken systematically. The following are especially important if poisoning is being considered in the differential diagnosis:

A. **Occupational Exposure:** Occupational hazards include the following types of poisoning:

1. **Arsenic–**Smelter workers, refinery workers, gardeners, agricultural workers, pest control operators.
2. **Benzene–**Rubber and plastic cement workers and users, dye makers, gasoline blenders, electroplaters, paint and paint remover manufacturers and users, painters, printers, varnishers, dry cleaners.
3. **Carbon monoxide–**Blacksmiths, furnace or foundry workers, brick or cement makers, chimney cleaners, filling-station attendants, parking attendants, garage workers, miners, refinery workers, plumbers, police officers, sewer workers.
4. **Chlorinated hydrocarbons (carbon tetrachloride, etc)–**Rubber cement and plastic cement workers or users, cobblers, leather workers, dry cleaners, painters (including varnish and lacquer painters), furniture finishers, cloth finishers, paint removers, rubber workers.
5. **Chromium–**Garage mechanics, dye makers, electroplaters, painters, pottery workers, printers, paper makers.
6. **Hydrogen sulfide–**Furnace workers, sewer workers, refinery workers, tannery workers, glass workers, miners.
7. **Lead–**Welders, steamfitters, plumbers, painters, ceramic workers, Babbitt metal workers, battery makers, brass polishers, burners, cable workers, miners, pottery makers, electroplaters, printers, enamel workers, filling-station attendants, junk-metal refiners.
8. **Mercury–**Amalgam makers, dentists and dental workers, detonator workers, felt hat makers, laboratory workers,

jewelers, thermometer manufacturers, radio equipment workers, electroplaters, printers.

9. **Methanol**–Bookbinders, bronzers, rubber and plastic cement users, dry cleaners, leather workers, printers, painters (including lacquer and shellac painters), wood workers.

10. **Nitro and amino aromatic compounds**–Dye makers, explosives workers, colored pencil makers, rubber workers, tannery workers, vulcanizers.

B. **Availability of Poisons in the Home:** Search the patient and the patient's home and immediate surroundings for poison containers.

1. Ingestion of food, drink, and medicines.
2. Contact with insecticides or other agricultural chemicals.
3. Exposure to fumes, smoke, or gases.
4. Skin contact with liquids such as insecticides or cleaning solvents.

System Examination
A. **General:**

1. **Weight loss**–Any chronic poisoning, but especially lead, arsenic, dinitrophenol, thyroid, mercury, and chlorinated hydrocarbons.

2. **Lethargy, weakness**–Lead, arsenic, mercury, chlorinated organic compounds, thiazide diuretics, organic phosphates, nicotine, thallium, nitrites, fluorides, botulism.

3. **Loss of appetite**–Trinitrotoluene.

4. **Blood pressure fall**–Nitrates, nitrites, nitroglycerin, *Veratrum,* cold wave neutralizer, acetanilid, chlorpromazine, quinine, volatile oils, aconite, disulfiram (Antabuse), iron salts, methyl bromide, arsine, arsenic, fluorides, phosphine, nickel carbonyl, stibine, pargyline (Eutonyl), ganglionic blocking agents, food poisoning, boric acid, phosphorus, carbon tetrachloride.

5. **Blood pressure rise**–Epinephrine or substitutes, *Veratrum,* ergot, cortisone, vanadium, lead, nicotine, tranylcypromine (Parnate), phencyclidine (PCP), iproniazid and related drugs.

6. **Fast pulse**–Potassium bromate, iron salts, atropine.

7. **Slow or irregular pulse**–*Veratrum, Zygadenus,* digitalis, mushrooms, oleander, nitrites.

8. **Hyperthermia**–Dinitrophenol or other nitrophenols, jimsonweed (stramonium), deadly nightshade (atropine), boric acid, salicylates, atropine, food poisoning, antihistamines, tranquilizers, camphor.

9. **Hypothermia**–Akee, barbiturates.

     10. Breath odor–Bitter almonds odor: cyanide; garlic odor: arsine, arsenic, phosphorus.

B. Skin:

    1. Cyanosis in the absence of respiratory depression or shock–Methemoglobinemia from aniline, nitrobenzene, acetanilid, phenacetin, nitrates from well water or food, bismuth subnitrate, cloth marking ink (aniline), chloramine-T, nitrites, chlorates, dapsone.

    2. Dryness–Atropine and related compounds.

    3. Corrosion or destruction–Acids or alkalies, permanganate.

    4. Jaundice from liver injury–Carbon tetrachloride, chlorinated compounds, arsenic and other heavy metals, chromates, mushrooms, phenothiazines, sulfonamides, chlorpromazine, trinitrotoluene, aniline, thiazide diuretics, iproniazid and related drugs, phosphorus, acetaminophen.

    5. Jaundice from hemolysis–Aniline, nitrobenzene, pamaquine, pentaquine, primaquine, benzene, castor beans, jequirity beans, fava beans, phosphine, arsine, nickel carbonyl.

    6. Redness and flushing–Atropine, antihistamines, tranquilizers, boric acid, cyanide.

    7. Rash–Bromides, sulfonamides, antibiotics, poison ivy or oak, hair preparations, photo developers, salicylates, trinitrotoluene, chromium, phenothiazines, indomethacin, gold salts, chlorinated compounds.

    8. Loss of hair–Thallium, arsenic, selenium.

    9. Edema–Adrenal glucocorticoids, androgens, estrogens, anabolic agents, antifertility agents, indomethacin.

    10. Burns–Lye, acids, hypochlorite, formaldehyde.

    11. Pallor–Lead, naphthalene, chlorates, favism, solanine plant poisons, fluorides.

    12. Sweating–Organic phosphate insecticides, muscarine and other mushroom poisonings, nicotine.

C. Central Nervous System:

    1. Psychosis–Thiazide diuretics, adrenal glucocorticoids, ganglionic blocking agents, bromides, atropine.

    2. Delirium or hallucinations–Alcohol, antihistamines, atropine and related drugs, camphorated oil, lead, *Cannabis sativa* (marihuana), cocaine, amphetamine, bromides, quinacrine, ergot, santonin, rauwolfia, salicylates, phenylbutazone, methyl bromide, DDT, chlordane, barbiturates, boric acid, aminophylline, scopolamine, phencyclidine (PCP).

    3. Depression, drowsiness, or coma–Barbiturates or other hypnotics, alcohols, solvents, kerosene, antihistamines, insecticides or rodenticides, atropine or related drugs, cationic detergents, arsenic, mercury, lead, opium and derivatives, paraldehyde, cyanides, carbon monoxide, phenol, salicylates, chlorpromazine, akee, hypoglycemia from oral hypoglycemic drugs, boric acid, naphthalene, digitalis, mushrooms.

4. **Muscular twitchings and convulsions**–Insecticides, strychnine and brucine, camphor, atropine, cyanides, ethylene glycol, nicotine, black widow spider, salicylates, aminophylline, amphetamine and other stimulants, boric acid, lead, mercury, phenothiazines, antihistamines, arsenic, kerosene, fluorides, nitrites, barbiturates, digitalis, solanine, thallium.

5. **Headache**–Nitroglycerin, nitrates, nitrites, hydralazine, trinitrotoluene, indomethacin, carbon monoxide, organic phosphate insecticides, atropine, lead, carbon tetrachloride, glutamates.

6. **Deafness or disturbances of equilibrium**–Streptomycin, neomycin, quinine, salicylates, aminoglycosides.

7. **Mental change or confusion**–Thallium, lead, mercury, alcohol, atropine, nicotine, antihistamines, carbon tetrachloride, digitalis, mushrooms, salicylates, barbiturates, tranquilizers.

8. **Paresthesias**–Lead, thallium, DDT.

9. **Ataxia**–Lead, organic phosphate insecticides, antihistamines, thallium, barbiturates.

D. **Head:**

1. **Eyes**–

   a. **Blurred vision**–Atropine, physostigmine, phosphate ester insecticides, cocaine, solvents, dinitrophenol, nicotine, methanol, indomethacin, botulism.

   b. **Colored vision**–Digitalis.

   c. **Double vision**–Alcohol, barbiturates, nicotine, phosphate ester insecticides, botulism.

   d. **Dilated pupils**–Atropine and related drugs, cocaine, nicotine, solvents, depressants, antihistamines, phenylephrine, mushrooms, thallium, oleander.

   e. **Contracted pupils**–Morphine and related drugs, phenothiazines, physostigmine and related drugs, phosphate ester insecticides, mushrooms and other plant poisons.

   f. **Pigmented scleras**–Quinacrine, jaundice from hemolysis or liver damage.

g. **Pallor of optic disk**–Quinine, nicotine, carbon disulfide.

h. **Papilledema**–Lead.

i. **Lacrimation**–Organic phosphate insecticides, nicotine, mushrooms.

j. **Ptosis**–Botulism, thallium.

k. **Strabismus**–Botulism, thallium.

2. **Ears**–

a. **Tinnitus**–Quinine, salicylates, quinidine, indomethacin.

b. **Deafness or disturbances of equilibrium**–Streptomycin, neomycin, quinine, salicylates, aminoglycosides.

3. **Nose**–

a. **Anosmia**–Phenol nose drops, chromium.

b. **Fetor nasalis**–Chromium.

c. **Perforated septum**–Chromium, cocaine.

4. **Mouth**–

a. **Loosening of teeth**–Mercury, lead, phosphorus.

b. **Painful teeth**–Phosphorus, mercury, bismuth.

c. **Dry mouth**–Atropine and related drugs, antihistamines, ephedrine.

d. **Salivation**–Lead, mercury, bismuth, thallium, phosphate ester insecticides, other heavy metals, mushrooms.

e. **Black line on gums**–Lead, mercury, arsenic, bismuth.

f. **Inflammation of gums**–Lead, mercury, arsenic, bismuth, other heavy metals.

g. **Stomatitis**–Corrosives, thallium.

E. **Cardiorespiratory System:**

1. **Respiratory difficulty, including dyspnea on exertion, chest pain, and decreased vital capacity**–Phosphate ester insecticides, salicylates, botulism, nickel carbonyl, black widow spider, scorpion, shellfish, fish, physostigmine, silicosis, other pneumoconioses, cyanide, carbon monoxide, atropine, strychnine, beryllium, dusts, chloramine-T, alcohol.

2. **Wheezing**–Phosphate ester insecticides, physostigmine, neostigmine, mushrooms *(Amanita muscaria)*.

3. **Rapid respirations**–Cyanide, atropine, cocaine, carbon monoxide, carbon dioxide, salicylates, chloramine-T, alcohol, amphetamine and other stimulants, mushrooms.

4. **Slow respirations**–Cyanide, carbon monoxide, barbiturates, morphine, botulism, aconite, magnesium, antihistamines, thallium, fluorides.

5. **Pulmonary edema**–Metal fumes, hydrogen sulfide, irritants, morphine and substitutes, methyl bromide, methyl chloride.
6. **Palpitations**–Nitrites, nitroglycerin, organic nitrates, potassium bromate.
7. **Cough**–Smoke, dust, silica, beryllium, hydrocarbons, mercury vapor.
8. **Aspiration pneumonia**–Kerosene, mineral oil, other hydrocarbons.

F. **Gastrointestinal System:**
1. **Vomiting, diarrhea, abdominal pain**–Caused by almost all poisons, particularly soaps and detergents, corrosive acids or alkalies, metals, phenols, medicinal irritants, solvents, cold wave neutralizer, food poisoning, black widow spider, boric acid, insecticides, phosphorus, nicotine, fluorides, thallium, solanine and other plant poisons, castor beans, mushrooms, digitalis, oleander.
2. **Activation of peptic ulcer**–Phenylbutazone, salicylates, indomethacin, adrenal corticosteroids.
3. **Blood in stools**–Coumarin anticoagulants, thallium, iron, salicylates, corrosives.
4. **Hematemesis**–Corrosive substances, coumarin anticoagulants, aminophylline, fluorides.

G. **Genitourinary System:**
1. **Anuria**–Mercurials, bismuth, sulfonamides, carbon tetrachloride, formaldehyde, phosphorus, ethylene chlorohydrin, turpentine, oxalic acid, chlordane, castor beans, jequirity beans, trinitrotoluene.
2. **Proteinuria**–Arsenic, mercury, phosphorus.
3. **Hematuria or hemoglobinuria**–Heavy metals, naphthalene, nitrates, chlorates, favism, solanine and other plant poisons.
4. **Myoglobinuria**–Phencyclidine (PCP), convulsants, amphetamines.
5. **Oliguria**–Lead.
6. **Menstrual irregularities**–Estrogens, lead, bismuth, mercurials, other heavy metals.
7. **Color of urine**–Coumarin anticoagulants (red), fava beans (red), hepatotoxins (orange).

H. **Neuromuscular System:**
1. **Muscular weakness or paralysis (muscle group or single muscle)**–Lead, arsenic, botulism, poison hemlock, organic mercurials, thallium, triorthocresyl phosphate (in gasoline), DDT, chlordane, shellfish, carbon disulfide, other insecticides.

      2. Muscle fasciculations–Phosphate ester and other insecticides, nicotine, black widow spider, scorpion, manganese, shellfish.

      3. Tremors, muscle stiffness–Phenothiazines.

      4. Muscle cramps–Thiazide diuretics, lead, black widow spider.

I. Endocrine System:

      1. Decreased libido–Lead, mercury, other heavy metals, sympathetic blocking agents.

      2. Breast enlargement–Estrogens.

Laboratory Examination

A. Blood:

      1. Leukopenia or agranulocytosis–See p 79.

      2. Anemia–Lead, naphthalene, chlorates, favism, solanine and other plant poisons, snakebite.

      3. Cherry-red color–Carbon monoxide, cyanide.

      4. Chocolate color (methemoglobin)–Nitrates, nitrites, aniline, dyes, chlorates.

B. Blood, Serum, or Plasma Chemistry: (See tables at the ends of chapters for toxic blood levels of chemicals and drugs.)

      1. Glucose (whole blood)–Increased after thiazide diuretics or adrenal glucocorticoids; decreased after salicylates, lead, or ethanol.

      2. Uric acid (serum)–Increased after thiazide diuretics or ethanol.

      3. Potassium (serum or plasma)–Decreased after salicylates, thiazide diuretics, adrenal glucocorticoids.

      4. Bromide–Serum chloride is spuriously increased in bromism because the standard tests (eg, AutoAnalyzer) measure total halides.

C. Special Chemical Examinations Useful in Diagnosis of Poisoning: Special chemical examinations for lead or other heavy metals, insecticides, cholinesterase, barbiturates, alkaloids, etc, may be necessary in the differential diagnosis of poisoning. The following laboratories are suggested for the performance of such analyses. (It is wise to make prior arrangements with the laboratory to ensure that it will accept samples for analysis.)

      1. County coroner's laboratory–Heavy metals, blood alcohol, barbiturates, alkaloids.

      2. City, county, or state police laboratory–Blood alcohol, barbiturates, other poisons.

      3. State toxicologist's office–As under 1. Analyses in connection with criminal poisonings.

4. **Federal Bureau of Investigation Laboratory, Washington, DC.** (Only through local police.)
5. **State departments of public health**–These offices usually perform analyses relating only to cases of occupational poisoning (eg, insecticides, heavy metals).
6. **County hospital laboratory**–Lead, barbiturates, alkaloids, blood alcohol.
7. **Private laboratories**–Heavy metals, barbiturates.
8. **Toxicology Laboratory, Pesticides Program, Food and Drug Administration, US Public Health Service, Atlanta 30333**–Insecticides in body fat, blood cholinesterase. (They will send sample containers on request by physicians.)
9. **Poisonlab/MetPath, 1469 South Holly Street, Denver 80222**–Laboratory determinations available 7 days a week. Call (303) 758–0430 for air freight pick-up.

For emphasis: "Toxic screens" should not be requested routinely. Many such screens are only intended to detect drugs of abuse, and even those with broader coverage may have poor sensitivity and specificity. However, specific laboratory tests for alcohols, acetaminophen, iron, lithium, salicylates, and some other drugs may be critical when poisoning with these drugs is suspected, because test results influence therapy. Remember that the most useful test is one whose result is likely to have an impact on therapy.

SUBSTANCE DEPENDENCY
(Drugs of Abuse)

The most notable drug of abuse is alcohol. Other commonly abused drugs are opiates; marihuana, LSD (lysergic acid diethylamide), PCP (phencyclidine), and other psychedelic drugs; stimulants, including amphetamines, cocaine, and the minor stimulants caffeine and phenylpropanolamine; sedatives, including barbiturates, benzodiazepines, and various hypnotics as well as alcohol; nicotine; and various gases and solvents that are sniffed or inhaled. The signs and symptoms common with each are described in the discussions of specific agents (see Index).

The signs and symptoms of drug abuse can be confusing, and correct diagnosis depends on a high index of suspicion. Confirmation of the diagnosis can be aided by increasingly sophisticated laboratory tests to detect various drugs in urine and blood, but in most cases, these tests do not help medical management. In most cases, immediate symptomatic medical management is simple but long-term management to prevent recurrence is far more difficult. Secondary complications, eg, subacute bacterial endocarditis, hepatic talc granulomatosis, wound botulism, and AIDS in association with intravenous drug abuse, may also be difficult to treat.

Adler GR et al: Narcotics control in anesthesia training. *JAMA* 1985;**253**:3133.

Anderson HR et al: Epidemiology: Deaths from abuse of volatile substances—A national epidemiological study. *Br Med J* 1985;**290**:304.

Fulminant hepatitis B among parenteral drug abusers—Kentucky, California. *MMWR* 1983;**33**:70.

Ghodse AH et al: Deaths of drugs addicts in the United Kingdom 1967–1981. *Br Med J* 1985;**290**:425.

Kandel DB et al: Patterns of drug use from adolescence to young adulthood. (3 parts.) *Am J Public Health* 1984;**74**:660, 668, 673.

Sourindrhin I: Solvent misuse. *Br Med J* 1985;**290**:94.

References

Arena JM: *Poisoning: Toxicology, Symptoms, Treatment,* 4th ed. Thomas, 1979.

Baselt RC: *Disposition of Toxic Drugs and Chemicals in Man.* Biomedical Publications, 1982.

Flanagan RJ et al: Value of toxicological investigation in the diagnosis of acute drug poisoning in children. *Lancet* 1981;**2**:682.

Gilman AG et al: *Goodman and Gilman's The Pharmacological Basis of Therapeutics,* 7th ed. Macmillan, 1985.

Goldfrank LR et al (editors): *Goldfrank's Toxicologic Emergencies,* 3rd ed. Appleton-Century-Crofts, 1986.

Haddad LM, Winchester JF: *Clinical Management of Poisoning and Drug Overdose.* Saunders, 1983.

Klaassen CD, Amdur M, Doull J (editors): *Casarett and Doull's Toxicology: The Basic Science of Poisons,* 3rd ed. Macmillan, 1985.

Loomis TA: *Essentials of Toxicology,* 3rd ed. Lea & Febiger, 1978.

Oehme FW: *Toxicity of Heavy Metals in the Environment.* Part 1 and Part 2. Vol 2 of: *Hazardous and Toxic Substances Series.* Marcel Dekker, 1978, 1979.

4 | Management of Poisoning

Apart from the specific measures directed at the poison itself (antidotes, lavage, demulcents, etc), the management of most severe cases of poisoning also involves control of the symptoms and effects of poisoning (pain, fluid imbalance, etc). These are discussed in the following paragraphs. Since poisoning requires emergency treatment, drugs and equipment for the following procedures must be readily available in the treatment center and the physician must be familiar with their use.

SUPPORTIVE MANAGEMENT

PAIN

Severe pain causes vasomotor collapse and reflex inhibition of normal physiologic functions.

Treatment
(1) Morphine sulfate, 5–15 mg subcutaneously, orally, intramuscularly, or slowly intravenously, is the most potent of the analgesics. It can cause nausea and vomiting, central nervous system depression, and slowing of respiration. It must be used cautiously or not at all in central nervous system depression, respiratory difficulty, hyperexcitability, and hepatic disease.
(2) Meperidine hydrochloride (Demerol, Dolantin), 50–150 mg orally or intramuscularly, causes less nausea and vomiting than morphine sulfate.

FLUID IMBALANCE

In the treatment of poisoning, careful attention must be paid to water metabolism. Excess of water or salt intake over loss in the presence of impaired kidney function leads to edema and pulmonary edema, whereas inadequate water intake impairs the ability of functioning kidneys to excrete toxic substances.

Daily Water Requirements

Imperceptible water losses may be calculated as 10–15 mL/kg/d, depending on the environmental and body temperatures. This amount plus the quantities lost daily in the urine, stools, and sweat represents the amount of fluid replacement necessary for 24 hours' maintenance. Water deficits should be replaced by administering water without electrolyte (5 or 10% dextrose in distilled water intravenously, or water by mouth).

Clinical Evaluation of Water Balance

A. Overhydration: Sudden weight gain, low urine specific gravity (< 1.010), high urine volume, low blood urea nitrogen. Opiates can produce the syndrome of inappropriate secretion of antidiuretic hormone (SIADH), in which typical symptoms of overhydration are associated with decreases in urine output and sodium concentration.

B. Dehydration: Sudden weight loss, decreased skin turgor, dry tongue and lips, elevated body temperature, high urine specific gravity (> 1.025), low urine volume (< 1 L/24 h), high blood nonprotein nitrogen or blood urea nitrogen, high hematocrit (> 55%).

Estimation of Fluid Needs

In addition to replacing the water loss from skin and lungs (10–15 mL/kg/d), adequate water must be given to permit renal excretion of electrolytes and metabolic wastes. These solids amount to 35–50 g/d for an individual at rest eating a normal diet, and 15–20 g/d for one at complete rest with no electrolyte intake and with all calories being supplied in the form of fats and carbohydrates. Renal excretion of 35 g of solids requires 400 mL of 1.030 specific gravity urine, 600 mL of 1.020 specific gravity urine, or 1200 mL of 1.010 specific gravity urine.

Table 4–1 indicates the approximate requirement for water in liters per 24 hours based on 1.6 L/m². This water requirement should contain at least 5% glucose to supply caloric requirements and reduce tissue catabolism.

Rodwell VW: Water. Chapter 2 in: *Harper's Review of Biochemistry*, 20th ed. Martin DW et al. Lange, 1985.

Table 4–1. Fluid requirements.

Weight (in kg)	3	6	10	20	30	40	50	60	70	80
Surface area (in m²)	0.21	0.30	0.45	0.80	1.05	1.30	1.50	1.65	1.75	1.85
Water for 24 hours (in L)	0.3	0.5	0.7	1.3	1.7	2.1	2.4	2.6	2.8	3.0

WATER & ELECTROLYTE IMBALANCE

Electrolyte imbalance after poisoning may be a result of vomiting, diarrhea, kidney damage, or other processes. An excess or deficit of water can also be present following poisoning episodes. If renal function is normal and the thirst mechanism is intact, water and electrolyte imbalances can be corrected relatively easily by administering "maintenance requirements" and replacements of deficits and concomitant losses either orally or intravenously. If levels of Na^+, K^+, Cl^-, HCO_3^-, etc, are known, approximations of necessary replacements can be calculated; likewise, serum or urine osmolality can be used to evaluate water status and adjust it if necessary. Normal concentrations of electrolytes in plasma and interstitial fluid are listed in Table 4–2.

For emphasis: Even though Na^+ and Cl^- are known to be distributed in the "extracellular compartment," which comprises 20% of body weight and 33% of the total body water (total body water = approximately 60% of total body weight), the practice in many centers is to replace Na^+ and Cl^- deficits as if these electrolytes occupied the total body water compartment. In others, the practice is to replenish the extracellular compartment by administering normal saline (140–150 meq of Na^+), 10–20 mL/kg body weight, to ensure adequate vascular perfusion, then to administer half of any remaining deficit in the next 8 hours and the final amount in the next 16 hours.

If the patient has a significant water excess (serum Na^+ ≤ 115 meq/L and symptoms are present, eg, convulsions), 3% NaCl solution (450 meq/L) should be given until the symptoms stop or the Na^+ level exceeds 125 meq/L. If the serum Na^+ level exceeds 155–165 meq/L, it should not be reduced rapidly by administration of free water; instead,

Table 4–2. Normal concentrations of electrolytes in plasma and interstitial fluid.

	Traditional Measurements	Conversion Factor*	SI Units
Cations			
Sodium	135–147 meq/L	1	135–147 mmol/L
Potassium	3.5–5 meq/L	1	3.5–5 mmol/L
Calcium	4.4–5.3 meq/L	0.5	2.2–2.7 mmol/L
Magnesium	1.6–2.4 meq/L	0.5	0.8–1.2 mmol/L
Anions			
Bicarbonate	22–28 meq/L	1	22–28 mmol/L
Chloride	95–105 meq/L	1	95–108 mmol/L
Phosphate	. . .	. . .	0.8–1.6 mmol/L
Miscellaneous			
Urea nitrogen	8–18 mg/dL	0.357	3–6.5 mmol/L
Creatinine	0.6–1.2 mg/dL	88.4	50–110 μmol/L

*For conversion of values in meq/L or mg/dL to SI units (mmol/L or μmol/L).

0.5 N saline (75 meq/L) should be given so that the serum Na^+ level does not fall precipitously.

Because most body K^+ is confined to the intracellular compartment and thus is not necessarily reflected in the serum K^+ level, it is almost impossible to calculate the amount of K^+ needed for replacement on the basis of the serum K^+ determination alone. The best way to correct a K^+ deficit is to first reestablish urine flow and then add 30 meq of K^+ to each liter of fluid administered to the patient; with normal kidney function, the K^+ level will be corrected.

ACIDOSIS

Acidosis occurs in association with poisoning by one of 2 mechanisms: (1) an increase in the production or retention of hydrogen ions, eg, conversion of methanol to formic acid; or inhibition of respiratory exchange, with retention of CO_2; or (2) loss of body buffering capacity due to renal losses or prolonged diarrhea.

Clinical Findings

During respiratory acidosis with CO_2 retention, respiratory inadequacy is obvious, and the patient may actually become cyanotic.

During metabolic acidosis, respirations usually increase in rate and depth, so that the respiratory effort is apparent.

Treatment

The primary goal of therapy should be to eliminate the cause of acidosis: in respiratory acidosis, ventilation must be improved in order to eliminate retained CO_2; in metabolic acidosis, the metabolic processes must be altered to reduce the production or retention of excess hydrogen ions. Administration of sodium bicarbonate is at best only a temporizing step and is unlikely to overcome the basic defect.

In salicylate poisoning, sodium bicarbonate is given not to overcome acidosis but instead to alkalinize the urine in order to permit ion trapping to occur: salicylate, being an acid, ionizes in alkaline urine; this prevents its reabsorption and allows it to be excreted. In poisoning due to tricyclic antidepressants, sodium bicarbonate, 1–3 meq/kg, is administered not to overcome any existing acidosis but rather to increase the blood pH; by an as yet unknown mechanism, this prevents the development of cardiac arrhythmias.

BODY TEMPERATURE REGULATION

Maintenance of normal body temperature is important in poisoning because hyperthermia increases the requirement of the body for O_2, food, minerals, and water and also increases the cardiac and renal loads. A body temperature rise of 0.8 °C increases the metabolism by about 10%.

Although hypothermia reduces the metabolic requirements, the detoxification and excretion of poisons is also correspondingly slowed and circulation is impaired.

If the patient's body temperature is above 40 °C or below 35 °C, it should be adjusted to normal concurrently with or immediately after attempts to remove the poison.

Treatment of Hyperthermia

Body temperatures up to 40 °C can be controlled by applying wet towels with adequate air circulation or a cooling blanket. Higher temperatures require the frequent application of towels wet with water at 10 °C or immersion of the extremities in water at approximately 25 °C. Antipyretics such as aspirin have no role in the treatment of poison-induced hyperthermia. For treatment of malignant hyperthermia, see p 316.

Treatment of Hypothermia

If the body temperature is below 35 °C, the patient should be warmed by immersion of the entire body or of the extremities in water not to exceed 42 °C. Peripheral warming can lead to pooling of blood and fall of blood pressure. Apply blankets or an electric blanket to avoid unnecessary chilling after the patient leaves the water. For more rapid warming, humidify and heat inspired air to 38 °C. Extracorporeal circulation of blood through a bath warmed up to 38 °C has been used. Warming by means of heat lamps, heating pads, or hot water bottles can be dangerous. If the skin temperature exceeds 42 °C, local tissue injury with capillary stasis and edema may cause circulatory collapse (see p 66). For less serious hypothermia, application of blankets will suffice. If intravenous solutions are given, they should be warmed to room temperature.

NUTRITION

In acute poisoning, the metabolic needs of the body should be supplied in order to minimize the breakdown of tissues and to reduce the catabolic load on the liver and kidneys.

Coma and esophageal injury are indications for intravenous or gastric tube feeding; hyperalimentation may occasionally be warranted.

Intravenous Feeding

Since a maximum of 3 L of 5 or 10% glucose can be given intravenously daily, intravenous feeding is generally unsatisfactory for more than a few days. The higher concentration tends to be associated with glycosuria. One liter of 5% glucose supplies 200 kcal. In order to avoid pulmonary edema, fluid intake should not exceed fluid loss.

Gastric Feedings

If the patient can tolerate an inlying gastric tube (3- to 4-mm polyethylene tubing intubated intranasally), nutritional needs can be supplied readily by tube feeding. A variety of commercial products are available, or a blended, strained preparation can be made from common foods.

Oral Feeding

A diet containing 50–100 g of protein, 50–100 g of fat, and sufficient carbohydrates to supply caloric needs is customary in the USA. Protein intake should be limited for patients with liver or kidney failure.

CENTRAL NERVOUS SYSTEM INVOLVEMENT

CONVULSIONS

Drugs cause convulsions by direct effect on the central nervous system, in response to the stimulation of peripheral receptors (eg, the carotid sinus), by O_2 deprivation, or by inducing hypoglycemia. The immediate treatment is the same for convulsions due to any cause, ie, to suppress the convulsion until a diagnosis can be made and specific treatment instituted.

Convulsions can be dangerous if accompanied by hypoxia; if hypoxia does not occur, secondary effects are rare. Because convulsions are often followed by coma and respiratory depression, antidotes that may also cause coma and respiratory depression must be used cautiously. Drugs that have easily controllable effects are preferable. Diazepam (Valium) is most commonly used, and phenobarbital is still popular; because either can be associated with acute respiratory arrest, resuscitative equipment must be available. Succinylcholine is also used, but ordinarily only by those trained in anesthesiology.

Clinical Findings

Substances that act primarily on the cerebrum (eg, amphetamine, caffeine, atropine) cause hyperactivity, restlessness, and mania. Substances such as pentylenetetrazol (Metrazol) and picrotoxin, which act primarily on the brain stem, cause clonic convulsions. Strychnine acts primarily on the spinal cord to produce typical tonic extensor spasms. Other agents such as veratrum, cyanide, and nicotine may cause convulsions by a combination of reflex, central nervous system, and anoxic effects.

Treatment
(Table 4–3)

A. Emergency Measures:

1. Restrain the patient during convulsions to prevent injury.

2. Consider administering an anticonvulsant.

3. Keep the patient in quiet, darkened surroundings and limit visitors and all nonessential nursing procedures.

4. Do not attempt emesis or gastric lavage while the patient is twitching or hyperirritable unless the airway is controlled and removal of drug is imperative.

B. General Measures:

1. Administer anticonvulsants (Table 4–3). Succinylcholine is the most powerful of the anticonvulsants, and minute-to-minute control of its effects is possible. However, this drug can only be used when complete control of respiration can be maintained. A tracheal catheter must be placed (see p 58) and artificial respiration with O_2 maintained for the duration of the action of succinylcholine.

2. Maintain hydration by oral or intravenous fluid administration. The urine output should be 1–3 L/d.

3. Maintain an adequate airway (see p 58). A mouth gag may occasionally be necessary.

4. Treat hypoglycemia by giving glucose.

5. Reduce elevated temperature by using tepid sponges.

6. Remove secretions from the pharynx by suction.

7. Give positive-pressure respiration with O_2 during convulsions.

COMA

Coma due to poisoning results from some interference with brain cell function or metabolism. The administration of stimulants to combat the effects of drugs that induce coma will not overcome the derangement of drug-induced coma and is contraindicated. The mechanism of action of cerebral stimulant drugs is also unknown, but these drugs presumably act by depressing some inhibiting function in the cell. There is no evidence that any stimulants specifically oppose the cellular effects induced by depressant drugs such as the barbiturates.

Table 4–3. Measures for the control of convulsions.

Method	Route and Method of Administration	Advantages	Disadvantages
Diazepam (Valium)	2–10 mg IV at 1 mg/min.	Little depression of respiration.	Not effective in all types of convulsions.
Phenytoin (Dilantin)	Give 0.1–0.5 g IV slowly. Maximum dose: 1 g.	Little depression of respiration. Effect lasts 12 hours.	Not effective in all types of convulsions.
Phenobarbital sodium	Give 1 mg/kg IM or orally. Maximum dose: 5 mg/kg.	Effect lasts 12–24 hours.	Causes severe persistent respiratory depression in overdoses.
Pentobarbital sodium	Give 5 mg/kg orally, rectally, or IV as sterile 2.5% solution at a rate not to exceed 1 mL/min until convulsions are controlled.	Good control of initial dose.	No control of effects after drug has been given. May produce severe respiratory depression.
Paraldehyde	Give 4–16 mL (0.05–0.2 mL/kg) orally, rectally, or, very rarely, IM.	Little depression of respiration. Effect lasts 12 hours.	Associated with gastrointestinal distress.
Thiopental sodium (Pentothal sodium)	Give 2.5% sterile solution IV slowly. Maximum dose: 0.5 mL/kg.	Good minute-to-minute control. Can be given during convulsions.	Doses larger than recommended may cause persistent respiratory depression.
Succinylcholine chloride	Give 10–50 mg IV slowly and give artificial respiration during period of apnea. Repeat as necessary.	Will control convulsions of any type. Effect lasts only 1–5 minutes. Circulation ordinarily not affected.	Artificial respiration must be maintained during use. No antidote. Apnea may persist for several hours.

Treatment

A. Emergency Measures:

1. Start intravenous drip for convenience in further intravenous administration of medication and for treatment of shock. Use an 18-gauge venous catheter and an administration rate of 50–100 mL/h if renal function is adequate. Avoid excessive fluid administration, which contributes to cerebral edema.

2. Maintain adequate airway–

a. Place the patient on one side or prone with the mouth to the side and the head well extended.

b. Aspirate mucus, vomitus, saliva, blood, etc, from nose and pharynx by means of a soft rubber catheter with a syringe or mechanical aspirator.

c. Consider inserting a pharyngeal airway if one is available.

d. Insert an endotracheal tube if necessary, or do tracheostomy.

3. Give artificial respiration if respiration is depressed (see p 60) or if arterial O_2 saturation is inadequate.

4. Give O_2 (see p 63). Use manual or mechanical resuscitation (see p 60) if respirations fall below 10 per minute.

5. Treat shock (see p 66).

6. Hospitalize the patient.

7. Perform gastric lavage with activated charcoal. If this is not done within 4 hours of poisoning, it is unlikely to be effective in preventing absorption of the poison but may hasten its excretion. If the patient is comatose, intubate the trachea (see p 58).

B. General Measures:

1. Record the following observations at 15- to 30-minute intervals: (The patient must be under observation constantly until consciousness returns.)

a. Temperature, pulse, respiration, blood pressure.

b. State of consciousness–Vocalization, laryngeal stridor.

c. Skin color–Cyanosis, pallor, lividity.

d. Auscultation of lung bases (pulmonary edema).

e. Reflexes (corneal, pupillary, gag, patellar, superficial pain).

f. Urine output–Catheterize if necessary.

2. Turn the patient every 30 minutes and massage skin and aspirate airway. Maintain the patient in the horizontal position unless low blood pressure indicates a need for the shock position.

3. Catheterize the patient if coma persists for longer than 4–12 hours and the patient fails to void. If necessary, insert an indwelling catheter. Save initial urine specimen.

4. Treat infections with organism-specific antibiotics.

5. Nutrition–

a. Unless cardiac failure or renal failure is present, give 1 L of 0.9% saline, with 5% dextrose intravenously every 24 hours plus 5%

dextrose in distilled water as necessary to maintain hydration. Do not overhydrate.

    b. If vomiting or diarrhea is present, replace the additional fluid loss with an equal quantity of 5% dextrose in 0.45% saline.

    c. If coma continues for more than 48 hours and renal function is adequate, tube-feed the patient (see p 50).

    d. If hypokalemia is suggested by muscle weakness and electro-cardiographic changes, give potassium chloride, starting with 30–40 meq/L of intravenous fluid and increasing the concentration only if an increased need for potassium is obvious. Do not give potassium in the presence of acute renal failure without laboratory determination of the precise degree of serum potassium deficiency.

    C. Special Measures: If coma persists as a result of drug ingestion, consider dialysis to remove the drug (see p 88).

HYPERACTIVITY, DELIRIUM, & MANIA

    Hyperactivity and delirium occur occasionally in severe poisoning and make treatment more difficult. Delirium is characterized by mental derangement (illusions, delusions, hallucinations) as well as physical hyperactivity. The patient is uncooperative and incoherent.

    Mania is characterized by wild activity with less mental disturbance than is characteristic of delirium.

Treatment
    A. General Measures:

    1. Protect the patient from physical injury. Lock screens, bar windows, and remove furniture. Avoid mechanical restraints.

    2. Reassure the patient by a calm, quiet manner.

    3. Avoid strange sensory stimuli. Absolute silence should be avoided, however.

    4. Use relatives and friends as attendants to reduce apprehension.

    B. Hydrotherapy:

    1. Tub baths at 33–36 °C for 30-minute periods or longer, if well tolerated, have a soothing effect on hyperactive patients. Adequate supervision must be maintained.

    2. Wet packs should be administered only by trained personnel. They are contraindicated in the presence of convulsions, respiratory difficulty, or fever. Vital signs must be observed at 15-minute intervals.

    C. Drugs: (Use one of the following.)

    1. Diazepam, 2–5 mg intravenously at a rate of 1 mg/min.

    2. Paraldehyde, 4–16 mL orally in cracked ice, milk, fruit juice,

or whiskey; or 8–32 mL in 2 volumes of vegetable oil rectally, can be used for alcoholics.

3. Chlorpromazine (Thorazine), 25–50 mg by deep intramuscular injection or orally. Repeat at intervals of 4–6 hours.

HYPOGLYCEMIA

Coma and convulsions resulting from hypoglycemia have been reported to occur occasionally as a result of exposure to toxic substances. Since the symptoms from exposure to toxic substances and from hypoglycemia are frequently the same, the possibility of hypoglycemia should be considered in the differential diagnosis.

The following substances have been reported to induce hypoglycemia: (1) Alcohol or anesthesia following starvation acts by depressing hepatic mechanisms for gluconeogenesis. (2) Akee and other plant toxins such as mushrooms act as hepatotoxins to depress glycogen storage and gluconeogenesis. (3) Acetylcholinesterase inhibitors act by increasing parasympathetic release of insulin from the pancreas. (4) In diabetic patients, edetate acts by chelating zinc in slow-release preparations of insulin, thus speeding the release of insulin into the bloodstream. (5) In periodic paralysis or after use of sympathomimetic agents, potassium acts by increasing the deposition of glycogen in the liver. (6) Salicylates act by increasing glucose utilization.

Treatment

Administration of glucose by any route will correct hypoglycemia immediately. In emergency rooms, 50% glucose is frequently used; for prolonged administration, 10–20% glucose should be used. Epinephrine and glucagon can also be effective.

RESPIRATORY TRACT INVOLVEMENT

The essentials of respiratory resuscitation are as follows:
A. **Adequate Airway:** See p 58.
1. Oropharyngeal–Tongue forward; use metal or plastic airway.
2. Tracheal–Catheter, tracheostomy, cricothyroid puncture.
B. **Adequate Pulmonary Ventilation:**
1. Mouth-to-mouth resuscitation.
2. Portable hand resuscitator.
C. **Oxygen Administration:** See p 63.
Emergency use of these procedures requires prior training and familiarity with the equipment.

HYPOXIA & DEPRESSED RESPIRATION

Hypoxia occurring during coma, unconsciousness, convulsions, or muscular paralysis with depressed or absent breathing requires immediate resuscitation, with the administration of air or O_2 until normal respiration returns. *Do not wait for the arrival of equipment before beginning artificial respiration.*

Resuscitation with oxygen equipment is becoming increasingly complex. Physicians should familiarize themselves with methods and equipment available in local hospitals, emergency rooms, or local rental agencies prior to the necessity for emergency use. The ability to use such methods and equipment quickly and surely in the event of respiratory failure may mean the difference between life and death.

Resuscitation requires adequate airway, artificial respiration, and O_2 administration if available.

The causes of hypoxia during poisoning and methods of treatment are outlined in Table 4–4.

Table 4–4. Hypoxia in poisoning: Causes and treatment.

Physiologic Classification	Type of Poisoning	Treatment
Normal lung and blood O_2 transport:		
Deficient atmospheric O_2	Natural gas suffocation; high nitrogen or methane concentrations in air (in mines).	Resuscitation in air or with O_2.
Airway obstruction	Edema of tongue, pharynx, larynx due to irritants or corrosives.	Ensure adequate airway.
Muscular paralysis	Curare, botulism, anesthesia, hemlock.	Resuscitation.
Respiratory center paralysis	Phosphate ester insecticides, triorthocresyl phosphate.	Resuscitation.
Abnormal lung with normal blood transport:		
Impaired diffusion	Pulmonary edema due to irritants.	Positive-pressure breathing; inhalation of O_2.
Normal lung with impaired blood transport:		
Inactive hemoglobin	Carbon monoxide poisoning; sulfhemoglobin formers.	100% O_2 by artificial respiration; hyperbaric O_2.
	Methemoglobin formers (eg, aniline, nitrobenzene, nitrites, acetanilid).	100% O_2 by artificial respiration; give methylene blue (see p 78).
Impaired O_2 exchange	Carbon dioxide poisoning.	Artificial respiration in air.
Low blood pressure	Shock.	O_2; positive-negative-pressure resuscitation.
Normal lung, normal blood transport, impaired tissue uptake:		
Cellular enzyme poisoning	Cyanide, fluoride, hydrogen sulfide.	100% O_2 by artificial respiration; hyperbaric O_2; treat cyanide poisoning (see p 254).

MAINTENANCE OF ADEQUATE AIRWAY

In coma, the airway is frequently impaired by oropharyngeal muscular relaxation, laryngeal spasm, laryngeal edema, or tracheobronchial secretions. Improving the airway helps to provide adequate oxygenation by increasing tidal exchange.

Equipment & Technique

Note: Use of equipment requires experience.

A. Oropharyngeal Airway: This consists of a curved and flattened plastic or rubber-covered metal tube that fits over the curve of the tongue and allows air to pass freely to the pharynx. Small, medium, and large sizes should be available.

B. Laryngoscopes: These are used for placement of endotracheal airways. They are obtainable in adult and child sizes.

C. Endotracheal Airways: (Fig 4–1.) Plain catheters and catheters with inflatable cuffs should be available. The smaller sizes can be used for tracheal suction to remove mucus and secretions. While the endotracheal airway is in place, constant supervision is necessary. Be certain that foreign bodies have been removed from the mouth and the pharynx before placing the endotracheal airway.

D. Suction Device: Use a mechanical suction machine with tubing and traps, or a hand-operated aspirator.

E. Syringe and Catheter for Aspiration: A glass or rubber syringe for clearing the airway should be used with a soft rubber catheter (size 12F). Aspiration should be done using sterile precautions and a fresh sterile suction catheter each time. Excessive suction from mechanical suction devices can cause tracheal injury.

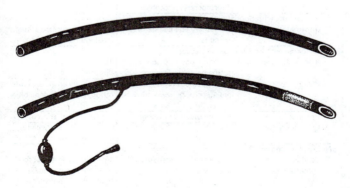

Figure 4–1. Magill catheter, alone and with inflatable cuff.

F. Mouth Gag: This is used during suction or placement of an endotracheal tube.

G. Tracheostomy: (Fig 4–2.) Tracheostomy can be performed with a minimum of equipment. A sharp scalpel or razor blade is used to divide the skin of the neck downward from the cricoid cartilage to the suprasternal notch. The trachea can then be exposed, the tracheal ring

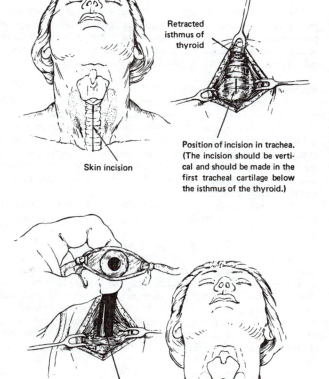

Retracted
isthmus of
thyroid

Skin incision

Position of incision in trachea.
(The incision should be vertical and should be made in the first tracheal cartilage below the isthmus of the thyroid.)

Tracheostomy tube

Figure 4–2. Technique of tracheostomy.

below the isthmus of the thyroid divided in the midline, the opening spread by means of a forceps or pair of scissors, and a tracheostomy tube inserted. Sutures around the tracheostomy tube should not be tight. Postoperative care includes (1) changing the tracheostomy tube daily; (2) frequent aspiration of tube and trachea, using sterile precautions and a sterile suction catheter; and (3) humidification of inspired air or O_2.

METHODS OF MANUAL ARTIFICIAL RESPIRATION

Artificial respiration methods vary considerably in their ability to provide adequate tidal air. The simple back pressure methods may not produce adequate tidal air in deep coma due to drug poisoning because of lack of chest and abdominal muscle tone. Direct inflation is considered to be superior to other types of artificial respiration.

Artificial Respiration by Direct Inflation

Direct inflation of the victim's lungs from the operator's mouth is especially useful when there is an obstruction to the free passage of air. The method also requires less effort than other methods of manual artificial respiration and allows the operator to appraise the patient's condition more readily. Mechanical aids improve the technique and at the same time prevent pharyngeal constriction by the victim's tongue when the mouth is opened. Inflation 15 times per minute is necessary to maintain adequate oxygenation.

A. Mouth-to-Mouth Insufflation: This method is used when no mechanical aids are available. Place the victim supine on a firm surface, preferably a table.

1. Take a position at the victim's head as shown in Fig 4–3.

2. If the victim is not breathing, take immediate steps to open the airway. In unconscious victims, the tongue becomes lax and may fall backward, blocking the airway. Gently tip the victim's head backward as far as possible by lifting up the neck, near the base of the skull, with one hand and pressing down on the forehead with the other hand (Fig 4–3). Avoid hyperextending the victim's neck in accident cases when there is a possibility of neck fracture. If necessary, keep the mandible displaced forward by pulling strongly at the angle of the jaw ("chin-lift").

3. Clear the mouth and pharynx of foreign material (eg, blood, vomitus) with the hooked index finger ("finger-sweep") but avoid undue probing. Do not remove dentures but leave them in the mouth to obtain a better seal around the lips.

4. If steps 2–3 fail to open airway, forcibly blow air through mouth (keeping nose closed) or nose (keeping mouth closed) and quickly and fully inflate the lungs 4 times. Watch for chest movement.

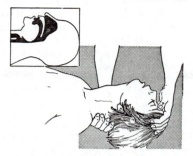

(1) Open airway by positioning neck anteriorly in extension. Inserts show airway obstructed when the neck is in resting flexed position and opening when neck is extended.

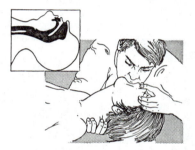

(2) Rescuer should close victim's nose with fingers, seal mouth around victim's mouth, and deliver breath by vigorous expiration.

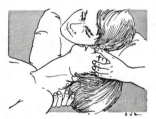

(3) Victim is allowed to exhale passively by unsealing mouth and nose. Rescuer should listen and feel for expiratory air flow.

Figure 4–3. Technique of mouth-to-mouth insufflation.

If this fails to clear the airway immediately, foreign body airway obstruction is possible; roll the victim onto one side and deliver a sharp blow between the shoulder blades. If this measure also fails, use the Heimlich procedure (Fig 4–4) or place an endotracheal tube. Perform a tracheostomy if other measures fail.

5. Feel the carotid or femoral artery for pulsations.

6. Give lung inflation by mouth-to-mouth breathing (keeping patient's nostrils closed) or mouth-to-nose breathing (keeping patient's

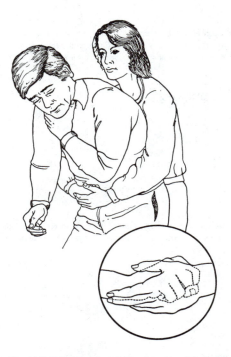

Figure 4–4. The Heimlich procedure is employed to dislodge an obstruction (frequently food) in the victim's throat. Place a fist with the thumb side against the victim's abdomen just above the navel and below the rib cage, and grasp the fist with the other hand. Give 4 quick, forceful upward thrusts. Repeat if necessary. If the victim is lying down, he or she should be turned to the supine position and straddled, and the rescuer should deliver the upward abdominal thrusts with one hand atop the other, the heel of the bottom hand pressing into the victim's abdomen. *If the victim is able to speak, even in a whisper, do not use the Heimlich procedure.*

mouth closed), 12 times per minute—allowing about 2 seconds for inspiration and 3 seconds for expiration—until spontaneous respirations return. The victim is allowed to exhale passively, or exhalation is assisted by pressure on the chest. The operator should be taking the next breath while listening to the sound of the victim's exhalation. Observe rise and fall of the chest, avoiding excessive pressure that may cause gastric distention.

B. Direct Inflation Using Anesthesia Mask: An oronasal anesthesia mask may be used as an aid for direct inflation. The victim's head must be extended and the jaw held anteriorly in order to keep the nasopharyngeal passage open. An oropharyngeal airway can also be used (see p 58).

OXYGEN ADMINISTRATION

Physiologic Basis for Oxygen Therapy
(Table 4–4)

Hypoxia develops when the blood is not carrying adequate amounts of O_2 and may only be evident by arterial gas analysis. Inadequate oxygenation or O_2 transport resulting from poisoning may be due to inadequacy or failure of respiration, pulmonary edema, laryngeal edema, laryngeal spasm or stridor, accumulation of tracheal or bronchial secretions, or combination of hemoglobin with substances that prevent O_2 exchange.

By increasing the percentage of O_2 in the inspired air, it is possible to greatly improve tissue oxygenation in anoxemia except when a portion of the lung is completely nonfunctioning or when the hemoglobin is in irreversible combination with interfering substances. However, even if most of the hemoglobin is unable to carry O_2, breathing 100% O_2 increases the amount of O_2 physically dissolved in the blood by 1.7 vol%; this may be sufficient to sustain tissue oxygenation.

At the same time increased amounts of O_2 are given in the air, CO_2 must be removed from the lungs. This can be accomplished by preventing rebreathing or by providing for the absorption of CO_2 with a soda-lime canister.

Adverse Effects of Oxygen Therapy
(See also p 455.)

A. Depression of Respiratory Centers: In anoxic comatose patients who have high blood CO_2 levels as a result of respiratory inadequacy, the respiratory center is not responsive to CO_2 and respiration is maintained by the chemoreceptor centers responsive to variations in O_2 tension. On rare occasions, a sudden increase in blood O_2 tension will cause a decrease in pulmonary ventilation, with further increase in retained CO_2. In such patients, O_2 therapy should be accompanied by artificial respiration to lower the blood CO_2 level and allow reestablishment of normal regulation of respiration. Maintenance of adequate blood oxygenation is of primary importance, and prolonged mechanical ventilation may be necessary.

B. Irritation From Improperly Humidified Oxygen: When O_2 is released from a tank it is completely dry; unless it is properly humidified, it will cause irritation.

C. Circulatory Embarrassment From Positive-Pressure Oxygen Therapy: Positive intrapulmonary pressures decrease venous return and may seriously lower blood pressure.

Devices for the Administration of Oxygen

Mechanical aids in the administration of O_2 vary greatly in complexity and require familiarity and practice for effective and safe use. The positive-pressure phase in resuscitation machines tends to be somewhat prolonged in relation to the expiratory phase, and the raised intrapulmonic pressure will limit venous return and lower blood pressure. Thus, use of these machines in the presence of cardiovascular collapse must be adequately supervised.

A. Inhalators: These are supplied with a tight-fitting face mask and a breathing bag. As a rule, no provision for reabsorption of CO_2 is supplied. O_2 concentration is variable from 50 to 100%, depending upon the rate of O_2 flow. With some types, resistance to exhalation can be increased in order to raise intratracheal pressure above atmospheric pressure. If a CO_2 absorber is used between the face mask and the breathing bag in the closed system, pressure applied to the breathing bag can be used for artificial respiration.

B. Automatic Cycling Positive-Pressure Oxygen Resuscitators: These are devices for the intermittent administration of O_2 at pressures as high as 25 mm Hg at a rate of 10–30 times per minute.

C. Automatic Cycling Positive-Negative–Pressure Oxygen Resuscitators: These utilize a cycling device operated by O_2 pressure and vary the pressure from 15 mm Hg positive to 10 mm Hg negative. The negative intratracheal pressure developed by these machines is dangerous in the presence of pulmonary edema, whereas in the presence of cardiovascular collapse the varying pressure tends to improve the circulation. Adjustment of these machines is critical, and O_2 consumption from the tank is considerably higher than that of resuscitators using positive pressure only.

PULMONARY EDEMA

Pulmonary edema resulting from poisoning is usually due to the inhalation of irritants, eg, chlorine gas, with injury to the pulmonary epithelium followed by exudation into the alveoli. Parasympathetic stimulants or cholinesterase inhibitors (phosphate esters) increase bronchial secretion and stimulate pulmonary edema. Overdoses of morphine analogs are also a common cause of pulmonary edema.

Pulmonary edema is dangerous because it interferes with O_2 exchange in the lungs. Patients eventually drown in their own secretions if the condition is not reversed.

Clinical Findings

Symptoms and signs of pulmonary edema include dyspnea, rales at the bases of or throughout both lungs, cyanosis, and rapid respiration. In extreme cases, gurgling respirations and foaming at the mouth may occur. The patient may be overwhelmed with anxiety.

Treatment

A. Emergency Measures:

1. Relieve anxiety. Give morphine sulfate, 10 mg, to decrease rate of rapid, inefficient respiration.

2. Give 40% O_2 by face mask.

3. Use intermittent positive-pressure O_2 resuscitator for short periods.

4. Give aminophylline, 0.5 g intravenously, to relieve associated bronchial constriction.

5. Treat pulmonary edema caused by morphine or morphine analogs by giving naloxone (see p 327) plus O_2.

B. General Measures:

1. Diuresis with ethacrynic acid (Edecrin), 25 mg orally or intravenously, or furosemide, 20–80 mg orally or intravenously, is helpful because it reduces fluid volume. Do not inject at a rate faster than 10 mg/min.

2. Give a corticosteroid anti-inflammatory agent in maximum doses.

3. If pulmonary edema is the result of heart failure, digitalize the patient (see p 68).

4. The semi-Fowler or sitting position may aid in relieving anxiety.

5. Reassurance is helpful to patients.

CIRCULATORY SYSTEM INVOLVEMENT

CIRCULATORY FAILURE, OR SHOCK

Clinical Findings

A. Primary Shock: (Fainting or collapse with low blood pressure.) This type of immediate collapse results from cerebral anoxia, which in turn is caused by circulatory insufficiency induced by painful stimuli, injury, unpleasant odors, nitrites, and local anesthetics. Response to treatment is usually rapid, but unless treatment is prompt there may be progression into secondary shock.

B. Secondary Shock: (Delayed or refractory shock.) Signs of secondary shock are cold, pale, cyanotic skin; sweating; rapid pulse; and low blood pressure. Secondary shock may develop in almost any type of severe poisoning but is especially common after poisoning with corrosive substances or depressant drugs.

Laboratory Findings

The hematocrit may reveal hemoconcentration. Proteinuria and hematuria may be present. Red blood count may be high or low.

The level of lactate in arterial blood may be used as an indication of the severity of circulatory failure: patients with levels under 2 mmol/L of blood are likely to survive, but those with levels above 4 mmol/L are not.

Treatment

A. Emergency Measures:

1. Place patient in the shock position, ie, supine with the feet elevated.

2. Establish and maintain an adequate airway (see p 58).

3. Maintain adequate body warmth by application of blankets, but do not apply external heat, since this may further aggravate shock.

4. Allay pain (see p 46). Give morphine sulfate, 10 mg/70 kg subcutaneously or intravenously, for otherwise uncontrollable pain. Morphine should not usually be given to children under 5 years of age or to unconscious or stuporous patients. Patients with depressed respiration should not be given morphine unless personnel and equipment to maintain respiration are immediately available.

5. Restore and maintain adequate circulating blood volume. Estimate requirements from the history and findings of vomiting, diarrhea, sweating, blood loss, and blood pressure. Elevated hematocrit indicates loss of plasma and requires administration of plasma or a plasma expander (see below). During fluid replacement, central venous pressure should not exceed 15 cm of water and pulmonary artery wedge pressure should not exceed 14 mm Hg.

a. Place an 18-gauge venous catheter and start intravenous administration of fluid with normal saline at a rate of 0.5–1 L/h if blood pressure is under 80 mm Hg. If systolic pressure is over 80 mm Hg, an infusion rate of 100–200 mL/h is sufficient. Dextrose in saline or 5% dextrose can also be used.

b. Plasma or plasma substitutes produce a more lasting rise in blood pressure. Give 500 mL immediately and repeat every 30 minutes up to a total of 2 L or until blood pressure response is adequate. Avoid serious hemodilution by monitoring hematocrit.

c. Whole blood must be properly typed and cross-matched; 1–4 L may be required.

d. Plasma expander–Dextran as a sterile, nonpyrogenic, nonantigenic solution in normal saline or 5% dextrose is used as an infusion colloid. Doses of 0.5–1 L may be given at a rate of 20–40 mL/min to maintain the systolic blood pressure at 80–85 mm Hg. The effect of a single dose will persist for 24–48 hours. Serious reactions to dextran are rare.

e. In patients with a severe fall of blood pressure, the administration of hydrocortisone, 10–25 mg/kg in the first 24 hours, has been suggested. Large volumes of plasma are then given until the central venous pressure reaches 12–14 cm of water. Of the vasopressor agents, dopamine appears to be least hazardous. Dopamine hydrochloride, 200 mg in 500 mL of 0.9% saline, is given at a rate of 0.5 mL/80 kg/min (2.5 μg/kg/min). It increases renal blood flow and cardiac output. Adverse effects include ventricular arrhythmias, precordial pain, and increase in blood urea nitrogen. In the presence of severe arteriolar constriction and reduction of blood flow to the kidneys, slow administration of phenoxybenzamine (Dibenzyline), 1 mg/kg intravenously, has also been suggested.

B. General Measures:

1. Correct anoxia (see p 57).
2. Correct acidosis (see p 49).
3. Correct dehydration or replace inadequate blood circulatory volume. Give 0.5–1 L of normal saline or 5% dextrose intravenously as necessary. Give fluids by mouth as soon as possible. Avoid giving more than 1 L of normal saline per day unless there is evidence of a need for sodium.
4. Observe constantly. Check pulse, respiration, and blood pressure every 15–30 minutes, and take rectal temperature every 2 hours. Repeat hematocrit frequently.

Chatton MJ: Shock syndrome. Pages 8–13 in: *Current Medical Diagnosis & Treatment 1986.* Krupp MA, Chatton MJ, Tierney LM Jr (editors). Lange, 1986.

CONGESTIVE HEART FAILURE

Poisons that produce myocardial damage will secondarily cause congestive heart failure.

Clinical Findings
Symptoms and signs include dyspnea, dependent edema, pulmonary edema, cardiac enlargement, and high venous pressure.

Treatment
A. General Measures:
1. Rest should be in bed or on a chair, with use of a bedside commode rather than a bedpan unless dyspnea is severe.
2. Diet should consist of frequent (4–6 per day) low-calorie, low-residue meals.
3. Sodium restriction aids in reduction of retained fluid. Rapid diuresis may be helpful. Give ethacrynic acid (Edecrin), 25 mg orally, or furosemide, 20 mg orally. Severe sodium restriction should not be instituted unless the ability of the kidneys to conserve sodium is known.

B. Digitalis:
Give digitalis cautiously intramuscularly unless there is definite evidence of myocardial failure. Intravenous administration of full digitalizing doses should never be attempted unless it is known that the patient has had no digitalis for the preceding 2 weeks.
1. Digoxin, 1 mg intravenously or orally, followed by 0.5 mg after 4 hours; then 0.25 mg every 4 hours until the desired effect is obtained. Maximal effect is reached in 1–2 hours; duration of effect is 3–6 days. Digoxin is becoming the preferred drug for digitalization.
2. Digitoxin, 0.6 mg intravenously, intramuscularly, or orally, followed by 0.2–0.4 mg every 4 hours until 1.2 mg has been given. Maximal effect is reached in 3–8 hours; duration of effect is 2–3 weeks.

CARDIAC ARREST

Cardiac arrest may occur as a result of general anesthesia, asphyxia from carbon monoxide or other gases, inhalation of chlorinated hydrocarbons, injection of local anesthetic agents, accidental ingestion or overdosage of cardiac drugs, asphyxia from pulmonary edema following the inhalation of irritants, and drug idiosyncrasy (especially quinidine, procaine or other local anesthetics, procainamide, aminophylline, and iodides). The possibility of cardiac arrest must be anticipated in order to give effective treatment. Practice in using lifesaving techniques is mandatory.

Clinical Findings
A presumptive diagnosis of cardiac arrest is made when pulse and

blood pressure suddenly disappear and no heart sounds are audible on auscultation. The ECG may indicate fibrillation or a normal rhythm.

Treatment *(Begin immediately!)*

   A. Emergency Measures: Do not wait for electrocardiographic confirmation.

   1. Place the patient supine with the operator above (Fig 4–5). For effective compression, the operator will need to kneel on the bed. A plywood board, $40 \times 60 \times 1$ cm ($16 \times 24 \times \frac{1}{2}$ inches), should be kept at each nursing station; this can be slipped under the patient's chest to improve the efficiency of compression when a soft mattress is used. Place the hands on the patient's sternum with the heel of one hand over the lower sternum, the second hand on top of the first. Rhythmically compress the heart by exerting body weight on the lower sternum. The force required is about 30 kg in an adult. Maintain the pressure for $\frac{1}{2}$ second and release. Repeat at a rate of 80 times a minute. The sternum should move 2.5–5 cm (1–2 inches) when pressure is applied. Do not exert pressure on the rib cage, epigastrium, or xiphoid process. With adequate compression, a femoral or carotid pulse should be easily pal-

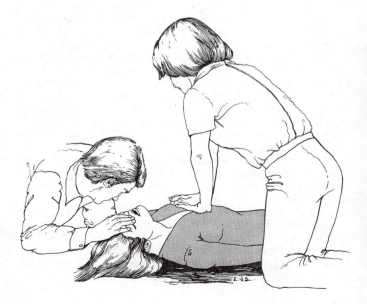

Figure 4–5. Technique of external cardiac massage.

pable simultaneously with chest compression. Use much less pressure in children to avoid rib fractures and separation of the sternum.

2. Maintain artificial respiration by either mouth-to-mouth, mouth-to-nose, or mouth-to-airway resuscitation at a rate of 2 quick inflations for each 15 chest compressions. Artificial respiration by means of a rebreathing bag, CO_2 absorber, and face mask using 100% O_2 is the most effective and controllable method, but instruction and practice in using this method are mandatory.

3. Maintain an adequate airway by means of a pharyngeal or endotracheal airway (see p 58).

4. Feel for the pulse and observe the pupils. If the circulation is maintained, the pulse will be palpable and the pupils will constrict if anoxia has been brief. (Pupils dilate with circulatory arrest.)

B. General Measures:

1. Start intravenous drip with 0.9% saline, 0.45% saline, or sodium bicarbonate.

2. Give epinephrine, 5 mL of 1:10,000 solution intravenously into arm vein (dilute 1 mL of 1:1000 solution to 10 mL). Repeat every 5 minutes as necessary.

3. If circulation is not restored in 5 minutes, give sodium bicarbonate, 1 mmol/kg body weight, to combat acidosis. Repeat half the initial dose every 10 minutes until spontaneous circulation is restored.

4. Give calcium chloride, 5 mL of 10% solution intravenously, to improve cardiac tone and contractions. Repeat every 10 minutes.

5. Defibrillation–If ventricular fibrillation is verified by electrocardiography, defibrillation should be performed if possible.

a. Use an external defibrillator. Prior instruction in its proper use is mandatory. Always maintain cardiac compression until immediately before defibrillation shock is applied. Only an oxygenated myocardium will defibrillate. Continue cardiac compression after defibrillation until a good pulse is maintained. The ECG may appear normal while the heartbeat is ineffective.

b. If ventricular fibrillation does not respond to electric shock, inject 1% lidocaine hydrochloride, 1 mg/kg intravenously. Procainamide, 1 mg/kg intravenously, or bretylium, 5 mg/kg intravenously, can also be tried.

6. Pacemaking in ventricular rhythm irregularity–In the presence of ventricular irregularities that can suddenly convert to ventricular fibrillation or other lethal rhythms, the use of a myocardial electrode and electrical pacemaker should be considered. Use an external electrical pacemaker with provision for internal electrode. Prior experience in its proper use is mandatory. During pacemaking, infusion of 0.1% lidocaine hydrochloride, 1 mL/min, may be necessary to suppress ventricular arrhythmias.

7. Give atropine sulfate, 0.5 mL of 1:1000 solution intra-

venously, to block vagal pacemaker inhibition and increase heart rate. Isoproterenol, 1 mg intravenously, can also be used.

8. Measure serum electrolytes and arterial pH. Correct hypokalemia by giving potassium chloride, 10–30 meq/h intravenously. Correct hyperkalemia by giving 50% glucose and insulin or potassium-adsorbing resin (sodium polystyrene sulfonate).

C. Equipment: The following items should be available at each nursing station, in each patient's room after cardiac surgery, and in every emergency room and operating room: electrocardiograph, pharyngeal airways of different sizes, O_2 tank, reducing valve, humidifier, tight-fitting face mask, CO_2 absorber, rebreathing bag, laryngoscope, mouth gag, and cuffed endotracheal tubes of various sizes, with adapters. For emergencies outside the hospital, a laryngoscope and several sizes of endotracheal tubes are most useful. Instructions in the use of this equipment should be given to physicians and nurses periodically.

Equipment that should be available on the operating floor and in the central supply room and emergency room includes the following:

1. Drugs–
   a. Epinephrine hydrochloride, 1:1000 solution.
   b. Lidocaine hydrochloride, 1-g ampules.
   c. Bretylium tosylate, 500-mg ampules.
   d. Procainamide, 1-g ampules.
   e. Calcium chloride, 10% solution.
   f. Atropine sulfate, 1:1000 solution.
   g. Potassium chloride, 15% solution (20 meq in 10 mL). Dilute to 1 L for use.
   h. Sodium bicarbonate, 7.5% (3.75 g in 50 mL).
   i. Saline, 0.45% and 0.9% solutions.
   j. Glucose, 50% solution.
   k. Insulin.
2. Syringes with needles.
3. Defibrillator unit, including sterile electrodes covered with gauze or felt, connecting wires, and jelly.
4. External electrical pacemaker with provision for internal electrode.

D. Complications During Closed-Chest Compression: These include pneumothorax, hemothorax, hemopericardium, fractured ribs, liver injury, bone marrow emboli, fractured sternum, ruptured spleen, and ruptured blood vessels, including abdominal, retroperitoneal, or intrathoracic vessels. Some of these can be avoided by observing the proper technique. Pressure should always be applied vertically just below the mid sternum and not over the rib cage or the abdomen.

Commerfield TJ, Lloyd EA: Arrhythmias in patients with drug toxicity, electrolyte, and endocrine disturbances. *Med Clin North Am* 1984;68:1051.

GENITOURINARY TRACT INVOLVEMENT

ACUTE RENAL FAILURE

Acute renal failure with oliguria or anuria may occur in poisoning from carbon tetrachloride, mercurials, arsenicals, sulfonamides, ethylene glycol, hemolytic substances (naphthalene, benzene, castor bean, etc), or substances that cause myoglobinuria (phencyclidine, convulsants, amphetamines). These substances either produce focal degenerative lesions in the tubule cells or block the tubules with hemoglobin or crystalline precipitates. Renal failure also occurs as a consequence of prolonged hypovolemia and hypotension.

Clinical & Laboratory Findings
A. Initial Period: The patient may be asymptomatic, with a daily urine output of up to 300–400 mL. Blood pressure may be normal or low. Urine examination reveals hemoglobin, protein, and red blood cells.

B. Period of Renal Shutdown: The patient may continue to be asymptomatic until signs of uremia appear, at which time weight gain, edema, and rales indicate fluid retention from overhydration. During this period, blood urea nitrogen rises rapidly and serum potassium also rises.

C. Recovery Period: The diuresis that accompanies recovery from renal shutdown can lead to dehydration and electrolyte imbalance. For example, muscular weakness can occur as a result of loss of potassium; tetany can also occur.

Treatment
A. Emergency Measures:
1. Treat shock (see p 66).
2. In hemolytic reactions, give sodium bicarbonate, 1–2 meq/kg every 6–12 hours; use it to supply the daily sodium requirement and to maintain an alkaline urine.

B. General Measures During Period of Renal Shutdown:
1. Weight monitoring–Weigh patient daily. Weight gain indicates fluid retention, which must be avoided. Weight loss of 0.3–0.5 kg/d represents tissue catabolic losses.
2. Fluid restriction–Restrict fluids to replacement of insensible water loss with glucose solutions. Increase the amount of water to replace fluid lost in diarrhea or vomiting.
3. Infection–Prevent infections by reverse isolation.
4. Blood chemistry–Serum sodium and potassium, blood urea ni-

trogen, blood creatinine, and blood pH should be determined daily and deficiencies corrected. Potassium should be avoided in most cases.

5. Digitalization–Cardiac failure is indicated by pulmonary venous congestion, cardiac enlargement, prolonged circulation time, tender enlargement of the liver, or increased venous pressure. If any of these develop, digitalize cautiously, because the half-life of digoxin is prolonged with renal impairment.

6. Dialysis–If the blood creatinine rises above 15 mg/dL or the serum potassium approaches 7–8 meq/L, consider hemodialysis or peritoneal dialysis (see p 88).

C. Period of Recovery: During this period, rapid blood electrolyte changes are likely to take place; daily serum electrolyte determinations are of great value in managing therapy.

The type of diuresis may vary from one patient to another. The following are examples:

1. If the return of tubular function is delayed, the patient's urine may be essentially a glomerular filtrate with large volume and low specific gravity. These patients continue to lose large amounts of potassium, sodium, and other ions. Adequate management requires analysis of daily 24-hour urine samples for total sodium and potassium losses and replacement as needed.

2. The diuresis may be accompanied by retention of sodium and a consequent rapid rise in serum sodium and chloride. Treatment in this case consists of providing sodium-free water.

3. Specific loss or retention of sodium, potassium, or calcium is best revealed by daily serum electrolyte determinations. Deficiencies are then corrected with appropriate salts.

D. Follow-Up: When recovery of renal function is complete, no further treatment is necessary but follow-up observation must be arranged.

URINE RETENTION

Irritant poisons excreted by the kidney may inflame the neck of the bladder sufficiently to cause urine retention, and poisoning can occasionally cause decreased bladder contractility. If urine is scanty, the size of the bladder should be determined by percussion or palpation. Catheterization can be performed if necessary. A self-retaining catheter may be advisable.

GASTROINTESTINAL TRACT INVOLVEMENT

VOMITING

Vomiting frequently accompanies poisoning and aids in the removal of ingested poisons. If vomiting is prolonged, however, symptomatic relief is desirable.

Treatment

A. Fluid Therapy: Fluid and nutritional balance must be maintained, although food and fluids must not be given orally until vomiting ceases. Administer 5–10% glucose in 0.3–0.5 N saline intravenously to maintain hydration until food can be given by mouth. When fluids can be given, clear broth, tea, and iced drinks are well tolerated. Resume oral feedings with dry foods in small quantities (eg, crackers or toast).

B. Drugs: Give chlorpromazine, 25–50 mg orally or by suppository as necessary every 4–6 hours. Chlorpromazine is contraindicated in central nervous system depression, jaundice, and liver disease; and many pediatricians prefer not to use it in children under age 6 years.

DIARRHEA

Diarrhea may be useful in aiding the removal of poisons from the body, but prolonged or severe diarrhea requires symptomatic relief to prevent fluid imbalance.

Treatment

A. Fluid Therapy: Fluid and nutritional balance must be maintained. Give 5–10% dextrose in 0.3–0.5 N saline or multiple electrolyte solution orally or intravenously. Food intake in the first 24 hours should be restricted to liquids or to low-residue foods, eg, broth, tea, rice gruel, precooked cereals, toast, or crackers. Later, bland foods can be added: cereals, strained soup, meat (not fried), bread, milk, milk products, and baked or boiled potatoes.

B. Drugs:

1. Pectin-kaolin mixtures, 15–30 mL after liquid bowel movements.

2. Atropine sulfate, 0.5 mg orally 3 times daily until liquid bowel movements cease, is occasionally employed.

ABDOMINAL DISTENTION

Intestinal atony is induced by some poisons and may be associated with hypokalemia.

Treatment
Colonic distention is relieved by passing a rectal or colonic tube (22–32F, 50–75 cm long) and eliminating the cause.

LIVER DAMAGE FROM DRUGS & CHEMICALS

Classification
The following types of liver damage can be distinguished:

A. General Cell Injury: Transaminase values are elevated, but alkaline phosphatase is low. Depending on the extent of damage, this type of injury may not be reversible.

1. Direct hepatotoxic effects (single dose, effect immediate, all individuals susceptible)–Acetaminophen, *Amanita phalloides*, arsenic, carbon tetrachloride, chloroform, phosphorus, stilbamidine, tannic acid, tetracyclines.

2. Delayed hepatotoxic effect (long exposure, all individuals susceptible)–Ethanol.

3. Hepatitislike reactions (sporadic, possible idiosyncrasy, response delayed)–Chloramphenicol, chlortetracycline, cinchophen, gold salts, halothane, iproniazid, isoniazid, methoxyflurane, novobiocin, penicillins, phenylbutazone, pyrazinamide, streptomycin, sulfamethoxypyridazine, trinitrotoluene, zoxazolamine.

4. Chronic hepatitislike reactions (slow onset, prolonged or repeated exposure)–Acetaminophen, aspirin, chlorpromazine, halothane, isoniazid, methyldopa, nitrofurantoin, oxyphenisatin.

B. Cholestatic Without Inflammatory Change: Transaminases and alkaline phosphatase are slightly elevated, and elevated bilirubin is obvious. This type of damage is dose-related and follows prolonged administration of methyltestosterone and progestational contraceptives.

C. Cholestatic With Portal Inflammation: Transaminases are slightly elevated and alkaline phosphatase and bilirubin are significantly elevated. This type usually occurs as a result of idiosyncrasy after prolonged or repeated administration. The damage occasionally progresses to biliary cirrhosis. The following drugs and chemicals have been implicated; aminosalicylic acid, chlorothiazide, chlorpromazine, phenindione, phenylbutazone, prochlorperazine, promazine, sulfadiazine, thiouracil, toluenediamine.

Clinical Findings
A. Acute Poisoning: Nausea and vomiting, anorexia, headache,

malaise, lethargy, abdominal pain, fever, jaundice, and enlarged, tender liver.

B. Chronic Poisoning: Weight loss, weakness, pallor, hematemesis, palmar erythema, enlarged or atrophic liver, jaundice, ascites, dependent edema, hemorrhoids, pruritus.

C. Laboratory Findings in Hemolytic Jaundice Due to Poisons: (Castor beans, naphthalene.) Hemoglobin is easily identified in the serum, and bilirubin is present in the urine. Urinary and fecal urobilinogen are increased. Serum bilirubin is increased, indicating the inability of the liver to remove bilirubin as fast as it is formed. The degree of the accompanying anemia indicates the severity of the process.

D. Laboratory Findings in Hepatic Cell Injury Due to Poisons:

1. Bilirubin is present in the urine.

2. Urinary urobilinogen is increased.

3. Fecal urobilinogen is decreased or unchanged.

4. Blood bilirubin is increased, indicating the inability of the liver to remove bilirubin as fast as it is formed. A gradual increase in bilirubinemia indicates progression of the lesion; reduction of the bilirubinemia indicates healing of the cellular injury.

5. Serum levels of liver cell enzymes—glutamic-oxaloacetic transaminase (SGOT), glutamic-pyruvic transaminase (SGPT), and lactate dehydrogenase (LDH)—are increased variably.

6. The synthetic and conjugative functions of the liver can be tested by a variety of methods. While reduced function indicated by these tests is important diagnostically, the presence of even severe liver injury cannot be excluded by a normal test. The following tests are used:

a. Altered serum albumin-globulin ratio can be shown by chemical tests. Serum albumin is decreased and serum globulin is normal or increased. These tests may show little correlation with clinical findings and are poor indicators of prognosis or of overall liver function. However, they are useful in monitoring the effect of treatment on impaired liver function or to indicate adverse effects of new drugs. Changes in serial tests are of more importance diagnostically and prognostically than are single tests.

b. A low plasma prothrombin concentration 24 hours after administration of phytonadione, 1 mg/kg intramuscularly, indicates that the liver is unable to synthesize prothrombin from vitamin K. Persistence of low plasma prothrombin in the absence of obstruction indicates a poor prognosis.

c. Diminished serum cholesterol or cholesteryl esters indicates severe injury to hepatic cells. Prognosis is poor if low levels persist. Serum cholesterol should be 150–240 mg/dL, of which 60% should be esterified.

E. Laboratory Findings in Bile Duct Obstruction With Cholestasis:
1. Serum bilirubin may rise over 30 mg/dL.
2. Serum alkaline phosphatase activity is increased.
3. Serum cholesterol is greatly increased.
4. Urine and fecal urobilinogen are decreased.

Treatment
A. Emergency Measures in Acute Liver Damage:
1. If possible, discontinue all drugs and chemicals, especially ethanol, barbiturates, sulfonamides, narcotics, salicylates, phenothiazines, steroids, arsenicals and other metals, and antihistamines.
2. Maintain complete bed rest.
3. Avoid anesthesia or surgical procedures.
B. General Measures in Acute or Chronic Liver Damage:
1. Avoid dehydration or overhydration. If vomiting is severe and oral fluids are not retained, replace vomitus with an equal quantity of 5–10% dextrose in 0.3–0.5 N saline. Administer maintenance fluids and electrolytes as necessary, depending on renal function.
2. Resume oral feedings as soon as the patient can tolerate them. Pay particular attention to the patient's appetite, and liberalize intake for a hungry patient. Control the amount of protein in the diet in order to correct the serum protein level.
3. Vitamin K–Give phytonadione, 2.5 mg daily.
4. Blood transfusion–If anemia is severe (hematocrit 10–15%), consider blood transfusion.

BLOOD & HEMATOPOIETIC SYSTEM INVOLVEMENT

METHEMOGLOBINEMIA

Methemoglobin is formed by oxidation of the ferrous (Fe^{2+}) iron of hemoglobin to the ferric (Fe^{3+}) form by the action of a number of chemicals, including nitrites, chlorates, and amino and nitro organic compounds. For example, sodium nitrite is used in meat curing; it may be present in excess in home-cured meat, or the meat-curing salt may be used accidentally as table salt. In infants or children, nitrates in well water contaminated from agricultural use of fertilizers or from bismuth subnitrate may be reduced to nitrites in the intestine and absorbed to cause methemoglobinemia. Organic nitrates and nitrites, including nitroglycerin, amyl nitrite, and other vasodilating nitrates, are all capable of causing methemoglobinemia. Acetanilid, phenacetin, aniline, nitrobenzene, and other nitro and amino organic compounds are also powerful methemoglobin formers.

The ferric iron of methemoglobin can be reduced to ferrous iron (hemoglobin) most promptly by administration of methylene blue. After administration, the colored methylene blue is rapidly converted to a leuko base by the coenzyme diphosphopyridine nucleotide (DPN). This leuko base rapidly reduces ferric iron (Fe^{3+}) to ferrous iron (Fe^{2+}). The reactions are as follows:

$$\text{Reduced DPN} + \text{Methylene blue} \rightarrow \text{DPN} + \text{Leuko methylene blue}$$

$$\text{Leuko methylene blue} + \underset{(Fe^{3+})}{\text{Methemoglobin}} \rightarrow \underset{(Fe^{2+})}{\text{Hemoglobin}} + \text{Methylene blue}$$

The reaction continues in the presence of reduced DPN. In the absence of methemoglobinemia, administration of methylene blue will convert a small portion of hemoglobin to methemoglobin.

Ascorbic acid is also capable of reducing the ferric iron of methemoglobin to the ferrous iron of hemoglobin, but the action is slower than that of methylene blue.

Clinical Findings

A. Symptoms and Signs: Cyanosis occurs when 15% of hemoglobin has been converted to methemoglobin, but symptoms of headache, dizziness, weakness, and dyspnea are not likely to occur until the concentration reaches 30–40%. At levels of 60%, stupor and respiratory depression occur, and blood is chocolate-colored. At levels above 60%, fatalities occur.

B. Laboratory Findings: Spectrophotometric analysis gives the concentration of methemoglobin in the blood.

Treatment

A. Emergency Measures:

1. Give 100% O_2 by mask to increase the O_2 saturation of plasma and unchanged hemoglobin if the patient shows dyspnea or air hunger.

2. Remove ingested poison by emesis or gastric lavage; terminate skin contact by removing contaminated clothing and washing the skin thoroughly with soap and water.

B. Antidote: (When methemoglobin concentration is 25–40% or in presence of symptoms.)

1. Give methylene blue, 1% solution, 0.1 mL/kg intravenously over a 10-minute period. Cyanosis may disappear within minutes or may persist longer, depending on the degree of methemoglobinemia. Intravenous administration of therapeutic doses of methylene blue may

cause a rise in blood pressure, nausea, and dizziness. Larger doses (> 500 mg) cause vomiting, diarrhea, chest pain, mental confusion, cyanosis, and sweating. Hemolytic anemia has also occurred several days after administration. These effects are temporary, and fatalities have not been reported.

2. If methylene blue is not available, give ascorbic acid, 1 g slowly intravenously.

3. Without treatment, methemoglobin levels of 20–30% revert to normal within 3 days.

C. General Measures:

1. Absolute bed rest must be enforced if methemoglobinemia is above 40%.

2. Continue O_2 therapy for at least 2 hours after methylene blue has been given.

AGRANULOCYTOSIS & OTHER BLOOD DYSCRASIAS

A large number of drugs, chemicals, and metals are capable of causing blood dyscrasias, including agranulocytosis, leukopenia, aplastic anemia, and thrombocytopenia. The incidence of these reactions varies from approximately one case in 100 to one in 1000 in patients receiving aminopyrine, phenylbutazone, thiouracil, apronalide (Sedormid), gold salts, and arsenicals; the incidence is less than one case in 10,000 users of antihistamines, antibiotics, anticonvulsants, and thiouracil derivatives (Table 4–5).

Almost all blood dyscrasias appear to occur because of sensitivity to a drug in concentrations that are ordinarily tolerated; a few are seen after obviously toxic drug concentrations have been achieved; and irreversible idiosyncratic responses to a drug occur rarely. With chloramphenicol, all 3 types of reactions have been seen.

Laboratory Findings

A. Agranulocytosis: Decrease or disappearance of granulocytes from peripheral blood. Myeloid cells are reduced or absent in bone marrow smears while red cell series and megakaryocytes are normal.

B. Aplastic Anemia: Bone marrow is deficient in all cellular elements.

C. Thrombocytopenia: Decrease or disappearance of platelets from blood.

Treatment

A. Emergency Measures: Discontinue the offending drug at the first symptom.

Table 4—5. Incidence of blood dyscrasias from drugs or chemicals.

Drug	Estimated Incidence per 100,000 Users	Type of Blood Dyscrasias Produced
Aminopyrine	1000	Agranulocytosis.
Benzene	1000	Aplastic anemia.
Phenylbutazone, dipyrone, oxyphen-butazone	1000	Leukopenia.
Thiouracil	1000	Agranulocytosis.
Apronalide (Sedormid)	1000	Thrombocytopenia.
Propylthiouracil	100	Agranulocytosis.
Gold salts	100	Agranulocytosis, aplastic anemia.
Arsenicals	100	Aplastic anemia, agranulocytosis.
Phenothiazine tranquilizers	100	Agranulocytosis.
Indomethacin	100	Leukopenia.
Sulfonamides, lindane, chlordane	10	Agranulocytosis, thrombocytopenia, aplastic anemia.
Trimethadione (Tridione)	10	Agranulocytosis, aplastic anemia.
Phenytoin (Dilantin), chlorpromazine, imipramine, methimazole	10	Agranulocytosis, thrombocytopenia.
Mephenytoin (Mesantoin)	10	Hemolytic anemia, aplastic anemia.
Quinidine, sulfamethoxypyridazine, chlorothiazide, hydrochlorothiazide, quinine	10	Agranulocytosis, thrombocytopenia.
Chloramphenicol	4–10	Any combination.
Antihistamines	1	Agranulocytosis.
Streptomycin	1	Agranulocytosis.

B. General Measures:

1. Chemotherapy–In the presence of fever, sore throat, pulmonary congestion, or other signs of infection, give organism-specific antibiotic therapy until infection is controlled.

2. Blood transfusion–Give transfusions of specific components needed.

3. Isolate the patient, if possible, to reduce exposure to infection.

HEMOLYTIC REACTIONS

A number of substances, including arsine, stibine, and dichloromethane, can cause acute hemolytic reactions by a direct effect on red cells. Many other hemolytic reactions occur on the basis of glucose-6-phosphate dehydrogenase (G6PD) deficiency, which occurs in approximately 11% of black American males, in a smaller proportion of the descendants of Mediterranean and Oriental ethnic groups, and in about 1% of others. More than 40 substances are capable of causing hemolysis on this basis. The list includes naphthalene, nitrofurantoin, salicylazosulfapyridine, sulfisoxazole, sulfamethoxypyridazine, aminosalicylic acid, sulfoxone, primaquine, antipyretics, water-soluble vitamin K (menadiol and menadione sodium bisulfite), and uncooked fava beans.

Clinical Findings

A. Symptoms and Signs: Onset is sudden, with chills, fever, nausea and vomiting, abdominal or back pain, jaundice, and red or black urine. Fall of blood pressure and shock may occur if the onset of anemia is severe and abrupt. Oliguria or anuria indicates acute renal failure as a result of renal ischemia and precipitation of hemoglobin in the renal tubules.

B. Laboratory Findings: The anemia is normocytic, but burr cells and red cell fragments are apparent on microscopic examination. Serum may contain hemoglobin or methemalbumin, and urine may contain hemoglobin and hemosiderin. G6PD deficiency can be identified by several tests: glutathione stability, cresyl blue reduction, methemoglobin reduction, and a commercially available dye reduction spot test. The red cell count is lowest several days after onset and then gradually returns to normal.

Treatment

A. Maintain Urine Output: In the presence of hemoglobinuria with normal kidney function, maintain urine output at 2–3 mL/kg/h. Furosemide, 20–80 mg orally or intravenously every 4–8 hours, may be helpful. Alkalinize the urine by giving sodium bicarbonate, 1–2 meq/kg every 12 hours. Monitor central venous pressure and electrolytes. Mannitol administration has been used to maintain urine output.

B. Exchange Transfusion: If serum hemoglobin exceeds 1.5 g/dL, total exchange transfusion may prevent renal failure.

C. Treat Methemoglobinemia: In the presence of methemoglobinemia with hemolysis, treat methemoglobinemia by giving methylene blue, 1 mg/kg.

DERMATITIS DUE TO CONTACT WITH CHEMICALS

Dermatitis due to chemicals may arise as a result of primary irritation or may be due to sensitization.

Diagnosis

    A. Primary Reactions: Dermatitis due to primary irritants is characterized by the following:

    1. The site of maximal involvement is the site of maximal exposure.

    2. The site of maximal exposure is the site of first appearance.

    3. Other exposed persons have similar involvement.

    4. The time relationship between the beginning of exposure and the onset of dermatitis is similar in all those exposed.

    B. Allergic Reactions: Dermatitis caused by sensitizing materials is characterized by the following:

    1. The site of maximal involvement may be different from the site of maximal exposure.

    2. The time relationship between the onset of exposure and the onset of dermatitis is variable.

    3. Other exposed persons may not have similar eruptions.

**Evaluation of Dermatitis Due to
Contact With Chemicals**

    A. Contact Dermatitis From Direct Irritants: About 80% of cases of contact dermatitis are due to primary irritants. A primary or direct irritant is an agent that is capable of injuring the skin at the site of the first application if the concentration and duration of exposure are sufficient. Examples of primary irritants are solvents, acids, alkalies, soaps, and other corrosives and irritants (see Chapters 14 and 29).

    B. Sensitization Dermatitis: Dermatitis due to sensitizers occurs only after repeated contact. The site of allergic contact dermatitis is often a clue to the diagnosis; for example, reactions on earlobes or around wrist or neck may be due to jewelry, and scalp reactions may be due to chemicals in hair dyes. However, the dermatitis is not necessarily limited to the site of contact; it may involve larger areas of skin. Patch tests may be helpful in the diagnosis of sensitization to a chemical, but they have serious limitations.

    Patch tests: Patch testing consists of applying a nonirritating (low) concentration of the suspected contact antigen to the patient's skin and covering it with an occlusive dressing. Sterile, unimpregnated gauze must surround the patch and separate it from the area where the adhesive tape touches the skin (to distinguish reactions to the patch from reactions to adhesive). The dressing is removed after 48 hours. An eczematous reaction at the site of the patch test constitutes a positive response. A positive response is more meaningful than a negative one, because false-negative results may occur for many reasons.

Prevention

    (1) Use of impervious gloves, masks, gauntlets, aprons, and

clothing if necessary may help to reduce the incidence of dermatitis.

(2) Workers should wash frequently with mild soap.

(3) The use of degreasing solvents, paint thinner, solvents, and harsh cleaning agents for cleaning the skin should be avoided.

(4) Protective creams or ointments may be useful preventives.

(5) A high incidence of dermatitis in a factory may require personal inspection of the workplace by the physician.

Treatment

A. Avoidance: Discontinue contact with any irritating or sensitizing medications. Sensitizers include all mercurial antiseptics, sulfonamides, antibiotics, local anesthetics, phenols, resorcinol, nitrofurazone, adhesive tape, various dyes, and many others. Ointments sometimes contain a mercurial as a preservative.

B. Mild Wet Dressings: Moist, oozing lesions are treated by application of mild wet dressings, which should be replaced every 2–3 hours. Impervious coverings prevent the cooling effects of evaporation and should not be used. The following medications can be used without fear of aggravating the irritation:

1. Aluminum acetate, 1% solution.

2. Magnesium sulfate, half-saturated (25%) solution.

3. Sodium bicarbonate, saturated (10%) or half-saturated (5%) solution.

4. Starch or oatmeal solution (can be used as a bath and repeated every 2–4 hours). A starch bath is prepared by mixing a cup of cornstarch in 2 quarts of water. The mixture is heated to boiling and then poured into a cool bath. The patient then sits in the bath for 10 minutes and pours the starch solution over the affected areas.

5. Normal saline solution (sodium chloride, 1 teaspoon per pint or 1 pound per 12 gallons).

6. Potassium permanganate, 1:10,000 solution (leaves a stain but otherwise is excellent).

C. Mild Ointments: Fissured, thickened, scaling eruptions are treated by mild ointments, of which the following are satisfactory:

1. Zinc oxide ointment.

2. Zinc oxide (Lassar's) paste.

3. Hydrophilic ointment (Aquaphor).

Mathias CGT, Maiback HI: Perspectives in occupational dermatology. *West J Med* 1982;**137**:486.

SPECIAL METHODS USED IN TREATMENT
OF POISONING

CHELATING AGENTS

Lead, ferric or ferrous iron, mercury, copper, nickel, zinc, cadmium, cobalt, beryllium, arsenic, and manganese can be effectively detoxified by the formation of stable ring compounds by the coordination of electrons from the metallic element with an unshared pair of electrons from an organic compound (chelation). These metal chelates are excreted from the body.

1. DIMERCAPROL (BAL)

Metals such as mercury and arsenic apparently combine with –SH groups in enzyme systems to cause inactivation. Dimercaprol serves as a metal acceptor to prevent or reverse this inactivation. It combines with metals as shown in Fig 4–6, forming cyclic combinations that are soluble in body fluids and appear to be more stable than the monothio compounds formed between metals and the cellular enzymes. The metals are thus removed from the plasma or from combination in or on cells and excreted.

Effects of Dimercaprol

The drug stimulates the central nervous system and constricts muscular arterioles, possibly by inhibiting cytochrome oxidase.

Overdose of dimercaprol causes a variety of symptoms depending on the dosage. At doses up to 3 mg/kg, about 20% of patients will have anorexia, restlessness, generalized aches and pains, itching, salivation, and elevation of blood pressure of 10–20 mm Hg. At doses up to 5 mg/kg, up to 60% of patients will have, in addition, fever and tachycardia, and blood pressure elevation may reach 30–40 mm Hg. At doses over 5 mg/kg, all patients are likely to have vomiting, convulsions, and stupor or coma, beginning within 30 minutes after injection. Such reactions

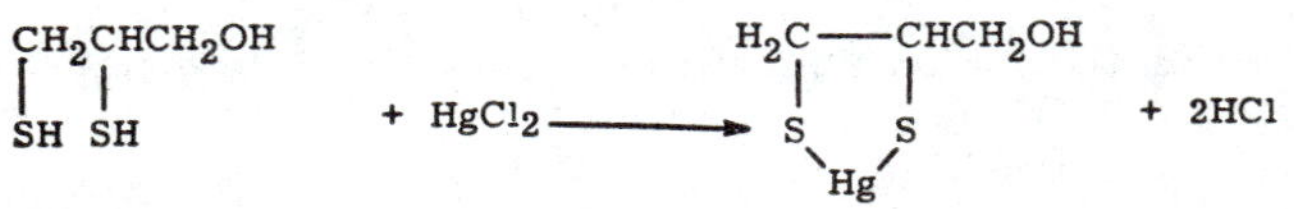

$$\begin{array}{c}\text{CH}_2\text{CHCH}_2\text{OH} \\ | \quad | \\ \text{SH} \quad \text{SH}\end{array} \quad + \quad \text{HgCl}_2 \longrightarrow \quad \begin{array}{c}\text{H}_2\text{C}———\text{CHCH}_2\text{OH} \\ | \qquad | \\ \text{S} \qquad \text{S} \\ \diagdown \quad \diagup \\ \text{Hg}\end{array} \quad + \quad \text{2HCl}$$

Dimercaprol

Figure 4–6. Dimercaprol in combination with metals.

have usually subsided in 1–6 hours, even after doses as large as 40 mg/kg. Fatalities have not been reported.

Treatment With Dimercaprol

A. Timing: Because dimercaprol is more effective in preventing combination of metals with enzymes than in reactivating enzyme systems, prompt use is important. It should be given within the first 4 hours after poisoning to obtain the maximum benefit.

B. Administration and Dosage: Dimercaprol is supplied as a 10% solution in oil for intramuscular administration. Each ampule contains 3 mL (300 mg). Give 3 mg/kg (0.3 mL/10 kg) every 4 hours for the first 2 days and then 2 mg/kg every 12 hours. A total of 10 days of treatment may rarely be necessary.

C. Precautions:

1. Maintain an alkaline urine during treatment, because the dimercaprol-metal complex is not acid-stable.

2. Since recent observations suggest that dimercaprol chelates can enter the central nervous system in significant amounts, patients should be monitored for central nervous system symptoms.

D. Contraindications:

1. Do not use in iron, cadmium, or selenium poisoning or when iron is being administered medicinally; the resulting chelates are more harmful than the metals alone.

2. Do not use in the presence of hepatic insufficiency unless this is due to arsenic poisoning.

3. Discontinue or do not use at all in the presence of acute renal insufficiency.

E. Ephedrine: If nausea and sweating are severe, give ephedrine sulfate, 25 mg orally prior to administration of each dose of dimercaprol. Diphenhydramine is also useful.

2. CALCIUM DISODIUM EDETATE
(EDTA)

Calcium disodium edetate (ethylenediaminetetraacetic acid) is an effective chelating agent that forms readily soluble, practically nonionized and nontoxic compounds with multivalent metals (Fig 4–7), but its usefulness as an antidote is limited to those metals which are bound more tightly than calcium. Lead, iron, zinc, manganese, beryllium, and copper form compounds with edetate that cannot be displaced by calcium. Edetate is given in the form of a calcium chelate in order to prevent the toxic effects of rapid removal of calcium from the body. Edetate does not appear to be metabolized by the body, and it is poorly absorbed by the gastrointestinal tract.

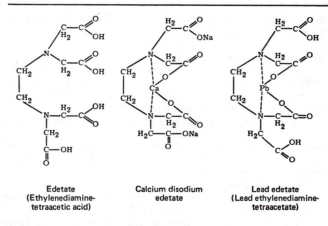

Edetate
(Ethylenediamine-
tetraacetic acid)

Calcium disodium
edetate

Lead edetate
(Lead ethylenediamine-
tetraacetate)

Figure 4–7. Forms of edetate. Dotted lines represent coordinate bonds.

Effects of Edetate

A. Adverse Effects: Administration of edetate in doses larger than those recommended has caused renal tubular damage with oliguria. The dose recommended below has caused only a transient fall in blood pressure without other signs of toxicity. Hypokalemia also occurs. A prolonged course of administration would remove other metals such as magnesium from the body, and it is advisable to interrupt treatment frequently so that mineral losses can be replaced.

B. Laboratory Findings: Studies on the use of edetate in lead poisoning indicate that a large increase in lead excretion occurs on the first day or so of administration. This indicates that the drug should be given in repeated short courses interrupted by rest periods.

Treatment With Edetate

Edetate is available in 5-mL ampules containing 200 mg/mL (20% solution).

A. Intravenous: Give 15–25 mg/kg (0.08–0.125 mL/kg body weight) in 250–500 mL of 5% dextrose intravenously over a 1- to 2-hour period twice daily. The maximum dose should not exceed 50 mg/kg/d. The drug should be given in 5-day courses with a rest period of at least 2 days between courses. After the first course, subsequent courses should not exceed 50 mg/kg/d. Daily urinalyses should be done during the treatment period. The dosage should be reduced if any unusual urinary findings appear.

B. Intramuscular: For intramuscular administration, give 12.5

mg/kg body weight every 4–6 hours. Dilute each dose with an equal volume of 1% procaine. Dose limitation is the same as that given above.

C. Dimercaprol (BAL): For severe intoxications, some experts urge simultaneous administration of dimercaprol during the first 48 hours of treatment.

3. DEFEROXAMINE
(Desferal)

Deferoxamine has a specific ability to chelate iron and is useful in treating acute iron intoxication. Its iron chelate, ferrioxamine, is water-soluble and is excreted in the urine. Effects on other metals have not been found. It is usually given only if the serum iron level exceeds 400–600 μg/dL 3–4 hours after ingestion and vomiting and diarrhea are present.

Adverse Effects

Adverse reactions include pain and induration at the site of injection, generalized erythema, urticaria, hypotension, other skin rashes, anaphylactic reactions, blurring of vision, abdominal discomfort, diarrhea, leg cramps, tachycardia, and fever.

Treatment With Deferoxamine

Neither oral nor intramuscular administration is now recommended. Deferoxamine should be given intravenously in a dose of 40 mg/kg over 4 hours, with the rate of administration not exceeding 15 mg/kg/h.

4. PENICILLAMINE
(Cuprimine)

Penicillamine, a hydrolysis product of penicillin, is readily absorbed after oral administration and rapidly excreted without metabolic change. It is useful for removing copper, lead, and possibly mercury from the body.

Adverse Effects

Anaphylaxis may occur in patients sensitive to penicillins. Other adverse effects include nausea, skin rash, fever, leukopenia, thrombocytopenia, aplastic anemia, nephrosis, purpura, lymph gland enlargement, pyridoxine deficiency, optic neuritis, and nephrotic syndrome. These reactions have occurred in patients being treated for copper storage disease, cystinuria, or scleroderma. Such reactions have not been reported in the treatment of lead poisoning.

Treatment With Penicillamine

Give up to 100 mg/kg/d (maximum 1 g/d), divided into 4 doses, for no longer than 1 week. If a longer administration period is warranted, dosage should not exceed 40 mg/kg/d. Give the drug orally half an hour before meals. For young children, empty capsule into small amount of fruit juice before giving.

OSMOTIC DIURESIS

Forced diuresis has been considered useful in increasing the excretion of some drugs, but it can be hazardous, and there is only limited evidence that it is significantly effective. Intravenous infusions of hypertonic solutions of dextrose, urea, and mannitol increase extracellular fluid volume, resulting in temporary diuresis. Osmotic diuretics are used as an aid in the treatment of cerebral edema resulting from lead poisoning.

Warren SE, Blantz RC: Mannitol. *Arch Intern Med* 1981;**141**:493.

DIALYSIS, HEMOPERFUSION, & "GUT DIALYSIS"

Hemodialysis and peritoneal dialysis can be useful in removing certain poisons from the body, especially if kidney function is impaired (Table 4–6). These techniques have been superseded by other easier, equally effective or more effective methods of managing many types of poisoning (eg, intensive supportive care for barbiturate overdoses, alkalinization of the urine for salicylate intoxication), but dialysis is still considered a useful back-up measure for such cases. In contrast, dialysis is the treatment of choice for acute management of seizures or tachyarrhythmias in some poisonings due to agents that are limited in distribution and not highly bound, eg, theophylline intoxications with blood drug levels of 60–70 mg% (adults) or 100 mg% (children).

Indications for dialysis include deep coma with low blood pressure, anuria, and apnea following severe poisoning with any agents for which dialysis is useful.

Lipid dialysis has been successfully used to remove the lipid-soluble agent camphor.

Hemoperfusion through resin or coated charcoal columns is also used in the treatment of toxic reactions.

"Gut dialysis" was originally developed to sterilize the bowel for colon surgery. The technique involves continuous flushing of the intestine with a hypotonic electrolyte-containing solution administered via a

Table 4–6. Toxic agents for which peritoneal dialysis or hemodialysis may be indicated.*

Sedative-hypnotics	Heavy metals	Miscellaneous
Alcohols	Arsenic (after dimercaprol)	Anilines
Chloral hydrate	Arsenicals	Antibiotics
Ethanol	Arsine	Borates
Ethchlorvynol (Pla-	Iron (after deferoxamine)	Boric acid
cidyl)	Lead (after edetate)	Carbon tetrachloride
Ethylene glycol	Mercury (after dimercaprol)	Chlorates
Methanol	**Other metals**	Dichromate
Barbiturates	Calcium	Ergotamine
Carbamates	Lithium	Isoniazid
Ethinamate (Valmid)	Magnesium	Mushroom *(Amanita*
Meprobamate (Equa-	Potassium	*phalloides)*
nil, Miltown)	**Halides**	Nitrobenzenes
Paraldehyde	Bromides	Nitrofurantoin
Nonnarcotic analgesics	Fluorides	Phenytoin (Dilantin)
Acetaminophen	Iodides	Sulfonamides
Aspirin	**Alkaloids**	Theophylline
Methyl salicylate	Quinidine	Thiocyanates
Phenacetin	Quinine	
Amphetamines	Strychnine	

*Dialysis is not usually useful for the following compounds:

Amitriptyline (Elavil)	Digitalis	Nortriptyline
Anticholinergics	Diphenoxylate (Lomotil)	(Aventyl)
Antidepressants	Glutethimide (Doriden)	Oxazepam (Serax)
Antihistamines	Hallucinogens	Phenelzine (Nardil)
Atropine	Heroin, other opiates	Phenothiazines
Chlordiazepoxide	Imipramine (Tofranil)	Propoxyphene
(Librium)	Methaqualone (Quaalude)	(Darvon)
Diazepam (Valium)	Methyprylon (Noludar)	

nasogastric tube. It has recently been used in the management of paraquat intoxications, but its effectiveness in such cases is not yet proved.

PHARMACOKINETICS & TOXIC CONCENTRATIONS
(See tables at end of Chapters 21, 22, 23, 24, 26, 27, 28, 31, and 32.)

Data concerning the distribution, metabolism, and elimination of drugs and chemicals can be of use in the management of poisoning. For example, if a pH gradient exists across a membrane, drugs and chemicals tend to be trapped in the compartment in which they are more ionized. Thus, aspirin, for which the dissociation constant (pK_a) of the carboxyl group is 3.16×10^{-4}, is half ionized at pH 3.5 ($pK_a = 3.5$) and even more ionized with higher pHs. Thus it is trapped on the more alkaline side of membranes. By alkalinizing the urine, the excretion of aspirin can be increased by a factor of 10–20. The excretion of phency-clidine, which has a pK_a around 9.0, can be increased 200-fold by acidifying the urine to pH 5.0 or less. However, it should be pointed out that excretion of phencyclidine in urine, unlike that of aspirin, accounts for elimination of only a small fraction of the drug present.

The **apparent volume of distribution** (V_d in L/kg) indicates the apparent body volume into which a substance is distributed after absorption. The V_d in L/kg is calculated by dividing the amount of a substance absorbed (mg/kg) by the plasma or serum level of the substance in mg/L.

$$V_d \text{ (L/kg)} = \frac{\text{Dose absorbed (mg/kg)}}{\text{Plasma concentration (mg/L)}}$$

Substances that have volumes of distribution appreciably greater than 1 L/kg, ie, are deposited widely in fat (for example, tricyclic antidepressants and digitalis) or that are 90% or more bound to plasma proteins, are not effectively dialyzable in practice.

For some drugs, such as salicylate and acetaminophen, the "zero time" concentration is most indicative of the toxic effect to be expected. Serial blood concentrations can be used to estimate zero time concentration by extrapolation (see disappearance half-times, below).

Disappearance half-times ($t_{\frac{1}{2}}$) indicate the length of time in hours required to reduce the plasma concentration of a substance by one-half. By graphing the serial plasma concentration on semilogarithmic paper, the resulting straight line can be used to determine the disappearance half-time in any particular patient. The rate of disappearance from plasma is often dose-dependent or varies depending on the concentration; this is referred to as "first-order" kinetics. Some compounds (eg, ethanol) rapidly saturate the enzymes involved, so that regardless of the drug concentration, a constant reduction in serum level is found (eg, 15 mg%/h for ethanol); this is called "zero-order" kinetics. In some instances, metabolism of a given drug will follow "first-order" kinetics when the drug is present in low concentrations but will revert to "zero-order" kinetics as the serum concentration of the drug rises. This situation is referred to as Michaelis-Menton kinetics or saturation kinetics.

Atkinson AJ, Kushner W: Clinical pharmacokinetics. *Annu Rev Pharmacol Toxicol* 1979;**19**:105.

Avery GS (editor): *Drug Treatment,* 2nd ed. Publishing Sciences Group, 1980.

Baselt RC: *Disposition of Toxic Drugs and Chemicals in Man,* 2nd ed. Biomedical Publications, 1982.

Burke MD: Principles of therapeutic drug monitoring. *Postgrad Med* (July) 1981;**70**:57.

Kalman SM, Clark DR: *Drug Assay: The Strategy of Therapeutic Drug Monitoring*. Masson, 1979.

Knoben JE, Anderson PO, Watanabe AS (editors): *Handbook of Clinical Drug Data*, 5th ed. Drug Intelligence Publications, 1983.

Ritschel WA: *Handbook of Basic Pharmacokinetics*, 2nd ed. Drug Intelligence Publications, 1982.

Rodwell VW: Water. Chapter 2 in: *Harper's Review of Biochemistry*, 20th ed. Martin DW et al. Lange, 1985.

Rowland M, Tozer JT: *Clinical Pharmacokinetics*. Lea & Febiger, 1980.

Williams RL, Benet LV: Drug pharmacokinetics in cardiac and hepatic disease. *Annu Rev Pharmacol Toxicol* 1980;**20:**389.

5 | Legal & Medical Responsibility in Poisoning

Responsibility for the consequences of poisoning has been shifting in recent years with the advent of legal action by consumers and workers against producers and sellers of toxic materials. For example, a class action suit on behalf of asbestos workers in one company was settled for $20 million, and thousands of other legal claims involving asbestos are still pending. Workers and consumers are beginning to assert their right to know what poisons are present in products they are exposed to.

Legal action for alleged mismanagement of poisoning cases has been taken against physicians and against at least one poison information center.

Written Records

In any case of poisoning in which there is a possibility of legal action at a later date, the physician must keep careful written records of all relevant observations and findings. A history obtained from another party must be carefully noted as such in the records. Since court action may begin several years later, written records are essential to maintain the physician's position as an accurate and unbiased observer.

Preservation of Evidence

If the physician suspects poisoning in any patient, care must be used to save evidence that may be important for identification of the poison. The bottles used for storing specimens should be clean and free from contamination by chemicals or metals. It is best not to use bottles that have been previously used for chemicals or for pathologic specimens. A clear glass bottle with a plastic or metal cap with a heavy waxed paper liner is adequate. The container should be sealed with a glue-paper label extending over the cover and down onto the jar. The physician's signature should be affixed to the label at the juncture between cap and bottle. Avoid using a seal such as adhesive tape, which can be removed and replaced. If analysis cannot be done immediately, the material should be stored in a freezer. Preservatives should not be used, since they may mask chemicals of toxicologic importance. If shipping is necessary, containers should be wrapped with paper and placed in cartons with dry ice.

A. Evidence to Be Saved in Nonfatal Poisoning:

1. Prescription containers or other containers from which the poison was obtained.
2. Urine (24-hour specimen).
3. Blood (10–50 mL).
4. Vomitus and first 2 gastric washings. (Indicates ingestion of poison but not necessarily systemic poisoning.)
5. Feces.
6. Body fat (obtained by biopsy).
7. Hair clippings.
8. Clippings of fingernails and toenails.
9. Food.

B. Evidence to Be Saved in Fatal Poisoning: Autopsy must be performed prior to embalming because blood collected at the time of embalming will be contaminated by embalming fluid. In taking pathologic specimens, be certain that gloves and instruments are not contaminated by disinfectants or chemicals which may be transferred to specimens. Specimens should be placed directly in containers known to be clean; do not allow them to become contaminated on a table or sink. Store the specimens in a frozen state without any chemical preservatives. In addition to the items listed above, the following should be collected and stored:

1. The stomach and contents.
2. Liver (at least one-half).
3. Kidneys (at least one).
4. Blood (50–100 mL; should completely fill container).
5. Bone (100 g).
6. Lung (at least one).
7. Brain (at least one-half).

C. Legal Chain of Custody: In cases of poisoning in which specimens are of medicolegal importance, the physician must use care to establish a legal chain of custody so that each person having responsibility for the material can state under oath that it has not been contaminated or tampered with.

SPECIAL PROBLEMS

Attempted Suicide

In treating a patient who has attempted suicide, the physician's main responsibility is to give immediate medical care and to prevent further attempts. The patient must be placed in quiet, protected surroundings, preferably away from the family. Hospitalization is frequently necessary. After the patient recovers from the immediate symptoms, a careful evaluation should be made, preferably by a psychiatrist, to minimize the possibility of further suicide attempts.

Successful Suicide

If a patient commits suicide, the physician is legally responsible for reporting the death to the police and to the coroner. Proof of suicide may have considerable legal importance, and the physician will be called upon to justify all statements by careful observations and written records.

Homicidal Poisoning

Although homicidal poisoning appears to be rare, in view of the frequent newspaper accounts of poisoners being discovered only after they have successfully poisoned as many as 6 or 8 of their relatives, many cases must go unrecognized even today. If attempted homicidal poisoning is considered as a possible cause of unexplained illness, the patient must be hospitalized until recovery. The circumstances should be reported to the police. Further proof of attempted homicidal poisoning must be left to the police. If a patient dies as a result of a suspected homicidal poisoning, the physician is legally bound to report the death to the police and to the coroner. Carefully written records of all observations will aid the physician in court appearances.

In the past decade, poisoning has been increasingly recognized as a form of child abuse. Both acute poisoning from single overdoses and chronic poisoning from multiple doses have been reported. The physician is required by law to report suspected cases of child abuse by poisoning or other means to the appropriate protective services agency.

Accidental Poisoning

In accidental poisoning, the first responsibility of the physician is to give proper treatment. The frequency of litigation involving poisoning indicates that treatment must be thorough and personal; instructions given over the telephone may not be sufficient even if the poisoning appears to be inconsequential. The physician may have to see the patient immediately, carry out the necessary emergency measures even if these seem superfluous, and continue observing the patient during the time when the maximum effects of the poison are calculated to occur. This may require 24 hours of observation. Absence of symptoms or presence of mild symptoms an hour or more after ingestion is not necessarily an indication for complacency.

Of all nonoccupational poisonings, food poisoning resulting from eating in a public restaurant or from eating contaminated commercial food is the only type that must be reported. Such cases must be reported to the local public health officer.

Fatalities from suspected accidental poisonings must be reported to the police and to the coroner.

Occupational Poisoning

If poisoning has resulted from occupational exposure, a report must be sent to the proper authorities if the poisoning is reportable. The local health department will have the name and address of the agency to which these reports should be sent.

References

Melville M: Risks on the job: The worker's right to know. *Environment* (Nov) 1981;**23**:12.

Provost GJ: Legal trends in occupational health. *J Occup Med* 1982;**24**:115.

Schroeder O Jr: Toxicology and law. In: *Legal Medicine–1980*. Wecht CH (editor). Saunders, 1980.

Schulte PA, Ringen K: Notification of workers at high risk. *Am J Public Health* 1984;**74**:485.

II. Agricultural Poisons

Halogenated Insecticides | 6

HALOBENZENE DERIVATIVES & ANALOGS

Halobenzene derivatives (Table 6–1) are synthetic chemicals that are stable for weeks to years after application. They are soluble in fat but not in water. Some of these chemicals decompose at high temperatures and possibly in the environment to 2,3,7,8-tetrachlorodibenzodioxin (TCDD, dioxin) or similar compounds (see p 106).

Commercial insecticide formulas consist of, variously, insecticides in technically pure form, dry mixtures of several insecticides, or solutions of one or more insecticides in various organic solvents, especially kerosene, toluene, or other petroleum derivatives. These organic solvents are themselves toxic (see Chapter 13).

DDT seems to be one of the most toxic of these chemicals, at least in experimental animals. In humans, ingestion of 20 g of DDT in the form of a 10% dry mixture with flour has induced severe symptoms that persisted for more than 5 weeks, with gradual recovery. Virtually all fatalities reported in the literature have resulted from purposeful ingestion of DDT in various solvents. The toxicity of these solutions is greater than that of either DDT or the solvent alone.

The tolerance of chlorobenzene derivatives in most foods is 0.05–7 ppm, with the exception of methoxychlor (14 ppm).

Fatal doses of the various halobenzene derivative insecticides as estimated on the basis of animal experiments are shown in Table 6–1.

The mechanism of poisoning by these agents is not known. The toxic action does not require metabolic alteration of their chemical structure.

DDT acts chiefly on the cerebellum and motor cortex of the central nervous system, causing a characteristic hyperexcitability, tremors, muscular weakness, and convulsions. The myocardium becomes sensitized so that, at least in experimental animals, injection of epinephrine may induce ventricular fibrillation. DDD and Perthane specifically depress the function of the adrenal cortex, and they have been used for this purpose in humans. Ovotran has caused skin irritation or skin sensitization in humans.

Inasmuch as most deaths from DDT are complicated by the presence of other insecticides and of solvents, data obtained at autopsy are not reliable. In DDT-poisoned animals, the findings are centrilobular necrosis of the liver, vacuolization around large nerve cells of the central nervous system, fatty change of the myocardium, and renal tubular degeneration. The most characteristic finding in experimental animals exposed to the other halobenzene derivatives is liver damage.

Clinical Findings

The principal manifestations of poisoning with these agents are vomiting, tremors, and convulsions.

A. Acute Poisoning: (Results only from ingestion.)

1. Ingestion of 5 g or more of dry DDT–Severe vomiting begins within 30 minutes to 1 hour; weakness and numbness of the extremities have a more gradual onset. Apprehension and excitement are marked, and diarrhea may occur.

2. Ingestion of more than 20 g of dry DDT–Twitching of the eyelids begins within 8–12 hours; this is followed by muscular tremors, first of the head and neck and then more distally, involving the extremities in severe clonic convulsions similar to those seen in strychnine poisoning. The pulse is normal; respiration is accelerated early and slowed later.

3. Effects of solvents–The organic solvents present in many commercial insecticides decrease the convulsive effects of DDT and increase the depression of the central nervous system. Onset of slow, shallow breathing within 1 hour after inhaling, ingesting, or absorbing a DDT solution through the skin implicates the solvent rather than the DDT.

B. Chronic Poisoning: Workers with a history of many months' exposure to DDT and having up to 648 ppm of DDT in their body fat have remained completely well, whereas most persons have body fat levels of halogenated insecticides below 15 ppm. These insecticides are all stored for long periods in body fat, but not in sufficient quantity to induce symptoms on starvation. Liver damage from DDT exposure might be expected from evidence obtained in experimental animals, but no such reports have appeared.

C. Laboratory Findings:

1. A high urine level of organic chlorine or especially of bis(*p*-chlorophenyl)acetic acid (DDA) indicates exposure to DDT or to one of the analogous compounds and is indicative of the severity of the exposure.

2. In suspected poisoning, analysis of serum or a fat biopsy is useful for diagnosis. A sample of fat can be taken from subcutaneous tissue by means of an 18-gauge disposable needle and disposable syringe. The sample should weigh at least 50 mg. Place sample in previously weighed glass-stoppered vial or vial with Teflon-lined cap and weigh to the nearest 0.1 mg. Prepare at least 5 mL of serum from blood

Table 6—1. Halobenzene derivative pesticides.

	LD50 (g/kg)
Acifluorfen, Blazer	0.4
Amiben (3-amino-2,5-dichlorobenzoic acid)	3.5
Bromopropylate, Acarol	5
Chlomethoxynil	10+
Chloranil, Spergon	4
Chlorbenside (*p*-chlorobenzyl-*p*-chlorophenyl sulfide)	0.3
Chlordimeform, Galecron	0.2
Chlorfenethol, Qikron	0.9
Chlorfenprop-methyl, Bidisin	1.1
Chlorfenson, Ovex, Ovotran	2
Chlorflurenol, Maintain	3.1
Chlorobenzilate (ethyl-4,4'-dichlorobenzilate)	1
Chloromethyl-*p*-chlorophenyl sulfone	1
Chloroneb, Demosan	11
p-Chlorophenylbenzenesulfonate, fenson	1.5
Chloropropylate, Acaralate	5
Chlorothalonil, Bravo, Daconil	10
Chlorotoluron, Dicuran	10+
Chloroxuron, Tenoran	3.7
Chlorpropham, ChloroIPC	1.5
Chlorsulfuron	3.4
Clofentezine	3.2+
Clopyralid	5+
Dacthal	3
DDD, TDE, Rhothane, mitotane	3
DDT, dichlorodiphenyltrichloroethane (exposure limit, 1 mg/m^3)	0.4
Dicamba, Banvel	3.5
Dicloran, DCNA	5+
Diflubenzuron, Dimilin	4.6+
Dimite, DMC, chlorfenethol	1
Fenarimol, Rubigan	2.5
Fenoxaprop-ethyl, Furore	2.3
Fenvalerate	0.45
Figaron, Ethychlozate	4.8
Flamprop-isopropyl, Barnon, Suffix BW	3
Flamprop-methyl, Mataven	5+
Fluorbenside (*p*-chlorobenzyl-*p*-fluorophenyl sulfide)	
Flutriafol	1.5
Fomesan, Flex	1.5
Fthalide, Rabcide	10
Fusarex, Tecnazene	7.5
Imazalil, Bromazil	5+
Ioxynil, Actril, Bantrol	0.1
Kelthane, Dicofol	0.5
Lactofen, Cobra	5+
Methoxychlor (trichloro-bis[*p*-methoxyphenyl] ethane) (exposure limit, 10 mg/m^3)	5
Mitran	0.9

Table 6–1 (cont'd). Halobenzene derivative pesticides.

	LD50 (g/kg)
Nuarimol, Trimidal	1.25
Pemonazole, Topaz	2
Perthane (di-[p-ethylphenyl] dichloroethane)	8
Plifenate, Baygon MEB	10
Ronilan, Vinclozolin	10+
Tetradifon, Tedion (tetrachlorodiphenylsulfone)	8
Tetrasul	10
Triclopyr, Garlon	0.63
Triflumizole, Trifmine	1
Triflumuron, Alsystin	5

taken after an overnight fast. The container should be carefully labeled with the patient's name, weight of sample, date of collection, and name and address of physician. Send frozen sample to Toxicology Laboratory, Pesticides Program, Food & Drug Administration, US Public Health Service, Atlanta 30333. Containers and further directions are obtainable from the same source. The local health department may also be able to arrange for analysis.

Prevention
See p 6.

Treatment of Halogenated Insecticide Poisoning (Acute)
A. Emergency Measures:
1. Emesis–Give syrup of ipecac (see p 21).
2. Give activated charcoal followed by gastric lavage with 2–4 L of tap water. Follow with saline cathartic. Do not give fats or oils. Intestinal lavage with 20% mannitol (200 mL) by stomach tube is also useful.
3. Scrub skin with soap and water to remove skin contamination.
4. Give artificial respiration with O_2 if respiration is slowed.
B. General Measures:
1. Anticonvulsants–Give diazepam, 10 mg slowly intravenously. If convulsions persist, use a neuromuscular blocking agent (Table 4–3) and controlled respiration. For hyperactivity or tremors, give phenobarbital sodium, 100 mg subcutaneously hourly until convulsions are controlled or until 0.5 g has been given.
2. *Do not give stimulants*, especially epinephrine, since they sometimes induce ventricular fibrillation.

Prognosis
Recovery has occurred except when DDT was ingested dissolved

in an organic solvent. If convulsions are severe and protracted, recovery is questionable. If symptoms progress only to tremors, recovery is complete within 24 hours. After convulsions, recovery may require 2–4 weeks.

BENZENE HEXACHLORIDE
(Gamma Isomer = Lindane)

Benzene hexachloride (hexachlorocyclohexane) is stable for 3–6 weeks after application. It is soluble in fat but not in water.

Wettable powders, emulsions, dusts, and solutions in organic solvents are available for use as insecticides. Both the technical preparation and the gamma isomer (lindane) are used in vaporizers, and serious poisoning has occurred from vapor exposure.

Ingestion of 20–30 g of technical benzene hexachloride will produce serious symptoms, but death is unlikely unless this amount was dissolved in an organic solvent. In the case of lindane, 3.5 g/70 kg is considered a dangerous dose. In a $2\frac{1}{2}$-year-old girl, ingestion of 50–100 mg/kg caused convulsions, with recovery in 24 hours. The tolerance of benzene hexachloride or lindane in food is 10 ppm or less. The exposure limit for lindane is 0.5 mg/m^3.

Reported instances of serious poisoning have been rare and have resulted from accidental or suicidal ingestion.

Technical benzene hexachloride and lindane stimulate the central nervous system, causing hyperirritability, ataxia, and convulsions. Pulmonary edema and vascular collapse may also be of neurogenic origin. Effects of lindane on experimental animals have their onset within 30 minutes and last up to 24 hours; with the technical product, onset of effects may be delayed 1–6 hours and then persist up to 4 days.

Benzene hexachloride is stored in the body fat and slowly lost through metabolism or excretion in urine, feces, or milk. Of the various isomers of benzene hexachloride, lindane is excreted most rapidly.

The most prominent feature of benzene hexachloride or lindane poisoning in animals is liver necrosis. Other changes seen in experimentally poisoned animals are hyaline degeneration of renal tubular epithelium and histologic changes in the brain, adrenal cortex, and bone marrow. Benzene hexachloride is a carcinogen in animals.

Clinical Findings
The principal manifestations of poisoning with benzene hexachloride or lindane are vomiting, tremors, and convulsions.

A. Acute Poisoning: (From ingestion or massive skin contamination with a concentrated solution in an organic solvent.) Symptoms begin 1–6 hours after exposure. Vomiting and diarrhea appear first and convulsions later. Recovery is likely unless the material contains an organic solvent, in which case dyspnea, cyanosis, and circulatory failure may progress rapidly.

Exposure to smaller amounts by skin contamination or by ingestion leads to dizziness, headache, nausea, tremors, and muscular weakness. In addition to these symptoms, exposure to vaporized benzene hexachloride or lindane produces irritation of the eyes, nose, and throat. Such symptoms disappear rapidly upon removal from exposure.

B. Chronic Poisoning: True systemic chronic poisoning has not been reported from any of the isomers of benzene hexachloride.

Dermatitis from skin contamination with benzene hexachloride has occurred but has improved rapidly upon elimination of exposure.

C. Laboratory Findings: Liver function may be impaired. Specific examination of feces, urine, or fat may reveal the presence of benzene hexachloride. For method of collection and analysis of fat specimens, see p 100.

Treatment

Treat as for halogenated insecticide poisoning (see p 102).

Prognosis

A. Acute Poisoning: In acute poisoning not complicated by ingestion of an organic solvent, complete recovery occurs in 1–2 weeks. Progression of symptoms to pulmonary edema and vascular collapse following ingestion of benzene hexachloride or lindane in an organic solvent may make recovery unlikely.

B. Mild Exposure: Symptoms from slight exposure to benzene hexachloride or lindane vaporizers or ingestion of small amounts of benzene hexachloride have lasted not more than 2 weeks.

Jaeger U et al: Acute oral poisoning with lindane-solvent mixtures. *Vet Hum Toxicol* 1984;**26**:11.

TOXAPHENE
(Chlorinated Camphenes)

Toxaphene consists of chlorinated terpenes with chlorinated camphene predominating. It is stable for 1–6 months after application and is fat-soluble and water-insoluble. Toxaphene is available for insecticidal use in the form of wettable powders, dusts, emulsion concentrates, and concentrated solutions in oil.

The fatal dose of toxaphene for an adult is estimated to be around 2 g. Several members of one family were nonfatally poisoned after eating greens contaminated with toxaphene to the extent of 3 g/kg of greens. The maximum dose ingested by one person was thought to be approximately 1 g. Several fatalities in children have followed ingestion of larger but undetermined amounts. The tolerance of toxaphene in foods is 7 ppm. At least 3 fatalities from toxaphene ingestion have been reported. The exposure limit for toxaphene is 0.5 mg/m^3.

Toxaphene induces convulsions by diffuse stimulation of the brain and spinal cord. These are clonic in character; salivation, vomiting, and auditory reflex excitability indicate medullary stimulation comparable to that induced by camphor.

Pathologic findings in acute poisoning are petechial hemorrhages and congestion in the brain, lungs, spinal cord, heart, and intestines. Pulmonary edema and focal areas of degeneration in the brain and spinal cord are also present. In experimentally induced chronic poisoning, degenerative changes were found in the liver parenchyma and renal tubules of animals.

Clinical Findings

The principal manifestations of toxaphene poisoning are vomiting and convulsions.

A. Acute Poisoning: (From ingestion or skin absorption.) Convulsions frequently begin without premonitory symptoms but may be preceded by nausea and vomiting. In fatal poisoning, convulsions occur at decreasing intervals until respiratory failure supervenes, almost always within 4–24 hours after poisoning. In nonfatal poisoning, cessation of convulsions is followed variably by a period of weakness, lassitude, and amnesia.

B. Chronic Poisoning: (From ingestion, inhalation, or skin absorption.) Instances of chronic poisoning have not appeared in the literature. Experiments in animals indicate that toxaphene is less apt to cause chronic toxicity than DDT but that similar changes in the liver and kidneys are possible.

C. Laboratory Findings: Liver function may be impaired. Analysis of body fat or serum for toxaphene indicates severity of exposure (see p 100).

Treatment

Treat as for halogenated insecticide poisoning (see p 102).

Prognosis

In acute poisoning, recovery is likely unless convulsions are progressive and cannot be controlled. The interval from 4 to 24 hours after poisoning is the most dangerous.

2,4-DICHLOROPHENOXYACETIC ACID & RELATED PESTICIDES

2,4-Dichlorophenoxyacetic acid (2,4-D); its esters and acetates; 2,4,5-trichlorophenoxyacetic acid (2,4,5-T); esters and acetates of 2,4,5-T; 2-methyl-4-chlorophenoxyacetic acid (MCPA); salts and esters of MCPA; and the propionate or butyrate analogs (MCPB, MCPP, 2,4-DB, Butyrac, Butoxone, Embutox, silvex, Tropotox) of these compounds are used as herbicides. Other herbicides that would be expected to have similar toxicities include erbon, Natrin, dichlorprop, Diphenex (chlomethoxynil), diclofop methyl, mecoprop, Methoxone, phenothiol, bifenox (Modown), fenac, and sesone (2,4-dichlorophenoxyethyl sulfate).

Tetrachlorodibenzo-p-dioxin (TCDD, dioxin), a contaminant and degradation product of 2,4,5-T and other chlorophenoxy herbicides, is a potent mutagen in experimental systems and is suspected of being mutagenic in humans at extremely low doses.

One fatality has occurred from an amount of 2,4-D not less than 6.5 g. Other fatalities have occurred from varying amounts up to 120 g. The LD50 for these compounds in animals ranges from 300 to 700 mg/kg. The exposure limit for 2,4,5-T and 2,4-D is 10 mg/m³. The exposure limit for sesone is 0.1 mg/m³.

The mechanism of poisoning has not been elucidated. No specific pathologic changes have been reported.

Clinical Findings

The principal manifestations of 2,4-D poisoning are weakness and fall of blood pressure.

A. Symptoms and Signs: (From ingestion or skin absorption.) Ingestion of amounts near the lethal dose causes burning pain in the tongue, pharynx, and abdomen; flushing of the skin; vomiting; painful and tender muscles with fibrillary twitching; fever or subnormal temperature; lethargy; weakness; and intercostal paralysis. Skin absorption has also caused muscle weakness. After a delay of a week, urine may become dark. Patients ingesting massive doses have had persistent irreversible fall of blood pressure. Convulsions and disturbances in cardiac rhythm have been reported but have not been a constant finding.

Effects of exposure to 2,3,7,8-tetrachlorodibenzodioxin (TCDD, dioxin) include a burning sensation in the eyes, nose, and throat followed by headache, dizziness, and nausea and vomiting. One to several days later, itching, redness, and swelling of the face that is more marked over the eyelids, nose, and lips develop. Within weeks, nodules as well as pustules appear on the face, forearms, shoulders, neck, and trunk, progressing to comedones and cysts. Acneiform eruptions appear after a month or more, and the skin becomes hyperpigmented. At the same time, aching muscles—mainly in the thighs and chest—are evident. The muscle pain is aggravated by exertion. Insomnia, extreme irritability, and loss of libido also occur. There may also be neuromuscular symptoms of weakness and pain with nerve conduction abnormalities. Porphyria cutanea tarda, hepatic dysfunction, hyperlipidemia, hirsutism, chronic eye irritation, emotional disorders, and neuropsychiatric syndromes have been observed. Personality changes may persist for years.

B. Laboratory Findings: Myoglobin and hemoglobin may be found in the urine. Elevations in lactate dehydrogenase (LDH), SGOT, SGPT, and aldolase indicate the extent of muscle damage. The ECG should be monitored for cardiac rhythm abnormalities.

Treatment

A. Emergency Measures:

1. Give syrup of ipecac. After emesis, perform gastric lavage with activated charcoal (see p 24). Follow with saline cathartic.

2. Remove skin contamination by scrubbing with soap and water.

B. Antidote: For muscle and cardiac irritability, give lidocaine, 50–100 mg intravenously, followed by 1–4 mg/min by intravenous infusion as necessary.

C. General Measures:

1. Treat convulsions (Table 4–3).

2. Reduce fever by cool (10 °C) applications. Raise subnormal temperature by applying warm packs at not more than 40 °C.

3. Replace electrolyte losses due to vomiting.

4. Maintain alkaline urine during myoglobinuria by the administration of sodium bicarbonate, 10–15 g daily.

Prognosis

Survival for more than 48 hours has been followed by complete recovery. Impotence may persist for several months.

Health-risk estimates for 2,3,7,8-tetrachlorodibenzodioxin in soil. *MMWR* 1984;**33**:25.

Kimbrough RD et al: Toxicity of chlorinated biphenyls, dibenzofurans, dibenzodioxins, and related compounds. *Environ Health Perspect* 1985;**59**:1.

National Institute of Occupational Safety and Health: 2,3,7,8-Tetrachlorodibenzodioxin. *Current Intelligence Bulletin* 1984;**40**:1.

POLYCYCLIC CHLORINATED INSECTICIDES: CHLORDANE, HEPTACHLOR, ALDRIN, DIELDRIN, ENDRIN, MIREX, THIODAN, & CHLORDECONE

These compounds are synthetic fat-soluble but water-insoluble chemicals. Aldrin is stable for 1–3 weeks after application The others are stable for months to a year or more.

These chemicals, either singly or in mixtures in the form of dusts, wettable powders, or solutions in organic solvents, are used as insecticides for the control of flies, mosquitoes, and field insects.

The toxicity of these polycyclic derivatives for rodents is considerably greater than that of the chlorobenzene derivatives. For example, the experimental fatal dose (LD50; see p 31) in rats for aldrin or endrin is 5 mg/kg; for dieldrin, it is 40 mg/kg; for heptachlor, 90 mg/kg; for chlordecone (Kepone), 65 mg/kg; for chlordane, 200 mg/kg; for mirex, 300 mg/kg; and for endosulfan (Thiodan), 30 mg/kg. In an average adult human, severe symptoms follow ingestion of or skin contamination with 15–50 mg/kg or 1–3 g of chlordane. Other indane derivatives are probably more toxic. In one instance, accidental skin contamination with 30 g of chlordane as a 25% solution in an organic solvent was fatal to an adult in 40 minutes.

Allowable residual tolerances of these indane chemicals in food range from 0 to 0.1 ppm. The exposure limit for chlordane and heptachlor is 0.5 mg/m³; for dieldrin and aldrin, 0.2 mg/m³; for endrin, 0.1 mg/m³; and for endosulfan, 0.1 mg/m³. No safe level has been established for chlordecone or mirex.

Pathologic changes include congestion, edema, and scattered petechial hemorrhages in the lungs, kidneys, and brain. The kidneys also show damage to tubular cells. In the liver, hepatic cell enlargement and peripheral margination of basophilic granules are induced by feeding experimental animals the various indane derivatives at levels of 10–200 ppm. At higher doses, degenerative changes are found in the hepatic cells and renal tubules.

Clinical Findings

The principal manifestations of poisoning with the indane derivatives are tremors and convulsions.

A. Acute Poisoning: (From ingestion or inhalation of or skin contamination by any indane derivative, even in the absence of solvent.) Symptoms of hyperexcitability, tremors, ataxia, and convulsions begin within 30 minutes to 6 hours and are followed by central nervous system depression that may terminate in respiratory failure. In one person who ingested chlordane, 25 mg/kg, evidence of renal damage was indicated by proteinuria and hematuria. Anuria has also been reported. Two years after exposure to endosulfan while cleaning vats, a patient had cognitive and emotional deterioration, severe impairment of memory, gross impairment of visual motor coordination, and inability to perform any but the simplest tasks.

B. Chronic Poisoning: (From ingestion, inhalation, or skin contamination.) Prolonged exposure to chlordecone has caused neurologic symptoms. Both chlordecone and mirex have been shown to be carcinogenic in animal experiments. Occasional epileptiform convulsions of the grand mal or petit mal type have occurred in workers from dermal absorption of endosulfan in powder form. Electroencephalographic findings in poisoning have been suggestive of epilepsy but have reverted to normal when exposure was discontinued. Symptoms may persist for more than 1 week after exposure is discontinued or after acute poisoning.

C. Laboratory Findings: Liver function may be impaired as revealed by appropriate tests (see p 75). A fat biopsy or serum test may reveal the presence of indane derivatives (see p 100 for method of collection).

Treatment

Treat as for halogenated insecticide poisoning (see p 102). Cholestyramine resin (Questran) can be administered to increase the elimination of chlordecone up to 7-fold. Personnel involved in therapy should wear neoprene gloves as protection against contamination.

Prognosis

If the liver has previously been damaged, the toxicity of the polycyclic halogenated insecticides is greatly increased. Recovery is likely if onset of convulsions is delayed more than 1 hour and if convulsions are readily controlled.

Kutz SW et al: A fatal chlordane poisoning. *J Toxicol Clin Toxicol* 1983;**20**:167.

7 | Cholinesterase Inhibitor Pesticides

Cholinesterase inhibitors are mostly used in agriculture for the control of soft-bodied insects. They consist of 2 distinct chemical groups of compounds: organophosphorus derivatives and carbamates. In both groups there are widely varying toxicities. The chemical difference is of interest, since antidotes useful in treating the organophosphorus type may not work or may be contraindicated in poisoning by carbamate type insecticides. Formulations containing from less than 1% to more than 95% of pure material are commonly available. The highest concentrations are mostly used to prepare dusts and wettable powders in factories, although TEPP and malathion concentrates have been available to the general public.

Tables 7–1 and 7–2 give fatal doses in experimental animals, and

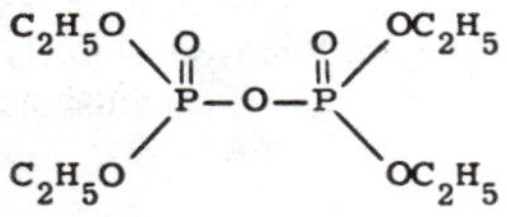

TEPP
(Tetraethyl pyrophosphate)
Liquid, water-soluble, decomposes within 6 hours.

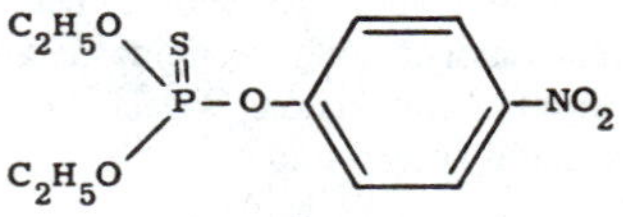

Parathion
Liquid, water-insoluble, stable for 1–3 weeks.

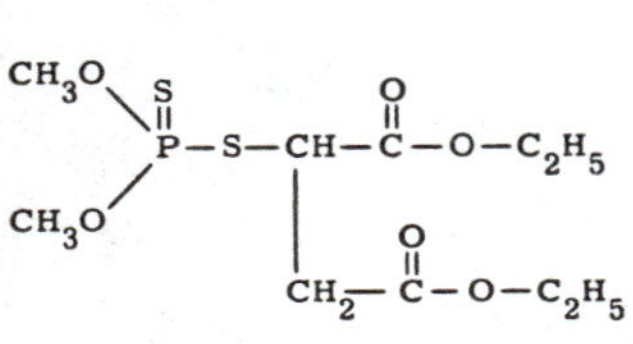

Malathion

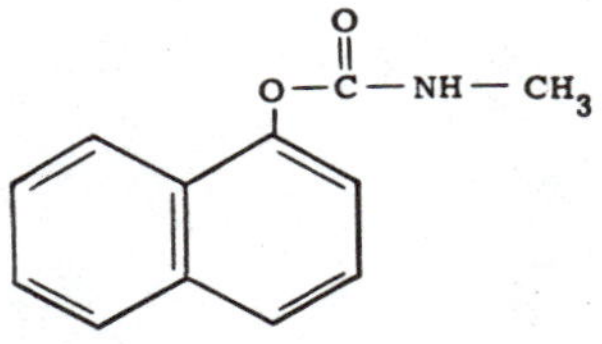

Carbaryl
(1-Naphthyl-N-methyl carbamate)

Figure 7–1. Cholinesterase inhibitors.

110

Table 7—1. Organic phosphate pesticides.

	Exposure Limit (mg/m^3)	LD50 (mg/kg)
Abate, temophos	10	2000
Acephate, Orthene		866
Acethion		100
Agritox, trichloronate		37
Akton		146
Amidithion, Thiocron		94
Aspon, tetra-n-propyl dithionopyrophosphate		890
Avirosan		324
Azinphos-ethyl		17
Azodrin, monocrotophos	0.25	8
Basta, Total		1620
Bensulide, Betasan, Prefar		271
Bidrin, dicrotophos		15
Bomyl, Swat		31
Bromophos, Nexion		3750
Bromophos-ethyl, Nexagan		52
Carbophenothion, Trithion		10
Chlorfenvinphos, Birlane, Supona, Vinylphate		10
Chlormephos		7
Chlorphoxim, Baythion C		1500
Chlorpyrifos, Lorsban		8
Chlorthiophos, Celathion		8
Ciodrin, crotoxyphos		125
Coroxon		12
Coumaphos, Co-Ral		13
Crufomate, Ruelene	5	770
Cyanofenphos, Surecide		44
Cyanophos		565
Cyolane, phosfolan		8.9
Cythioate, Cyflee, Proban		160
DEF, S,S,S-tributyl phosphorotrithioate		200
Delnav, dioxathion		23
2,4-DEP, Falone		850
Dialifor, Torak		43
Diazinon	0.1	100
Dibrom, naled	3	430
Dichlofenthion, Mobilawn		270
Dichlorvos, DDVP, dimethyl-2,2-dichlorovinyl phosphate	0.1	56
Dimefox, bis-(dimethylamino)-fluorophosphine oxide*		1—2
Dimethoate		215
Di-Syston, disulfoton	0.1	12
Ditalimphos, Plondrel		1000
Dyfonate, fonofos	0.1	8
Dymet		2000
Edifenphos, Hinosan		212
Efosite, Aliette, Fosetyl		5800

*May cause delayed paralysis of extremities.

Table 7—1 (cont'd). Organic phosphate pesticides.

	Exposure Limit (mg/m³)	LD50 (mg/kg)
EPN, O-ethyl-O-*p*-nitrophenyl benzenethionophosphonate*	0.5	14
Ethion, bis(diethoxyphosphinothioylthio)methane		27
Ethoate-methyl, Fitios		340
Ethoprop, Mocap		61
Etrimfos		1800
Famphur, Famfos		36
Fenitrothion, Agrothion, Folithion		500
Fensulfothion, Dasanit	0.1	2
Fenthion, Baytex	0.2	15
Folex, merphos, tributyl phosphorotrithioite		5
Formothion, Anthio, Aflix		365
Guthion, azinphos-methyl	0.2	6
Heptenophos, Hostaquick		96
Iodofenphos, jodfenphos, Nuvanol N		2100
Isophenphos, Oftanol, Amaze		28
Isothioate, Hosdon		60
Isoxathion, Karphos		112
Kitazin, IBP		490
Korlan, Ronnel	10	400
Kremite, fosamine		24,000
Malathion	10	1375
Mecarbam, Murfotox		36
Menazon		1950
Mephosfolan, Cytrolane		8.9
Metasystox-R, oxydemeton-methyl		56
Metasystox-S		105
Methamidophos, Monitor		19
Methidathion, Supracide, Ultracide		65
Methyl demeton	0.5	50
Methyl parathion, Metacide	0.2	10
Mipafox, Isopestox		1
Miral, isazophos		40
Nemacur, Fenamiphos	0.1	8
Nem-A-Tak, fosthietane		4
Omethoate, Folimat		50
Oxydisulfoton, Disyston-S		3.5
Parathion, O,O-diethyl-O-(*p*-nitrophenyl)phosphorothioate*	0.1	3
Phencapton		182
Phenthoate, Cidial, Papthion		300
Phorate, Thimet	0.05	1.1
Phosalone, Zolone		120
Phosdrin, mevinphos	0.01	3.7
Phosfon, chlorphonium		178
Phosmet, Imidan		300
Phosphamidon, Dimecron		17

*May cause delayed paralysis of extremities.

Table 7—1 (cont'd). Organic phosphate pesticides.

	Exposure Limit (mg/m³)	LD50 (mg/kg)
Phosvel, leptophos		53
Phoxim, Baythion		1845
Pirimiphos-ethyl, Primicid		140
Pirimiphos-methyl		2000
Profenofos, Curacron		400
Propetamphos, Safrotin		82
Prothiophos, Tokuthion		925
Prothoate, Fac, Fostion		8
Pyrazophos, Afugan		286
Pyridaphenthion, Ofunack		850
Quinalphos, Bayrusil		66
Salithion		91
Schradan, OMPA, octamethyl pyrophosphoramide	0.004	10
S-Sevin, EPBP		274
Sulfotepp, Bladafume, tetraethyl dithionopyrophosphate	0.2	5
Sulprofos, Bolstar	1	107
Systox, Demeton	0.01	2.5
TEPP, tetraethyl pyrophosphate†	0.004	1
Terbuphos, Counter		3
Tetrachlorvinphos, Gardona, Rabon		4000
Thiometon, Ekatin		100
Triazophos, Hostathion		82
Trichlorfon, Dipterex, Dylox		450
Vamidothion		100

†TEPP decomposes in about 6 hours in the presence of moisture. The rest of these compounds are stable from 1 week to 1 month after spraying.

the data can be used as an indication of hazard to humans. Thus, exposure to Chlorthion, DEF, malathion, or Phostex is unlikely to cause fatal poisoning, whereas EPN, parathion, Di-Syston, and Bidrin can be dangerous to life. Humans may also be more sensitive to some of the cholinesterase inhibitors than are experimental animals.

Among the organic phosphates, fatalities have resulted from 2 mg (0.1 mg/kg) of parathion in 5- and 6-year-olds and 120 mg in a man. Five grams of malathion were fatal to a 75-year-old man, but ingestion of 4 g by a child was followed by recovery. Fatalities have also occurred following exposure to concentrated preparations of Diazinon, DDVP, Systox, TEPP, and carbophenothion.

Among the carbamates, a single dose of carbaryl, 2.8 mg/kg, caused moderate symptoms with recovery in 2 hours. Carbofuran in dust has also caused mild symptoms with recovery in 2 hours.

Organophosphorus derivatives act by combining with and inacti-

Table 7—2. Carbamate pesticides.

	Exposure Limit (mg/m^3)	LD50 (mg/kg)
Aldicarb, Temik		0.9
Allyxycarb, Hydrol		90
Baygon, propoxur	0.5	95
Bendiocarb, Ficam		143
Benomyl, Benlate	10	10,000
BPMC, Baycarb, Osbac		340
Bufencarb, Bux		170
Butacarb		4000+
Butocarboxim		158
Butoxycarboxim		458
Butylate, Genate		3500
Carbaryl, Sevin	5	89
Carbofuran, Furadan	0.1	5
Carbosulfan, Advantage		209
Cloethocarb, Lance		35.4
Cosban, Macbal, XMC		542
Dacamox, Thiofanox		100
Desmedipham, Betanex		2000
Dimetan		50
Dimetilan		50+
Dioxacarb, Elocron		72
Ethiofencarb, Croneton		411
Etrofol, Hopcide, CPMC		648
Formetanate, Carzol		20
Isocarb		128
Isoprocarb, Etrofolan, MIPC		485
Matacil, aminocarb		21
Meobal, MPMC		380
Mesurol, methiocarb		15
Methomyl, Lannate	2.5	17
Mexacarbate, Zectran		19
Orbencarb, Lanray		1832
Oxamyl, Vydate		5
Pirimicarb, Pirimor		147
Promecarb, Carbamult		74
Rowmate, Sirmate		1879
Swep		4197
Tandex, karbutilate		3000
Terbucarb, Azak		34,000
Thiodicarb, Darvin		66
Trimethacarb, Broot		566
Tsumacide, MTMC, Metacrate		268

vating the enzyme acetylcholinesterase (AChE). For example, the phosphate esters appear to combine as follows:

$$\text{AChE} + \begin{array}{c} \text{RO} \\ \text{R}'\text{O} \\ \text{R}''\text{O} \end{array}\!\!\!\!\text{P}{=}\text{O} \longrightarrow \text{ROH} + \begin{array}{c} \text{AChE} \\ \text{R}'\text{O} \\ \text{R}''\text{O} \end{array}\!\!\!\!\text{P}{=}\text{O}$$

$$\begin{array}{c} \text{HO} \\ \text{R}'\text{O} \\ \text{R}''\text{O} \end{array}\!\!\!\!\text{P}{=}\text{O} + \text{AChE} \qquad \text{This reaction may occur.}$$

The rapidity of the reaction and the stability of the final cholinesterase-phosphate combination are influenced markedly by the structure of the phosphate ester. Pralidoxime, a substance capable of reversing the phosphate ester–cholinesterase combination, is available.

The carbamate insecticides combine similarly with cholinesterase, but the combination is reversible with time. Thus, the hazard is not increased by daily exposure to amounts less than those required to produce immediate symptoms. If symptoms develop, they do not persist for more than 8 hours. Pralidoxime increases the hazard from carbaryl but apparently not from other carbamates.

The inactivation of cholinesterase by cholinesterase inhibitor pesticides allows the accumulation of large amounts of acetylcholine, with resultant widespread effects that may be conveniently separated into 4 categories:

(1) Potentiation of postganglionic parasympathetic activity. The following structures are affected: pupil (constricted), intestinal muscle (stimulated), salivary and sweat glands (stimulated), bronchial muscles (constricted), urinary bladder (contracted), cardiac sinus node (slowed), and atrioventricular node (blocked).

(2) Persistent depolarization of skeletal muscle, resulting in initial fasciculations followed by neuromuscular block and paralysis.

(3) Initial stimulation followed by depression of cells of the central nervous system, resulting in inhibition of the inspiratory center (depression of phrenic discharge) and convulsions of central origin.

(4) Variable ganglionic stimulation or blockade, with rise or fall in blood pressure and dilation or constriction of pupils.

No specific anatomic changes are found in acute poisoning. The usual postmortem findings are pulmonary edema and capillary dilatation and hyperemia of lungs, brain, and other organs.

Parathion, DFP, EPN, malathion, and mipafox cause paralysis in the extremities of chickens.

Clinical Findings

The principal manifestations of poisoning with the cholinesterase inhibitor pesticides are visual disturbances, respiratory difficulty, and gastrointestinal hyperactivity.

A. Acute Poisoning: (From inhalation, skin absorption, or ingestion.) The following symptoms and signs, listed in approximate order of appearance, begin within 30–60 minutes and are at a maximum in 2–8 hours:

1. Mild–Anorexia, headache, dizziness, weakness, anxiety, substernal discomfort, tremors of the tongue and eyelids, miosis, and impairment of visual acuity.

2. Moderate–Nausea, salivation, tearing, abdominal cramps, vomiting, sweating, slow pulse, and muscular fasciculations.

3. Severe–Diarrhea, pinpoint and nonreactive pupils, respiratory difficulty, pulmonary edema, cyanosis, loss of sphincter control, convulsions, coma, and heart block. Hyperglycemia and possible acute pancreatitis have occurred.

B. Chronic Poisoning: The cholinesterase inhibition from organophosphorus cholinesterase inhibitors sometimes persists for 2–6 weeks. Thus, an exposure that would not produce symptoms in a person not previously exposed might produce severe symptoms in a person previously exposed to smaller amounts. Phosvel, Dipterex, and Divipan are reported to cause peripheral nerve damage with persistent muscular weakness.

C. Laboratory Findings:

1. The usual clinical laboratory tests are noncontributory.

2. Cholinesterase levels of red blood cells and plasma are reduced markedly, as determined by special techniques. Levels 30–50% of normal indicate exposure, although symptoms may not appear until the level falls to 20% or less. Because the normal variation of the cholinesterase level is wide, a determination should be made upon all individuals prior to occupational exposure. Repeated determinations should then be made at weekly intervals during exposure.

Samples for cholinesterase level determination may be sent after inquiry to the Toxicology Laboratory, US Public Health Service, Atlanta 30333.

Treatment

A. Acute Poisoning:

1. Emergency measures–

a. Establish airway (see p 58).

b. Artificial respiration and O_2–Treat convulsions and respiratory difficulty by mouth-to-mouth insufflation. When equipment is available, this type of ventilation can also be carried out by applying intermittent compression to a rubber rebreathing bag attached to a tight-fitting face mask of the anesthesia type. Air or O_2 must be supplied continuously. A resuscitator, bellows respirator, or face mask and demand flow regulator may also be used. All such equipment must be fitted with a safety valve limiting the maximum pressure developed to 20 mm Hg. Be prepared to maintain artificial respiration for many hours. The patient must be watched constantly so that artificial respiration may be administered when necessary. Necessary equipment must be at hand for the first 48 hours after poisoning.

c. Give atropine in large doses (see Antidote, below).

d. Wash skin—Before symptoms appear or after they are controlled by atropine, the skin and mucous membranes are decontaminated by washing with copious amounts of tap water and soap. Emergency care personnel should wear gloves and avoid contamination.

e. Lavage or emesis—If symptoms have not appeared, remove ingested material by lavage with tap water or emesis induced by syrup of ipecac (see p 21).

2. Antidote—

a. Atropine—In the presence of symptoms, give atropine sulfate, 2 mg intramuscularly, and repeat every 3–8 minutes until signs of parasympathetic toxicity are controlled: eyelid and tongue tremors, miosis, salivation, sweating, slow pulse, muscular fasciculations, respiratory difficulty, pulmonary edema, heart block. Repeat 2 mg of atropine frequently to maintain control of symptoms. As much as 12 mg of atropine has been given safely in the first 2 hours. Interruption of atropine therapy may be rapidly followed by fatal pulmonary edema or respiratory failure.

b. Cholinesterase reactivator—Do not use in the presence of carbaryl intoxication. Use only with maximum atropine administration. Give pralidoxime (Protopam, pyridine-2-aldoxime methochloride, 2-PAM), 1 g in aqueous solution, intravenously slowly. Repeat after 30 minutes if respiration does not improve. This dose may be repeated twice within each period of 24 hours. Obidoxim (Toxogonin) is available in some countries and is used similarly.

3. General measures—Pulmonary secretions are removed by postural drainage or by catheter suction. Avoid morphine, aminophylline, barbiturates, phenothiazines, and other respiratory depressants. Treat convulsions (see Table 4–3).

B. Chronic Poisoning: Absorption of phosphate esters as detected by a decrease in blood cholinesterase (see above) indicates the need to avoid further exposure until the cholinesterase level is normal.

Prognosis

The first 4–6 hours are most critical in acute poisoning. Improvement of symptoms after treatment is instituted means that the patient will survive if adequate treatment is continued.

Combined therapy with atropine and artificial respiration is theoretically capable of protecting a patient against 50–100 times the dose that would be fatal without treatment.

References

Barrett DS et al: A review of organophosphorus ester-induced delayed neurotoxicity. *Vet Hum Toxicol* 1985;**27**:22.

Lotti M, Becker CE: Treatment of acute organophosphate poisoning: Evidence of a direct effect on central nervous system by 2-PAM (pyridine-2-aldoxime methyl chloride). *J Toxicol Clin Toxicol* 1982;**19**:121.

Mahieu P: Severe and prolonged poisoning by Fenthion: Significance of the determination of the anticholinesterase capacity of plasma. *J Toxicol Clin Toxicol* 1982;**19**:425.

Miscellaneous Pesticides | 8

BARIUM

Absorbable salts of barium such as the carbonate, hydroxide, or chloride are used in pesticides. The sulfide sometimes is used in depilatories for external application. A soluble barium salt such as the carbonate or hydroxide may be present as a contaminant in the insoluble barium sulfate used as a radiopaque contrast medium.

The fatal dose of absorbed barium is approximately 1 g. The exposure limit for barium and its soluble or insoluble salts is 0.5 mg/m³.

Barium ion presumably induces a change in permeability or polarization of the cell membrane that results in stimulation of all muscle cells indiscriminately. This effect is not antagonized by atropine but is antagonized by magnesium ions. No specific histologic changes are seen.

Clinical Findings

The principal manifestations of barium poisoning are tremors, convulsions, and cardiac arrhythmias plus hypokalemia.

A. Symptoms and Signs: (From ingestion or, rarely, from inhalation.) Symptoms and signs include tightness of the muscles of the face and neck, vomiting, diarrhea, abdominal pain, fibrillary muscular tremors, anxiety, weakness, difficulty in breathing, cardiac irregularity, convulsions, and death from cardiac and respiratory failure. Inhalation of barium sulfate or barium oxides has caused benign pneumoconiosis.

B. Laboratory Findings: The ECG shows ectopic beats. The red blood cell count may be increased as a result of dehydration from vomiting and diarrhea. Serum potassium may be reduced, and respiratory acidosis may be present.

Prevention

Orders for radiologic barium sulfate should never use abbreviated terms. Users must be certain that barium sulfate is not contaminated by soluble barium salts. A convenient test is to shake up a portion with water and, to the clear supernatant portion, add a small amount of a solution of magnesium sulfate or sodium sulfate in water. Appearance of a precipitate indicates the presence of a soluble barium salt.

Treatment of Acute Poisoning

A. Emergency Measures:

1. Give soluble sulfates orally (see Antidote).

2. If respiration is affected, give artificial respiration, using O_2 if available, until a sulfate antidote can be given and normal respiration has returned.

B. Antidote:
Give 30 g of sodium sulfate in 250 mL of water orally and repeat in 1 hour. Give by gastric tube if symptoms have appeared. The administration of sulfate salts intravenously is hazardous, since they induce the precipitation of barium sulfate in the kidney, with subsequent renal failure. Administration of potassium is critical.

C. General Measures:

1. In persistent paralysis that does not respond to sulfate administration, begin infusion of normal saline at a rate of 1 L every 4 hours to induce saline diuresis. Give furosemide, 10–40 mg intravenously every 4–6 hours or as necessary to maintain diuresis for 24 hours.

2. In the presence of hypokalemia, potassium should be supplemented. Give 1–2 meq/kg body weight intravenously initially; if hypokalemia persists, give additional potassium.

3. Give morphine, 5–10 mg subcutaneously, for severe colic.

Prognosis

If a soluble sulfate (eg, magnesium sulfate or sodium sulfate) is given before symptoms become severe, the patient will recover. Patients who have survived for more than 24 hours have always recovered.

DINITROPHENOL, DINITRO-*o*-CRESOL

Dinitro derivatives of phenol and cresol are used as insecticides and herbicides. Dinitrophenol was formerly used medically as a metabolic stimulator to aid in weight reduction.

The acute fatal dose of dinitrophenol is approximately 1 g; the acute fatal dose of dinitro-*o*-cresol (DNOC) is 0.2 g. Other compounds with similar toxicities include dinitro-6-sec-butylphenol (dinoseb), binapacryl (Morocide), dinitrocyclohexylphenol, dinitramine (Cobex), dinobuton (Acrex), Amex, dinoprop, dinoterb, and dinocap (Karathane). Danger is greatest during hot weather, when loss of body heat is impaired. The exposure limit for dinitro-*o*-cresol and dinitrophenol is 0.2 mg/m^3.

The dinitro derivatives of various phenols apparently act by inhibiting the synthesis of certain phosphate bonds that are important in conserving energy utilization in the cell. In the absence of the mechanism, cellular respiration is markedly increased.

In patients who die from exposure to dinitro derivatives, post-mortem examination reveals degenerative changes of the heart, liver, and kidneys.

Clinical Findings

The principal manifestation of poisoning with the dinitro derivatives is fever.

A. Acute Poisoning: (From skin contamination, ingestion, or inhalation.) Symptoms are frequently of sudden onset up to 2 days after cessation of exposure and include high fever, prostration, thirst, nausea and vomiting, excessive perspiration, and difficulty in breathing. Later, symptoms progress to anoxia with cyanosis and lividity, and finally muscular tremors and coma. Oliguria, hematuria, and jaundice may appear later from kidney and liver injury.

B. Chronic Poisoning: Chronic poisoning has not been reported following agricultural exposure. Medicinal use to induce weight loss has been accompanied by the following toxic reactions: skin eruptions, peripheral neuritis, liver damage, kidney damage, granulocytopenia, and, rarely, cataract formation.

C. Laboratory Findings: In exposed workers, blood concentrations of dinitro derivatives should not exceed 10 μg/g. (See Harvey: *Lancet* 1962;**1**:796.) Take a white blood count if the exposed person has unexplained persistent fever.

Prevention

Persons who show decreases in the white blood count should avoid further exposure.

Treatment

A. Emergency Measures: Remove ingested poison by thorough gastric lavage with saturated bicarbonate solution. If gastric lavage cannot be accomplished immediately, give syrup of ipecac to induce emesis (see p 21), and follow with saline cathartic (see p 27). Remove skin contamination by scrubbing with soap and water after removal of clothing. If body temperature is elevated, reduce to 37 °C by immersion in cool water or by applying cooling blanket. If body temperature is above 40 °C, ice water is necessary. In respiratory distress or cyanosis, maintain airway and respiration (see p 58).

B. General Measures:

1. Glucose–Administer 5% glucose in saline intravenously or orally at the rate of 1 L every 2 hours until body temperature is controlled.

Table 8—1. Miscellaneous pesticides.

Possible Symptoms and Signs*

	Skin Sensitivity Reactions	Convulsions or Coma	Irritant: GI-Skin-Respiratory Tract	Liver and/or Kidney Damage	Blood Pressure Fall	LD50 (mg/kg)
Rodenticides:						
Castrix (see Strychnine, p 418)		+				1
a-Naphthylthiourea, ANTU (0.3 mg/m³)†				+		10
Repellents:						
9,10-Anthraquinone, Corbit						5000
Deet, N,N-diethyl-m-toluamide		+	+			2000
Dibutyl phthalate (5 mg/m³)†‡		+	+	+		8000
Dibutyl succinate, Tabatrex		+		+		8000
Dimethyl carbate, Dimelone		+				1000
Dimethylphthalate (5 mg/m³)†‡		+	+	+		8000
2-Ethylhexanediol-1,3; 612		+	+	+		6500
MGK-11						2500
2-Octylthioethanol, MGK-874						8530
Herbicides and fungicides:						
Alanap, naptalam						1700
Alloxydim, Clout						2322
Alopex						723
Ametryn, Evik						1110
3-Amino-1,2,4-triazol, amitrole (0.2 mg/m³)†	+					25,000
Aralon, Isoproturon						1800
Arsenal			+			5000+
Asulam, Asulox						5000
Atrazine, Aatrex (10 mg/m³)†		+		+		1869
Azide, sodium salt						37
Banrot						5000
Benalaxyl, Galben						4200
Benazolin						3000
Benefin, Balan						10,000
Benodanil, Calirus						6400+
Benquinox, Ceredon						100
Bentazone, Basagran			+			2063
Bentranil						1600
2-Benzanilide, Benodanil						6400+
Benzomarc						5000
Benzoylprop Ethyl, Suffix						1555
Benzthiazuron, Gatnon						1280
Bipertanol, Baycor						500+

*Treatment: Lavage and catharsis; artificial respiration if respiration is depressed.

†Exposure limit.

‡Teratogen in animals.

Table 8—1 (cont'd). Miscellaneous pesticides.

	Skin Sensitivity Reactions	Convulsions or Coma	Irritant: GI-Skin-Respiratory Tract	Liver and/or Kidney Damage	Blood Pressure Fall	LD50 (mg/kg)
Possible Symptoms and Signs*						
Herbicides and fungicides (cont'd):						
Bladex, cyanazine		+				182
Blasticidin-S						50
Bromacil (1 ppm)†						5200
Bromofenoxim, Faneron						1217
Bromoxynil, Brominal						190
Bronopol						400
Bupirimate, Nimrod						4000+
Butachlor, Machete		+	+			3120
Buthidazole, Ravage						1581
Butrizol, Indar						90
Buturon, Arisan, Eptapur						5800
Captafol, Difolatan (0.1 mg/m³)†	+		+			5000
Carbendazim, Derosal						15,000
Carbetamide						1100
Carboxin, Vitavax		+		+		3280
CDAA, Randox		+	+			700
Chinosol, 8-hydroxyquinoline			+			1200
Chlorthiamid, Prefix						757
Cycloheximide, Actidione		+	+			2.5
Cymoxanil, Curzate						1100
Cyometrinil, Concep	+					2277
Cyprazine, Outfox						1200
Cyprex, dodine		+	+			660
Dazomet, Mylone	+	+				650
Desmetryn, Semeron						1390
Devrinol, napropamide			+			500+
Dichlobenil, Casoron						3160
Dichlofluanid, Euparen						1000
Diclobutrazol, Vigil						4000
Dichlozolinate, Serinal						4500+
Diethatyl ethyl, Antor						2300
Difenoxuron, Lironion						7750+
Dimefuron						1000
Dimethachlon, Ohric						1250
Dimethirimol, Milcurb						2350
Dimethyl dixanthogen, dimexan						240
Diphenamid, Dymid		+	+			700
Dipropetryn, Sancap		+		+		5000
Dithianon, Delan						610

*Treatment: Lavage and catharsis; artificial respiration if respiration is depressed.
†Exposure limit.

Table 8—1 (cont'd). Miscellaneous pesticides.

	Skin Sensitivity Reactions	Convulsions or Coma	Irritant: GI-Skin-Respiratory Tract	Liver and/or Kidney Damage	Blood Pressure Fall	LD50 (mg/kg)
Possible Symptoms and Signs*						
Herbicides and fungicides (cont'd):						
Diuron, Dynex, Vonduron						3400
Dodemorph, Meltatox						4180
Drazoxolon, Ganocide						126
Dymron						6500+
Dyrene, anilazine			+			2700
Endothall		+	+			50
Etaconazole, Vangard						1343
Ethirimol, Milcurb						6340
Ethofumesate, Nortron						1200
Fenaminosulf, Lesan		+				60
Fenpropimorph, Corbel, Mistral						4300
Fentiazon, Celdion						10,000
Fenuron, Dybar						6400
Fluazifop-butyl, Fusilade						3000
Fluchloralin, Basalin						1550
Fluometuron, Cotoran, Lanex		+	+		+	7880
Flurecol-n-butylester						5000+
Fluridone, Sonar						250+
Fongarid						940
Fuberidazol, Voronit						1100
Gesaran, Methoprotryne						5000
Glyodin						4600
Glyphosate, Roundup		+	+			4300
Glytac						7000
Goltix, metamitron						3343
Guazatine, Panoctine						327
Herbisan, ethyl xanthic disulfide		+	+			600
Hymexazol, Tachigaren						1968
Indar, Butrizol						90
Isocarbamid, Merpelan						2500
Isopropalin, Paarlan						5000+
Isoprothiolane, Fuji-One						1190
Kasugamycin, Kasumin						20,000
Koban						4000
Kumulan, nitrothal-isopropyl						9400
Lasso, alachlor						1200
Lenacil, Venzar						11,000+
Linuron, Lorox						1500
Maloran, chlorbromuron		+	+			2150
Mepronil, Basitac						10,000

*Treatment: Lavage and catharsis; artificial respiration if respiration is depressed.

Table 8—1 (cont'd). Miscellaneous pesticides.

	Skin Sensitivity Reactions	Convulsions or Coma	Irritant: GI-Skin-Respiratory Tract	Liver and/or Kidney Damage	Blood Pressure Fall	LD50 (mg/kg)
Possible Symptoms and Signs*						
Herbicides and fungicides (cont'd):						
Metalaxyl, Ridomil						669
Metazaclor, Butisan-S						2150
Methylmetiram, Basfungin						5200
Methyl thiophanate, Fungo						9700
Metobromuron, Patoran						2700
Metolachlor, Dual						2780
Metoxuron, Dosanex						3200
Metribuzin, Sencor						1936
Molinate, Ordram		+	+	+		680
Monalide, Potablan						4000+
Monolinuron, Aresin						1800
Monuron		+			+	3600
Naproanilide, Uribest						15,000+
Neburon, Kloben, Neburex						11,000
Nitralin, Planavin						2000+
Nitrofen, TOK						2630
Norflurazon, Evital, Zorial						8000+
Ofurace						2600
Ornitrol, diazacosterol						92
Oryzalin, Surflan						10,000+
Oxadiazon, Ronstar						8000+
Oxadixyl						3480
Oxycarboxin, Plantvax						2000
Oxyfluorfen, Goal						5000+
Panoram, fenfuram			+			12,900
Parinol, Parnon						5000
Pendimethalin, Prowl						1250
Perfluidone, Destun						920
Phaltan, captan, folpet (5 mg/m³)†	+		+			9000
Phenazine						3310
Phenisopham, Verdinal, Diconal						4000+
Phenmedipham, Betanal						8000
Picloram, Tordon (10 mg/m³)†						8200
Piperalin, Pipron						2500
Potassium cyanate					+	840
Preforan, Fluorodifen						9000
Probe, methazole						1350
Procyazine, Cycle						290
Profluralin, Tolban						2200

*Treatment: Lavage and catharsis; artificial respiration if respiration is depressed.
†Exposure limit.

Table 8—1 (cont'd). Miscellaneous pesticides.

	Skin Sensitivity Reactions	Convulsions or Coma	Irritant: GI-Skin-Respiratory Tract	Liver and/or Kidney Damage	Blood Pressure Fall	LD50 (mg/kg)
Possible Symptoms and Signs*						
Herbicides and fungicides (cont'd):						
Prometone, Pramitol		+				2950
Prometryne, Caparol		+		+		3750
Pronamide, Kerb						8350
Propachlor, Ramrod, Bexton		+	+			1200
Propanil, Rogue						1384
Propazine, Gesamil, Milogard		+		+		5000
Propham, IPC						5000
Prothiocarb, Previcur						1300
Prynachlor, Basamaize						1177
Pyracarbolid, Sicarol						5613
Pyramin, Chloridazone						3600
Pyridate						2000
Scepter						5000
Secbumeton, Sumitol		+		+		1000
Sethoxydim, Poast						2676
Siduron, Tupersan			+			5000
Simazine, Princep		+		+		5000
Simetryn						1830
Sonalan, ethalfluralin						10,000
Sulfamate, Ammate (10 mg/m³)†		+	+			3900
Sumilex, procymidone						6800
Tantizon, isomethiozin						10,000+
Tebuthiuron, Spike						644
Terbacil, Sinbar						5000
Terbumeton, Caragard						485
Terbuthylazine, Gardoprim						2160
Terbutryn, Igran		+	+			2500
Terrazole, Truban						2000
Thiophanate, Cercobin, Topsin						15,000+
Tilt, propiconazole						1517
Tolylfluanid, Euparen M						1000+
Tomilon, tetrafluoron						1265
Triadimefon, Bayleton						400
Triadimenol, Baytan						700
Tribunil						2500+
Tricyclazole, Bim						250
Tridemorph, Calixin						1112
Trietazine, Gesafloc						2830
Trifluralin, Treflan			+			10,000

*Treatment: Lavage and catharsis; artificial respiration if respiration is depressed.
†Exposure limit.

Table 8–1 (cont'd). Miscellaneous pesticides.

	Skin Sensitivity Reactions	Convulsions or Coma	Irritant: GI-Skin-Respiratory Tract	Liver and/or Kidney Damage	Blood Pressure Fall	LD50 (mg/kg)
Insecticides (cont'd):						
Pyrethrin (5 mg/m³)†	+	+				1500
Resmethrin, Chryson, Synthrin						4240
Rotenone (5 mg/m³)†	+	+				132
Ryania		+	+			1200
Sabadilla**			+		+	300 (est)
Sulfoxide, Sulfoxyl						2000
Sumithrin (D-phenothrin)						10,000+
Tetramethrin, Phthalthrin						4640
Tetrasul, Animert						10,000+
Thiocyclam						310
Thiophanate-methyl						7500
Tropital, heliotropin acetal						4400
Vendex, fenbutatin					◦	2631
Fish, worm, and mollusk toxicants:						
Antimycin		+	+		+	10
Lamprecide, TFN						370
Niclosamide, Yomesan, Bayluscid						5000+
Trifenmorph, Frescon						1200
Plant growth regulators:						
Alsol, etacelasil						2066
Ancymidol, A-Rest						4500
Atrinol, dikegulac						18,000
6-Benzylaminopurine, Bap						5000+
Butralin, Amex						12,600
Dehydroacetic acid, DHA						1000
Dimethepin, Harvade						1180
Ethephon, Florel						4229
Gibberellic acid	+					1500+
Glyoxime, Pik-Off						180
Glyphosine, Polaris						3925
Maleic hydrazide		+				3800
Mefluidide, Embark						1920
Mesoranil, Aziprotryn						3600
Nitrapyrin, N-Serve (10 mg/m³)†						500

*Treatment: Lavage and catharsis; artificial respiration if respiration is depressed.
†Exposure limit.
**Sabadilla also requires atropine, 2 mg intramuscularly, and repeat as necessary.

Table 8—1 (cont'd): Miscellaneous pesticides.

Possible Symptoms and Signs*						
	Skin Sensitivity Reactions	Convulsions or Coma	Irritant: GI-Skin-Respiratory Tract	Liver and/or Kidney Damage	Blood Pressure Fall	LD50 (mg/kg)
Herbicides and fungicides (cont'd):						
Triforine, Saprol, Funginex						16,000+
Ustilan						5000+
Validamycin, Validacin						20,000+
Velpar, hexazinone						1690
Vinicur, cyprofuram						174
Insecticides:						
Allethrin	+	+				920
Altosid, methoprene						35,000
Amdro						1131
Amitraz, Baam						200
Azacyclotin, Peropal						99
Barban, Carbyne			+			600
Benzomate						15,000
Bensultap, Bancol			+			1105
Buprofezin, Applaud						2188
Cartap, Padan						250
Cycloprate, Zardex						12,200
Cyfluthrin, Baythroid						590
Cyhexatin, Plictran						540
Cypermethrin, Ripcord						25
Cyromazine						3387
Dalapon, Dowpon			+			970
Deltamethrin, Decis						128
Dimethrin						15+
Eradex, thioquinox		+			+	3400
Esbiol, S-bioallethrin						680
Fluvalinate, Maverik			+			6000+
Gossyplur						15
Hexythiazox, Nissorun						5000+
Iprodione, Rovral						3500
Kinoprene, Enstar						4900
Octacide, MGK264		+				2800
Oxythioquinox, Morestan						2500
Pay-Off						67
Pentac, dienochlor						3160
Permethrin, Ambush, Talcord						430
Phenothiazine §			+	+		300
Piperonyl butoxide		+				11,500
Propargite, Omite, Comite						2200

*Treatment: Lavage and catharsis; artificial respiration if respiration is depressed.
§For phenothiazine poisoning, also force fluids to 2—4 L/d.

Table 8–1 (cont'd). Miscellaneous pesticides.

Possible Symptoms and Signs*						
	Skin Sensitivity Reactions	Convulsions or Coma	Irritant: GI-Skin-Respiratory Tract	Liver and/or Kidney Damage	Blood Pressure Fall	LD50 (mg/kg)
Plant growth regulators (cont'd):						
Phyomone, NAA, α-naphthalene acetic acid			+	+		1000
Succinic acid-2, 2-dimethyl hydrazide, Alar, Kylar, Daminozide		+	+	+		6810
Thidiazuron, Dropp						4000+
TIBA, Floraltone						813
Tomaset, Duraset						5230

*Treatment: Lavage and catharsis; artificial respiration if respiration is depressed.

2. Feedings–Administer readily digested food frequently to aid in maintaining an adequate source of energy for the increased metabolism.

Prognosis

Recovery from severe poisoning is likely if the body temperature can be kept below 40 °C and if adequate nutrition is supplied.

FLUOROACETATE

The sodium salt of fluoroacetic acid ($CH_2FCOONa$; 1080) is a water-soluble, synthetic chemical used in the past as a rodenticide. Fluoroacetate is no longer marketed in the USA, but fluoroacetamide is still available.

The fatal dose is estimated to be 50–100 mg. At least 13 deaths from sodium fluoroacetate have occurred. Fluoroacetamide and fluoroacetanilide have similar toxicities. The LD50 of fluoroacetic acid in rats is 0.22 mg/kg; that of fluoroacetamide is 15 mg/kg. The relative toxicity in humans is not known. The exposure limit for sodium fluoroacetate is 0.05 mg/m³.

Fluoroacetate in the body forms fluorotricarboxylic acid, which blocks cellular metabolism at the citrate stage. The relationship between this metabolic effect and poisoning has not been elucidated. All body cells, and especially those of the central nervous system, are affected by fluoroacetate as shown by depression of O_2 consumption of isolated tissues.

No specific histologic changes are seen in fluoroacetate poisoning. Findings include pulmonary and cerebral edema, congestion of the kidneys and lungs, and mediastinal emphysema.

Clinical Findings

The principal manifestations of acute fluoroacetate poisoning from ingestion or inhalation are vomiting and convulsions. Chronic poisoning does not occur. Symptoms begin within minutes to 4–5 hours, with vomiting, excitability, tonic-clonic convulsions, irregular heartbeat and respiration, exhaustion, coma, and respiratory depression. Death is from respiratory failure associated with pulmonary edema and bronchial pneumonia.

Prevention

Fluoroacetate is too toxic for use as a household rodenticide.

Treatment of Poisoning

A. Emergency Measures:

1. Lavage–Remove ingested poison by thorough gastric lavage with tap water. Follow with saline catharsis.

2. Emesis–Give syrup of ipecac (see p 21).

B. General Measures: Control convulsions (see Table 4–3).

Prognosis

Complete recovery may follow repeated convulsions. Rapid progression of symptoms within 1–2 hours after poisoning is likely to result in death. Survival for more than 24 hours indicates a favorable outcome.

Trabes J et al: Computed tomography demonstration of brain damage due to acute sodium monofluoroacetate poisoning. *J Toxicol Clin Toxicol* 1983;**20**:85.

TOBACCO & NICOTINE

Exposure to nicotine occurs during processing or extraction of tobacco; during the mixing, storage, or application of insecticides containing nicotine; or during smoking. Nicotine is available in concentrates as a free base, which is volatile, or as the sulfate. Both are liquids, even in pure form. In addition to concentrates, nicotine is also present in a large number of insecticide mixtures in concentrations of 1% or more. Additional less toxic compounds with similar actions are anabasine, nornicotine, and lobeline. The less toxic nicotine polacrilex (Nicorette) is used as a tobacco substitute.

The fatal dose of pure nicotine is about 40 mg (0.6 mg/kg, 1 drop), the quantity contained in 2 g of tobacco (2 cigarettes). However, because of diminished bioavailability, tobacco is much less poisonous than would be expected on the basis of its nicotine content. When tobacco is smoked, most of the nicotine is burned, but a number of carcinogens are produced. After ingestion of tobacco, nicotine is poorly absorbed. The exposure limit for nicotine is 0.5 mg/m^3. The fatal dose of lobeline, which is used in tobacco substitutes, could be as low as 5 mg/kg.

Nicotine first stimulates, then depresses and paralyzes the cells of the peripheral autonomic ganglia, brain (especially midbrain), and spinal cord. Skeletal muscle, including the diaphragm, is paralyzed.

No specific histologic changes are found after nicotine poisoning. After ingestion, the mouth, pharynx, esophagus, and stomach may show evidence of the caustic effect of nicotine.

Clinical Findings

The principal manifestations of nicotine poisoning are respiratory stimulation and gastrointestinal hyperactivity.

A. Acute Poisoning:

1. Small doses–(From skin contamination or inhalation of tobacco smoke, tobacco dust, or insecticide sprays.) Respiratory stimulation, nausea and vomiting, dizziness, headache, diarrhea, tachycardia, elevation of blood pressure, sweating, and salivation. Gradual recovery follows a period of weakness.

2. Large doses–(From ingestion or skin contamination with insecticide concentrates.) Initially there is burning of the mouth, throat, and stomach, followed by rapid progression of the above symptoms, proceeding to prostration, convulsions, respiratory slowing, cardiac irregularity, and coma. Death occurs within 5 minutes to 4 hours.

B. Chronic Poisoning: No cumulative effect from exposure to small amounts of nicotine insecticides has been noted. Tobacco smoking increases the incidence of coronary heart disease and oral, urinary bladder, and respiratory tract cancer.

Treatment

A. Acute Poisoning:

1. Emergency measures–

a. Wash skin–Remove nicotine from the skin by flooding with water and scrubbing vigorously with soap.

b. Emesis–Patient is likely to be already vomiting. If possible, give activated charcoal orally to adsorb any nicotine not expelled (see p 25).

c. Lavage–Remove ingested nicotine by thorough gastric lavage with tap water containing activated charcoal, if readily available (see p 25).

    d. Give artificial respiration, using O_2 if available.

    2. Antidote–Give atropine in maximum doses (see p 117) to control the signs of parasympathetic overstimulation, or give phentolamine, 1–5 mg intramuscularly or intravenously, to control signs of sympathetic hyperactivity, such as hypertension.

    3. General measures–Control convulsions (see Table 4–3).

    B. Chronic Poisoning: Remove from further exposure to dust or smoke.

Prognosis

    Survival for more than 4 hours is usually followed by complete recovery.

Manoguerra AS, Freeman D: Acute poisoning from the ingestion of *Nicotiana glauca*. *J Toxicol Clin Toxicol* 1982;**19**:861.

Smoking and cardiovascular disease. *MMWR* 1983;**32**:677.

THALLIUM

    Thallium has been used as a rodenticide and an ant killer. Its use as a pesticide is now prohibited. Poisoning has most frequently resulted from the accidental ingestion of thallium rodent or ant baits, which consisted of thallium sulfate or acetate mixed with grain, cookie crumbs, cracker crumbs, honey, or sweetened water.

    The most commonly available salts of thallium are the sulfate, acetate, and carbonate. Thallium sulfide and iodide are appreciably less soluble than the other salts.

    The fatal dose is approximately 1 g of absorbed thallium. The exposure limit for thallium and its compounds is 0.1 mg/m^3.

    Pathologic findings include pneumonitis and vacuolization and degenerative changes in the cells of the hair follicles, adrenal cortex, thyroid, and central nervous system.

Clinical Findings

    The principal manifestations of thallium poisoning are loss of hair and pains in the extremities.

    A. Acute Poisoning: (From ingestion or skin absorption.) Evidence of poisoning appears in 1–10 days and includes pains and paresthesias of the extremities, bilateral ptosis, ataxia, loss of hair, fever, coryza, conjunctivitis, abdominal pain, and nausea and vomiting. Progression of poisoning is indicated by the appearance of lethargy, jumbled speech, tremors, choreiform movements, convulsions, and cyanosis. Signs of pulmonary edema and bronchopneumonia may precede death in respiratory failure. Anuria with renal damage has also been reported.

B. Chronic Poisoning: (From ingestion or skin absorption.) If absorption of thallium occurs over an extended period, the earliest indications of poisoning are alopecia, atrophic changes in the skin, and occasionally salivation and a blue line on the gums. Gastrointestinal symptoms are also common. If absorption continues, renal damage and functional changes of the endocrine system (amenorrhea and aspermia) may appear along with symptoms and signs as in acute poisoning.

C. Laboratory Findings: Examination of urine may reveal proteinuria and an increase in red cells and cellular casts. Increase in eosinophils, lymphocytes, or polymorphonuclear leukocytes may occur.

Prevention

The sale of thallium for any household purpose should be banned.

Treatment

A. Acute Poisoning:

1. Emergency measures–

a. Remove ingested thallium by prompt emesis with syrup of ipecac. Follow by gastric lavage with activated charcoal. Leave 50 g of activated charcoal in the stomach.

b. Consider oral administration of a cathartic.

c. Remove skin contamination by scrubbing with soap and water.

2. Antidote–No specific antidote is known to be effective.

3. General measures–

a. Forced diuresis with furosemide and mannitol, hemoperfusion using activated charcoal, and hemodialysis can remove up to 40% of absorbed thallium.

b. Maintain blood pressure by administering 5% glucose in saline intravenously.

c. Maintain warmth and adequate fluid intake and nutrition.

d. Maintain urine output at 1000 mL or more daily. If renal insufficiency appears, give only enough fluid to replace losses (see p 72).

B. Chronic Poisoning: Remove from further exposure.

Prognosis

If the progression of signs of cerebral damage (lethargy, delirium, and muscular twitchings) can be halted, recovery is possible. Complete recovery may require 2 months or more.

DeGroot G et al: Thallium concentrations in body fluids and tissues in a fatal case of thallium poisoning. *Vet Hum Toxicol* 1984;**27**:115.

Heath A et al: Thallium poisoning: Toxin elimination and therapy in 3 cases. *J Toxicol Clin Toxicol* 1983;**20**:451.

Mayfield SR et al: Acute thallium poisoning in a 3-year-old child. *Clin Pediatr* 1984;**23**:461.

Nogué S et al: Acute thallium poisoning: An evaluation of different forms of treatment. *J Toxicol Clin Toxicol* 1982;**19**:1015.

THIOCYANATE INSECTICIDES: THANITE, LETHANE

Thiocyanate insecticides are ordinarily available in mixtures as concentrated solutions in an organic solvent, as emulsion concentrates, or in combination with other insecticides.

The toxicity of these compounds is moderate compared with that of nicotine. One adult died after ingesting a mixture containing approximately 5 g of Lethane-384 and 14 g of lauryl thiocyanate. Other fatalities have been reported following ingestion of similar quantities. The toxicities of ethyl and methyl thiocyanate are considerably greater, reaching 10 mg/kg in experimental animals, because they are converted to cyanide in the body. In rats, Thanite has an LD50 of 1600 mg/kg.

The thiocyanate insecticides induce coma, cyanosis, dyspnea, and tonic convulsions in rats at doses ranging from 90 mg/kg (Lethane-384) to 1 g/kg (Thanite).

Pathologic examination of animals poisoned by thiocyanate insecticides has not revealed organ damage.

Clinical Findings

The principal manifestation of acute poisoning with the thiocyanate insecticides is convulsions. Chronic poisoning does not occur.

A. Symptoms and Signs: (From ingestion or excessive skin contamination.) Convulsions with respiratory difficulty.

B. Laboratory Findings: The blood thiocyanate level is likely to be high.

Treatment

A. Emergency Measures: Remove skin contamination by scrubbing with soap and water. Remove swallowed poison by thorough gastric lavage with tap water. If gastric lavage cannot be accomplished immediately, give syrup of ipecac, 15 mL, and 250 mL of tap water or milk (see p 21). Maintain artificial respiration during convulsions or respiratory difficulty.

B. Antidote: Treat methyl and ethyl thiocyanate as for cyanide (see p 254).

C. General Measures: Give anticonvulsants (see Table 4–3).

Prognosis

If adequate gastric lavage and catharsis can be accomplished before onset of symptoms, recovery is likely. Progression of symptoms after gastric lavage indicates a poor outcome.

VACOR

Vacor—N-3-pyridylmethyl-N′-*p*-nitrophenylurea (PNU)—is used as a rodenticide. No longer commercially available in the USA, it was formerly marketed in 39-g packets containing 2% vacor in a dry bait. Fatalities have occurred following ingestion of 0.78 g of vacor, the amount contained in one packet. Most deaths have been the result of suicidal ingestion.

The chief pathologic finding is destruction of the B islet cells of the pancreas. Vacor may interfere with nicotinamide metabolism.

Clinical Findings

The principal manifestations of poisoning with vacor are hypotension and hyperglycemia.

A. Symptoms and Signs: (From ingestion.) Nausea and vomiting, diffuse abdominal pain, lightheadedness, chest pain, weakness, blurred vision, polyuria, thirst, numbness of the legs, lethargy, ataxia, hypotension, tremor, muscle cramps, sluggish pupillary responses, areflexia, loss of muscle stretch reflexes, dysphagia, postural hypotension, gastrointestinal hypomotility, bladder atony, impaired intellect, disturbances of balance, and delirium or stupor.

B. Laboratory Findings: The ECG shows ischemic changes in the myocardium. Blood analysis reveals hyperglycemia and hyponatremia. Ketotic acidosis may be present.

Prevention

Vacor is too dangerous for use as a household rodenticide. It has far more serious effects on humans than on rodents.

Treatment of Acute Poisoning

A. Emergency Measures: Remove vacor by emesis induced by syrup of ipecac followed by gastric lavage with activated charcoal (see p 24). Follow with a saline cathartic.

B. Antidote: Give nicotinamide parenterally within 30 minutes after vacor ingestion. Nicotinamide may not be effective if given several hours after ingestion of vacor.

C. General Measures:
1. Treat hyperglycemia with insulin.
2. Control orthostatic hypotension with elastic stockings.

Prognosis

Removal within the first 30 minutes has been followed by recovery. If symptoms develop, diabetes mellitus caused by vacor is permanent. Spontaneous recovery from orthostatic hypotension after a year or more is possible. The peripheral neuropathy also improves gradually for at least 1 year.

PARAQUAT & DIQUAT

Paraquat or methyl viologen (1,1'-dimethyl-4,4'-dipyridylium dichloride), diquat, chlormequat (Cycocel), mepiquat (Pix), morfamquat, and difenzoquat (Avenge) are water-soluble quaternary ammonium herbicides supplied in concentrations of 20–50%. They are inactivated by contact with soil, presumably as a result of combination with clay particles in the soil, and are also subject to rapid photodecomposition.

More than 80 fatalities from paraquat have been reported in the literature. One individual died after ingesting $\frac{3}{4}$ teaspoon of 19% solution, or an amount less than 10 mg/kg. The fatal dose for humans has been estimated to be as small as 4 mg/kg, although the oral LD50 in rats is 120 mg/kg. At least 4 fatalities have occurred following diquat ingestion. The smallest fatal dose was 30 mg/kg. The oral LD50 for diquat in rats is 200–300 mg/kg; for difenzoquat, it is 270 mg/kg; for chlormequat, it is 670 mg/kg; and for mepiquat, it is 1420 mg/kg. The exposure limit for paraquat is 0.1 mg/m^3; for diquat, it is 0.5 mg/m^3. Contaminated marihuana has contained from 3 to 2264 mg of paraquat per kilogram, and 0.03% of paraquat from burned marihuana appears in the smoke (0.6 μg of paraquat inhaled from 1 g of marihuana containing 2 mg of paraquat). Rabbits develop lung fibrosis from 10 μg of paraquat instilled into the lung. Morfamquat causes reversible renal tubular damage in dogs and rats.

Although the mechanism of poisoning has not been fully elucidated, it is believed to involve inhibition of superoxide dismutase in the lungs, making the lungs particularly susceptible to oxygen toxicity. Pathologic findings after paraquat fatalities include focal myocardial necrosis, pulmonary hemorrhages and edema, eosinophilic alveolar hyaline membrane formation, proliferation of fibroblasts in alveolar septa, necrosis of the adrenal cortex (mostly in fasciculata and reticularis), renal tubular necrosis, and centrilobular biliary stasis. In experimental studies, diquat has not produced the lung lesion found with paraquat. Pathologic findings after death from diquat include hemorrhagic necrotic areas in the brain, distention of the intestines, severe renal tubular necrosis, pulmonary edema and congestion, and bronchopneumonia.

Clinical Findings

The principal manifestations of paraquat poisoning are gastrointestinal distress (nausea, vomiting, and pain) and respiratory distress and cyanosis.

A. Symptoms and Signs: (From ingestion, skin contamination, or inhalation.) Ingestion of paraquat causes burning in the mouth and throat and vomiting. After 2–5 days, hemoptysis, oliguria, and ulceration of the tongue, pharynx, and esophagus appear. After 5–8 days, severely poisoned patients show jaundice, fever, tachycardia, respiratory distress, and cyanosis. Heavy skin contamination has caused corrosive damage and subsequent fatal lung damage. Inhalation of 1–100 μg of paraquat could cause delayed fibrosis of the lungs without immediate symptoms.

Diquat ingestion has caused abdominal cramps, vomiting, diarrhea, coma, oliguria and progressive renal failure, ventricular arrhythmias including fibrillation, and impaired pulmonary diffusion.

B. Laboratory Findings: A urinary paraquat excretion rate above 1 mg/h or a plasma paraquat level above 0.1 μg/mL indicates severe poisoning. Paraquat may continue to appear in the urine for more than a month after poisoning. The alveolar/arterial O_2 gradient is markedly increased. Elevation of blood urea nitrogen, serum alkaline phosphatase, and serum bilirubin indicates the severity of damage to liver and kidneys. A decrease in the level of serum trypsin inhibitor has been found; this may be an indicator of the extent of damage to the lungs.

Treatment

A. Emergency Measures: Give activated charcoal followed by gastric lavage with repeated 200-mL volumes of 1% bentonite solution (1 part of bentonite magma diluted with 4 parts of water), or give 200 mL of 30% suspension of fuller's earth in water. The administration of fuller's earth or bentonite should be repeated twice daily for the first 48 hours. The addition of a saline cathartic to fuller's earth or bentonite solution is also useful. If fuller's earth or bentonite is not available, activated charcoal should be given.

B. General Measures:

1. Whole gut lavage with a solution containing 6 g of sodium chloride, 0.75 g of potassium chloride, and 3 g of sodium bicarbonate per liter at a rate of 1 mL/kg/min by gastric tube has been suggested. Administer 200 mL of 20% mannitol into the gastric tube hourly and 60 g of fuller's earth or activated charcoal in 200 mL of water into the gastric tube every 2 hours. Continue gut lavage until only fuller's earth or charcoal is passed, usually 2–6 hours.

2. Maintain urine output at 200 mL/h by giving 4–8 L of fluid intravenously daily if renal function is not impaired. Furosemide, 20 mg intravenously every 4–8 hours, may be necessary.

3. Hydrocortisone, 200 mg intravenously every 6 hours, may be helpful early, but corticosteroids are useless later. Large doses of vitamins C and E as antioxidants may be helpful early.

4. Hemodialysis or hemoperfusion is most effective if begun within the first 12 hours. Patients with plasma paraquat levels more than 10 times the usual lethal level have recovered when hemoperfusion over charcoal was performed 8 hours per day for 2–3 weeks.

Prognosis

Patients have died of lung dysfunction up to 3 weeks after poisoning.

Bismuth C et al: Prognosis and treatment of paraquat poisoning: A review of 28 cases. *J Toxicol Clin Toxicol* 1982;**19**:461.

Gaudreault P et al: Efficacy of activated charcoal in the treatment of oral paraquat intoxication. *Ann Emerg Med* 1985;**14**:123.

Landrigan PJ et al: Maraquat and marihuana: Epidemiologic risk assessment. *Am J Public Health* 1983;**73**:784.

Okonek S et al: Successful treatment of paraquat poisoning: Activated charcoal per os and "continuous hemoperfusion." *J Toxicol Clin Toxicol* 1982;**19**:807.

Onyeama HP et al: A literature review of paraquat toxicity. *Vet Hum Toxicol* 1984;**26**:494.

Tungsanga K et al: Paraquat poisoning: Evidence of systemic toxicity after dermal exposure. *Postgrad Med J* 1983;**59**:338.

III. Industrial Hazards

Nitrogen Compounds | 9

ANILINE, DIMETHYLANILINE, NITROANILINE, TOLUIDINE, & NITROBENZENES

Aniline is used in printing inks, cloth-marking inks, paints, and paint removers and in the synthesis of dyes. Dimethylaniline, nitroaniline, toluidine, and nitrobenzene are used in the synthesis of other chemicals.

Ingestion of 1 g of aniline has caused death, although recovery has followed ingestion of 30 g. The toxicity of nitrobenzene is similar. The fatal dose (LD50) in animals for aniline is 400 mg/kg, and for nitrobenzene it is 700 mg/kg. The toxicities of aniline derivatives are given in Table 9–1. Infant deaths have been caused by absorption of aniline from diapers stenciled with cloth-marking ink containing aniline as the vehicle for dyes. The residual pigment is safe after washing.

Aniline and nitrobenzene act through an intermediate to change hemoglobin to methemoglobin. In one subject, 65 mg of aniline increased the methemoglobin level by 16% within 2 hours. The intense methemoglobinemia produced by all these chemicals may lead to asphyxia severe enough to injure the cells of the central nervous system. These compounds sometimes cause hemolysis.

Pathologic findings in acute fatalities from aniline and nitrobenzene derivatives include chocolate color of the blood; injury to the kidney, liver, and spleen; and hemolysis. Bladder wall ulceration and necrosis may also occur. β-Naphthylamine, which contaminates commercial aniline, causes bladder papillomas after 1–30 years' exposure. These papillomas become malignant if not removed.

Clinical Findings

The principal manifestations in poisoning with these compounds are cyanosis and jaundice.

A. Acute Poisoning: (From inhalation, skin absorption, or ingestion.) Symptoms and signs include cyanosis at methemoglobin levels above 15%; headache, shallow respiration, and dizziness at methemoglobin levels of 40–50%; confusion, blood pressure fall, lethargy, and stupor at 60%; and convulsions, coma, blood pressure fall, and possibly death at methemoglobin levels of 70% or higher. Jaundice, pain on urination, and anemia may appear later.

Table 9–1. Nitro and amino compounds and miscellaneous nitrogen compounds. (For treatment, see p 146.)

	Exposure Limit (ppm)	LD50 (mg/kg) or LC (ppm, ppb)	Forms Methemoglobin	Sensitization	Irritation, Corneal Damage	Bladder Irritation	Kidney and Liver Damage	CNS Effects	Carcinogen	Other Adverse Clinical Effects
Acetamide		360			+				+	
2-Acetylaminofluorene (AAF)	0	1000							+	
Acridine		500			+					
Acrylamide	0.3*	126								Neuropathy
2-Aminoanthraquinone									+	
3-Amino-9-ethylcarbazole		144					+		+	
4-Aminodiphenyl	0	500			+	+	+	+	+	Debility
p-Aminophenol		375	+	+	+		+	+		
1-Amino-2-propanol		4000								
2- or 4-Aminopyridine	0.5	20	+					+		Convulsions
2-Aminothiazole		120		+	+			+		
Aniline	2	400	+		+					
Anisidine, o- or p-	0.1	1400	+	+	+		+			
Azobenzene		1000					+		+	
Benzidine	0	200		+		+			+	
Bone oil		800	+					+		
ε-Caprolactam	5, 1*	2140		+	+			+		Convulsions
p-Chloroaniline		100	+	+						
Chloronitrobenzenes	0.05*	135	+	+	+		+	+		Hyperthermia
1-Chloro-1-nitropropane	2	50			+		+			
Chloronitropropanes	20	200			+		+	+		
Chloropicrin	0.1	250			+					Heart damage
Chlorotoluidines		2	+			+				
Clopidol	10*	8000+								
Cyclohexylamine	10	710			+			+		
Diallylamine		516			+			+		
4,4'-Diaminodiphenylmethane	0.1	347					+		+	
Diazomethane	0.2	100			+			+	+	Lung damage
3,3'-Dichlorobenzidine	0	4740							+	
Dichloronitroanilines		1500	+	+	+	+				
1,1-Dichloro-1-nitroethane	2	150			+	+	+			
Dimethylacetamide	10	2240			+		+	+		Teratogen

*mg/m^3.

Table 9–1 (cont'd). Nitro and amino compounds and miscellaneous nitrogen compounds. (For treatment, see p 146.)

	Exposure Limit (ppm)	LD50 (mg/kg) or LC (ppm, ppb)	Forms Methemoglobin	Sensitization	Irritation, Corneal Damage	Bladder Irritation	Kidney and Liver Damage	CNS Effects	Carcinogen	Other Adverse Clinical Effects
p-Dimethylaminoazo-benzene	0	300							+	
N,N-Dimethyl aniline	5	1400	+		+					
2,6-Dimethyl aniline		700	+		+					
3,3'-Dimethylbenzi-dine	0?	404				+			+	
Dimethylcarbamyl-chloride	0?	10 ppm		+	+				+	
Dimethylformamide	10	4000			+		+	+		
Dimethylhydrazines	0.5	100			+		+		+	Convulsions
Dimethylnitrosamine	0	20			+		+	+		
Dinitrobenzenes	0.15	30	+		+					
Dinitrotoluamide	5*	560	+							
Dinitrotoluene	1.5*	200	+				+	+	+	Anemia
N,N-Diphenylamine	10	2000		+	+	+	+			Heart damage
1,2-Diphenylhydra-zine	0?	301							+	
Diphenylnitrosamine		1650			+				+	
2,4-Dithiobiuret		20						+		
Ethylenimine	0.5	15		+	+				+	Lung damage
N-Ethylmorpholine	5	1780			+					Corneal damage
Formamide	20	6100			+		+	+		
Hexamethyl phos-phoramide	0?	400 ppb					+		+	
Hydrazine	0.1	60			+		+	+	+	Hemolysis
Hydrazoic acid	0.1	23						+		Hypotension
Hydroxylamine		400	+	+	+					Teratogen
Imidazolidinethione		0.2							+	Teratogen
Isophorone diisocy-anate	0.01			+	+					
N-Isopropyl aniline	2		+		+					
N-Methyl aniline	0.5	280	+		+		+			
4,4'-Methylene-bis(2-chloroaniline)	0.02								+	
Methylene bis(4-cyclo-hexyl isocyanate)	0.01			+	+					
Methylene bisphenyl isocyanate (MDI)	0.02			+	+					

*mg/m^3.

Table 9–1 (cont'd). Nitro and amino compounds and miscellaneous nitrogen compounds. (For treatment, see p 146.)

	Exposure Limit (ppm)	LD50 (mg/kg) or LC (ppm, ppb)	Forms Methemoglobin	Sensitization	Irritation, Corneal Damage	Bladder Irritation	Kidney and Liver Damage	CNS Effects	Carcinogen	Other Adverse Clinical Effects
Methyl hydrazine	0.2	33	+		+				+	Convulsions
Methyl isothiocyanate		97		+			+			
o-Methylnitrobenzene		890	+		+			+		
N-Methyl-N'-nitro-N-nitrosoguanidine		90							+	
N-Methyl-N-nitro-sourea		110			+				+	Pancreatic damage
N-Methyl-2-pyrroli-done		3000			+					
Morpholine	20	1000			+		+			
α- or β-Naphthylamine	0	700			+	+	+		+	
Naphthylamine mustard		1000							+	
Nitrilotriacetate (NTA)		680			+					
Nitroanilines	0.5	300	+	+			+			
Nitrobenzene	1	700	+	+	+					
4-Nitrodiphenyl	0	1970			+		+		+	
Nitroethane	100	500			+		+	+		
Nitromethane	100	125			+		+	+		Convulsions
Nitrophenols		467	+		+		+	+		Hyperthermia
1-Nitropropane	25	250	+		+		+	+		
2-Nitropropane	10	500	+		+		+	+	+	
Nitropropanes	25	250	+		+		+			
N-Nitrosodimethyl-amine	0	26					+		+	
Nitrotoluenes	2	330	+		+		+			Anemia
Pentachloronitro-benzene		1650		+	+		+		+	
p-Phenylenediamine	0.1*	100	+	+	+		+	+		
Phenylhydrazine	5	80		+	+		+	+	+	Anemia
Phenylhydroxylamine		500 est	+	+	+		+			
p-Phenyl-β-naphthyl-amine	0								+	
2-Picoline	5*	674			+		+			Lymph nodes
Picric acid	0.1*	120		+	+		+	+		Hyperthermia
Piperidine		400						+		Vomiting
Polyamides		1500			+					Caustic
Propylene imine	2	19			+			+	+	
n-Propyl nitrate	25	100 IV	+		+			+		Hypotension

*mg/m^3.

Table 9–1 (cont'd). Nitro and amino compounds and miscellaneous nitrogen compounds. (For treatment, see p 146.)

	Exposure Limit (ppm)	LD50 (mg/kg) or LC (ppm, ppb)	Forms Methemoglobin	Sensitization	Irritation, Corneal Damage	Bladder Irritation	Kidney and Liver Damage	CNS Effects	Carcinogen	Other Adverse Clinical Effects
Pyridine	5	891			+		+	+		Heart damage
Quinoline		460	+		+		+			
Sulfanilic acid		1000 est	+				+			
Tetrachloronitro-benzene		250	+	+	+		+		+	
Tetramethylsuccinoni-trile	0.5	60 ppm			+			+		Convulsions
Tetranitromethane	1	33 ppm	+		+			+		Heart damage
Tetryl	1.5*	500 est			+					
o-Tolidine		400			+		+		+	
Toluenediamine		100	+	+	+		+	+		
Toluene diisocyanate (TDI)	0.005	12 ppm		+	+					Asthma
Toluidines	2	5	+		+				+	
Triallylamine		492			+		+			
Trinitrotriazine	1.5*	100					+	+		Anemia
Triphenylamine	5*	1600								
m-Xylene-a,a'-diamine	0.1*	930	+	+	+		+			
Xylidines	2	5	+				+	+		

*mg/m^3.

B. Chronic Poisoning: (From inhalation or skin absorption.) Nervous system, liver, kidneys, and bone marrow may be affected. Weight loss, anemia, weakness, and irritability occur.

C. Laboratory Findings:

1. Blood methemoglobin, determined photometrically, is the best measure of the seriousness of poisoning with these substances.

2. Red blood cells may be reduced to 20–30% of normal, with accompanying poikilocytosis and anisocytosis. Erythrocyte inclusion (Heinz) bodies are common.

3. Hepatic cell function impairment may be indicated by the appropriate tests (see p 75).

4. N-Acetyl-*p*-aminophenol in urine indicates chronic exposure. Gross or microscopic hematuria may be present as a result of bladder or kidney irritation or hemolysis. Renal function may also be impaired.

Treatment

A. Acute Poisoning:

1. Emergency measures–

a. Remove poison from skin by washing thoroughly with soap and water.

b. If poison was swallowed, remove by emesis or gastric lavage and consider using activated charcoal (see pp 21–28).

c. Give O_2 if respiration is shallow or anoxia is present.

2. Antidote–For severe methemoglobinemia, give methylene blue, 1% solution, 0.1 mL/kg (1 mg/kg) slowly intravenously, to reduce methemoglobin to normal hemoglobin (see p 78).

3. Other measures–If methemoglobinemia does not respond to methylene blue, hemodialysis or exchange transfusion is useful.

B. Chronic Poisoning:

1. Remove from exposure.

2. Treat liver damage (see p 77).

Prognosis

Survival for 24 hours is usually followed by complete recovery.

Beauchamp RO Jr et al: A critical review of the literature on nitrobenzene toxicity. *CRC Crit Rev Toxicol* 1982;**11**:33.

Gilsanz V et al: Evolution of the alimentary toxic oil syndrome due to the ingestion of denatured rape seed oil. *Arch Intern Med* 1984;**144**:254.

TRINITROTOLUENE & TRINITROBENZENE

Trinitrotoluene (TNT) and trinitrobenzene are used as explosives.

The acute fatal dose is estimated to be 1–2 g. The exposure limit is 0.5 mg/m³. At least 22 fatalities from trinitrotoluene absorption occurred in the USA during World War II.

Trinitrotoluene and trinitrobenzene injure almost all cells, especially those of the liver, bone marrow, and kidney. Trinitrobenzene damages the central nervous system.

Pathologic findings are acute yellow atrophy of the liver, bone marrow aplasia, petechial hemorrhages, and toxic nephritis.

Clinical Findings

The principal manifestation of trinitrotoluene poisoning is jaundice.

A. Acute or Chronic Poisoning: (From inhalation, skin absorption, or ingestion.) Jaundice, dermatitis, cyanosis, pallor, nausea, loss of appetite, aplastic or hemolytic anemia, and oliguria or anuria occur variably. The liver may be enlarged early or atrophic later. Convulsions or coma may occur.

B. Laboratory Findings:

1. The blood methemoglobin level is the best measure of the seriousness of poisoning (see p 141).

2. In chronic poisoning, hepatic cell injury will be revealed by appropriate tests (see p 75).

3. The red blood cell count may be depressed, with anisocytosis and poikilocytosis. There may be relative lymphocytosis.

4. Urine may show protein and casts prior to the onset of anuria.

Treatment

A. Emergency Measures: Terminate skin contamination by thorough washing with soap and water. Remove swallowed trinitrotoluene by gastric lavage or emesis (see pp 21–28).

B. Other Measures: Treat failure of liver function (see p 77). Treat hemolytic reactions (see p 80).

Prognosis

Approximately 50% of patients with severe liver damage die of acute yellow atrophy. The others recover completely.

Rickert DE et al: Dinitrotoluene: Acute toxicity, oncogenicity, genotoxicity, and metabolism. *CRC Crit Rev Toxicol* 1984;**13**:217.

References

Diem JE et al: Five-year longitudinal study of workers employed in a new toluene diisocyanate manufacturing plant. *Am Rev Respir Dis* 1982;**126**:420.

Omae K: Two-year observation of pulmonary function in workers exposed to low concentrations of toluene diisocyanate. *Int Arch Occup Environ Health* 1984;**55**:1.

10 | Halogenated Hydrocarbons

CARBON TETRACHLORIDE

Formula: CCl_4; bp: 76.7 °C; vapor pressure at 20 °C: 91 mm Hg. Carbon tetrachloride decomposes to phosgene ($COCl_2$) and hydrochloric acid on heating.

Carbon tetrachloride is used as a solvent and intermediate in many industrial processes. Less toxic solvents should be used for such purposes as removal of adhesive tape.

The adult fatal dose by ingestion or inhalation is 3–5 mL. The exposure limit is 5 ppm (NIOSH 2 ppm) or 30 mg/m³ (1.5 g evaporated in a room $10 \times 10 \times 8$ ft = 10 ppm).

Carbon tetrachloride depresses and injures almost all cells of the body, including those of the central nervous system, liver, kidney, and blood vessels. Toxicity appears to result from the intracellular breakdown of carbon tetrachloride to more toxic intermediates, including epoxides, particularly in the liver. The heart muscle may be depressed, and ventricular arrhythmias may occur. Concomitant ethanol ingestion increases the effect of carbon tetrachloride on all organs.

On postmortem examination, the kidneys show marked edema and fatty degeneration of the tubules. The liver shows centrilobular necrosis and fatty degeneration and may be enlarged. The heart may also show fatty degeneration. The endothelium of blood vessels may be injured, with resultant petechiae or larger hemorrhages.

Clinical Findings

The principal manifestations in poisoning with carbon tetrachloride are coma, oliguria, and jaundice.

A. Acute Poisoning: (From inhalation, skin absorption, or ingestion.) The immediate effects are abdominal pain, nausea and vomiting, dizziness, and confusion, progressing to unconsciousness, respiratory slowing, slowed or irregular pulse, and fall of blood pressure. If consciousness is regained, the patient may have mild symptoms of nausea and anorexia or be free of symptoms for 1 day to 2 weeks until evidence of liver or kidney damage appears. Liver damage is indicated by nausea and vomiting, jaundice, and a swollen, tender liver; kidney damage is indicated by decreased urine output, edema, sudden weight gain, and azotemia progressing to uremia. Coma, liver damage, or kidney damage may appear independently, or all may occur in the same individual at different times.

B. Chronic Poisoning: (From inhalation or skin absorption.) The above occur after repeated exposures to low concentrations but are less severe. Vague symptoms suggestive of poisoning include fatigue, anorexia, occasional vomiting, abdominal discomfort, anemia, weakness, nausea, blurring of vision, memory loss, paresthesias, tremors, and loss of peripheral color vision. Dermatitis follows repeated skin exposure. Carbon tetrachloride is a potential carcinogen.

C. Laboratory Findings:

1. Serum glutamic-oxaloacetic transaminase (SGOT) is markedly elevated in the first 3 days after exposure.

2. Liver function impairment may be revealed by appropriate tests (see p 75).

3. Casts, protein, and red blood cells may appear in the urine prior to oliguria.

4. Renal damage with nitrogen retention is indicated by increase in blood nonprotein nitrogen, urea, and creatinine.

5. The ECG may show ventricular premature beats.

Prevention

Carbon tetrachloride workers must not drink alcoholic beverages and should have a twice-yearly physical examination, including laboratory evaluation of liver function.

Carbon tetrachloride should not be used as a fire extinguisher, since heat decomposes it to phosgene.

Treatment

A. Acute Poisoning:

1. Emergency measures–

a. If carbon tetrachloride is inhaled, give artificial respiration until consciousness returns.

b. Remove clothing contaminated with carbon tetrachloride.

c. If carbon tetrachloride is ingested, remove by emesis or gastric lavage (see pp 21–28).

2. General measures–

a. Maintain blood pressure by giving 5% glucose intravenously.

b. *Do not give stimulants.* Epinephrine or ephedrine may induce ventricular fibrillation.

c. If urine output is normal, maintain urine output at 1–2 L daily by osmotic diuresis or by giving fluids orally. Do not give diuretics.

d. Give a high-carbohydrate diet to attempt to restore optimal liver function.

3. Special problems–

a. Acute renal shutdown is treated as described on p 72. The oliguric phase of carbon tetrachloride intoxication is likely to last 7–10 days and is followed by a diuretic phase that may last up to 3 weeks before normal kidney function returns.

b. Treat hepatic coma by controlling blood ammonia levels. Useful measures include reducing protein intake to 20–30 g daily, preventing ammonia absorption from stool by daily administration of milk of magnesia or sodium sulfate, giving 8 g of neomycin daily to reduce ammonia formation in the bowel, avoiding chlorothiazide and acetazolamide, and using peritoneal dialysis.

c. Hemodialysis may be necessary to control blood electrolytes.

B. Chronic Poisoning: Remove from exposure and treat as indicated for acute poisoning.

Prognosis

In anuria, spontaneous return of kidney function may begin 2–3 weeks after poisoning. Complete return of liver and kidney function requires 2–12 months.

Ruprah M et al: Acute carbon tetrachloride poisoning in 19 patients: Implications for diagnosis and treatment. *Lancet* 1985;1:1027.

METHYL BROMIDE, METHYL CHLORIDE, & METHYL IODIDE

Formula: Methyl bromide, CH_3Br; methyl chloride, CH_3Cl; methyl iodide, CH_3I; all are gaseous or have high vapor pressure at ordinary temperatures.

Methyl bromide, methyl chloride, and methyl iodide are used as refrigerants, in chemical synthesis, and as fumigants. Methyl bromide is used with carbon tetrachloride in fire extinguishers.

The exposure limit is 5 ppm for methyl bromide, 50 ppm for methyl chloride, and 2 ppm for methyl iodide.

The fat-soluble methyl bromide, methyl chloride, and methyl iodide enter cells, where hydrolysis to methanol and halogen ion occurs.

Pathologic findings are congestion of the liver, kidneys, brain, and lungs, with degenerative changes in the cells. Bronchial pneumonia and pulmonary edema are common. These substances damage almost all body cells.

Clinical Findings

The principal manifestations of poisoning with these agents are coma and convulsions.

A. Acute Poisoning: (From inhalation or skin absorption.) If the concentration of methyl bromide, iodide, or chloride is high, nausea and vomiting, blurred vision, vertigo, weakness or paralysis, oliguria or anuria, drowsiness, confusion, hyperactivity, blood pressure fall, coma, convulsions, and pulmonary edema progress over 4–6 hours after a latent period of 1–4 hours. After exposure to lower concentrations, symptoms may not appear for 12–24 hours. Pulmonary edema and bronchial pneumonia are most often the cause of death. Skin contact causes irritation and vesiculation.

B. Chronic Poisoning: (From inhalation or skin absorption.) Repeated exposure to concentrations slightly higher than the exposure limit will cause blurring of vision, papilledema, numbness of the extremities, confusion, hallucinations, somnolence, fainting attacks, and bronchospasm. Methyl iodide is a potential carcinogen.

C. Laboratory Findings:

1. Hepatic cell function impairment may be indicated by appropriate laboratory tests (see p 75).

2. Urine may contain casts, red blood cells, and protein.

3. Blood pH may be reduced.

4. Blood methanol level may reach toxic concentrations.

Prevention

Gas masks are relatively ineffective because methyl bromide and methyl chloride penetrate the skin readily. Safety dispensers must always be used when applying methyl bromide as a fumigant.

Treatment

A. Acute Poisoning:

1. **Emergency measures**–Remove from further exposure and observe carefully for the first 48 hours. Restrain hyperactive patients.

2. **General measures**–

a. Treat pulmonary edema (see p 65).

b. Control convulsions by the cautious use of diazepam (see Table 4–3).

3. **Special problems**–

a. Bronchospasm complicating pulmonary edema or bronchial pneumonia is treated by aminophylline given intravenously (see p 65); repeat as necessary.

b. Treat renal failure (see p 72).

c. Treat acidosis (see p 49).

d. Treat methanol intoxication if necessary (see p 169).

e. Treat bacterial pneumonia with organism-specific chemotherapy.

B. Chronic Poisoning: Remove from further exposure.

Prognosis

Patients who survive 48–72 hours usually recover completely, but neurotoxic effects may persist for months.

TRICHLOROETHYLENE

Formula: $CHCl:CCl_2$; bp: 88 °C; vapor pressure at 20 °C; 60 mm Hg. Tetrachloroethane (see p 157) may be present as an impurity in technical products.

Trichloroethylene is used as an industrial solvent; in typewriter correction fluids; and in household cleaners for walls, clothing, and rugs. It has been used as an inhalation anesthetic or analgesic but is too dangerous for this use.

The exposure limit is 50 ppm. The adult fatal dose by ingestion or inhalation is estimated to be 5 mL.

Trichloroethylene decomposes to dichloroethylene, phosgene, and carbon monoxide on contact with alkalies such as soda lime.

The most striking effect of trichloroethylene is depression of the central nervous system. Other areas affected (in order of decreasing severity of involvement) include the myocardium, liver, and kidney. Trichloroethylene will induce acute ventricular arrhythmias, including ventricular fibrillation, or these may be precipitated by the administration of epinephrine while the heart rate is slowed. Trichloroethylene is suspected to be carcinogenic.

Findings in fatalities from exposure to commercial trichloroethylene include degenerative changes in the heart muscle, central nervous system, liver, and renal tubular epithelium. The presence of tetrachloroethane as a contaminant in commercial trichloroethylene may contribute to the cellular damage.

Clinical Findings

The principal manifestation of acute trichloroethylene poisoning is unconsciousness.

A. Acute Poisoning: (From inhalation, skin absorption, or ingestion.) Depending on concentration, symptoms progress more or less rapidly through dizziness, headache, nausea and vomiting, and excitement to loss of consciousness. Irregular pulse may indicate ventricular arrhythmia, which may progress to ventricular fibrillation. Recovery of consciousness is rapid, but nausea and vomiting may persist for several hours. Pulmonary edema may occur.

B. Chronic Poisoning: (From inhalation or skin absorption.) Symptoms and signs include weight loss, nausea, anorexia, fatigue, visual impairment, painful joints, dermatitis, and wheezing. Jaundice is uncommon.

C. Laboratory Findings:

1. The ECG may reveal ventricular irregularities during acute poisoning.

2. Trichloroethylene metabolites in urine can be used as an indicator of absorption. A level of more than 20 mg of metabolites per 24 hours indicates improper control of exposure.

3. Tests to evaluate liver damage are described on p 75.

Prevention

Cross-ventilation should be sufficient to prevent any noticeable odor when trichloroethylene is used as a cleaner in the home.

Treatment

A. Acute Poisoning: Move the patient to fresh air and give artificial respiration. Remove contaminated clothing. Do not give epinephrine or other stimulants that may cause ventricular arrhythmias. If symptoms are severe, treat as for carbon tetrachloride poisoning (see above). Treat pulmonary edema (see p 65).

B. Chronic Poisoning: Remove the patient from further exposure. If liver function is impaired, give a high-carbohydrate diet.

Prognosis

Survival for 4 hours is ordinarily followed by complete recovery.

1,1,1-TRICHLOROETHANE

Formula: CCl_3CH_3; bp: 74.1 °C.

1,1,1-Trichloroethane (methylchloroform) is used as a solvent for cleaning and degreasing, in paint removers, in typewriter correction fluids, and in crafts. Potential carcinogens such as vinylidene chloride may be present in technical grades as contaminants.

The exposure limit is 350 ppm. The adult fatal dose by ingestion or inhalation is estimated to be 5 mL.

The main effect of 1,1,1-trichloroethane is central nervous system depression. The myocardium is sensitized to catecholamine-induced arrhythmias. Kidney and liver damage are minimal in experimental animals and have not occurred after use of 1,1,1-trichloroethane as an anesthetic agent. Repeated exposure of guinea pigs to a state of anesthesia has produced reversible hepatitis.

Fatalities have occurred when workers have entered unventilated tanks or from use in restricted areas. In one fatality from exposure to an estimated 60,000-ppm concentration of 1,1,1-trichloroethane, the only significant pathologic findings related to the exposure were petechial hemorrhages in the lungs and brain.

Clinical Findings

A. Acute Poisoning: (From inhalation or ingestion.) Symptoms progress through headache, dizziness, nausea, fainting, unconsciousness, respiratory depression, arrhythmias, and fall of blood pressure. Kidney and liver damage may appear after severe exposure.

B. Laboratory Findings:

1. Infrared spectroscopy or gas chromatography can be used to quantitate 1,1,1-trichloroethane in expired air.

2. Elevation of urinary urobilinogen has occurred several days after exposure insufficient to alter SGOT or SGPT levels.

Treatment

Treat as for acute trichloroethylene poisoning (see above).

Prognosis

Patients who survived the initial anesthetic effects have recovered completely.

King GS et al: Sudden death in adolescents resulting from the inhalation of typewriter correction fluid. *JAMA* 1985;**253**:1604.

Jones RD, Winter DP: Two case reports of deaths on industrial premises due to 1,1,1-trichloroethane. *Arch Environ Health* 1983;**38**:59.

Poynter J: Typewriter correction fluid inhalation: A new substance of abuse. *J Toxicol Clin Toxicol* 1982;**19**:493.

TETRACHLOROETHYLENE

Formula: $CCl_2{:}CCl_2$; bp: 121 °C: vapor pressure at 20 °C: 15 mm Hg.

Tetrachloroethylene (perchlorethylene) is used as a solvent in commercial dry cleaning and degreasing. About 300 million kilograms are used annually in the USA.

The exposure limit is 50 ppm, and toxic effects occur at 230 ppm. The blood level in one fatality was 4.4 mg/dL, and the brain level was 36 mg/100 g. Pathologic findings include central fatty necrosis and fatty infiltration in the liver and moderate cloudy swelling of renal tubular epithelium.

Clinical Findings

The principal manifestation of acute tetrachloroethylene poisoning is unconsciousness.

A. Acute Poisoning: (From inhalation or ingestion.) Symptoms and signs include headache, dizziness, irresponsible behavior, loss of inhibitions, and ventricular premature beats. Physical activity and catecholamines exacerbate ventricular arrhythmias. Peripheral nerve damage is indicated by tingling, numbness, and muscle weakness.

B. Laboratory Findings:

1. The ECG reveals ventricular arrhythmias during acute poisoning.

2. Blood tetrachloroethylene levels above 0.4 mg/dL have been associated with cardiac effects.

3. Tests to evaluate liver damage are described on p 75.

Prevention

The exposure limit should not be exceeded.

Treatment

Treat as for trichloroethylene poisoning (see above).

Prognosis

Patients who survived the initial effects have recovered completely.

Worker exposure to perchlorethylene in commercial dry-cleaning operations— United States. *MMWR* 1983;**32**:269.

DICHLOROMETHANE

Formula: CH_2Cl_2; bp: 40 °C; vapor pressure at 25 °C: 440 mm Hg.

Dichloromethane (methylene dichloride, methylene chloride) is used as an ingredient in paint removers and as an industrial solvent. It has been used as an anesthetic agent, but fatalities occurred.

The exposure limit is 100 ppm. The adult fatal dose by ingestion or inhalation is estimated to be 25 mL.

The main effect of methylene chloride is central nervous system depression. Kidney and liver damage have not occurred after its use as an anesthetic agent or after toxic exposures. It is decomposed by heat to phosgene and is metabolized in the body to carbon monoxide, with release of chloride ion resulting in acidosis. In one experiment, the carboxyhemoglobin level increased 14% in 3 hours in one subject exposed to 986 ppm of methylene chloride. In massive exposures, intravascular hemolysis can occur. Pathologic findings are not specific.

Clinical Findings

A. Acute Poisoning: (From inhalation or ingestion.) Symptoms progress rapidly to unconsciousness and lack of response to painful stimuli. Respiration is at first fast, then slowed. Liquid methylene chloride spilled on the skin can cause erythema and blistering. Pulmonary edema can occur. One individual died of acute coronary insufficiency during exposure, possibly as a result of the stress of increased carboxyhemoglobin. Toxic encephalopathy has occurred after repeated exposures to levels above 500 ppm. One individual had painful joints, swelling of the extremities, mental impairment, diabetes, and skin rash after exposure to a paint stripper containing dichloromethane. Some of the symptoms persisted up to 6 months.

Gross hematuria occurs as a result of intravascular hemolysis. The swallowing mechanism may be disturbed by pharyngeal erosions, with resulting aspiration pneumonia.

B. Chronic Poisoning: Chronic poisoning with dichloromethane has not been reported.

C. Laboratory Findings:

1. Hemoglobin products in the urine indicate intravascular hemolysis.

2. The carboxyhemoglobin level may be increased and the blood pH reduced.

3. Radiographic examination reveals the extent of ulceration of the duodenum and jejunum.

4. Blood in the stools indicates gastrointestinal injury.

Treatment

A. Inhaled Dichloromethane: Treat as for acute trichloroethylene poisoning (see above).

B. Ingested Dichloromethane:

1. Emergency measures–Remove by gastric lavage or emesis using activated charcoal (see pp 21–28).

2. General measures–

a. Treat hemolytic reaction (see p 80).

b. Give hydrocortisone, 200 mg every 4 hours.

3. Special problems–

a. Treat aspiration pneumonia with antibiotics.

b. Blood transfusions may be necessary if gastrointestinal bleeding is excessive.

c. Treat acidosis.

d. Treat pulmonary edema (see p 65).

Prognosis

Patients who have ingested dichloromethane may have narrowing of the intestinal lumen as a result of erosions.

TETRACHLOROETHANE

Formula: $CHCl_2CHCl_2$; bp: 146 °C; vapor pressure at 20 °C: 11 mm Hg.

Tetrachloroethane is used as a solvent in industry and occurs as a contaminant in other chlorinated hydrocarbons. It is occasionally present in household cleaners.

Tetrachloroethane is the most poisonous of the chlorinated hydrocarbons. The exposure limit is 1 ppm.

Tetrachloroethane causes a long-lasting narcosis with delayed onset and severe damage to the liver and kidneys. The pathologic findings include acute yellow atrophy of the liver. If death has been immediate, congestion of lungs, kidneys, brain, and gastrointestinal tract may be the only evidences of poisoning.

Clinical Findings

The principal manifestations of tetrachloroethane poisoning are coma, jaundice, and oliguria.

A. Acute Poisoning: (From inhalation, ingestion, or skin absorption.) Initially tetrachloroethane causes irritation of the eyes and nose, followed by headache and nausea. Cyanosis and central nervous system depression progressing to coma appear after 1–4 hours.

Liver and kidney damage, after apparent recovery or after repeated exposures to amounts less than necessary to cause acute symptoms, is indicated by nausea and vomiting, abdominal pain, jaundice, and oliguria with uremia. The relative damage to the liver or kidneys varies.

B. Chronic Poisoning: (From inhalation or skin absorption.) Headache, tremor, dizziness, peripheral paresthesia, hypesthesia, or anesthesia.

C. Laboratory Findings:

1. An increase in the large mononuclear cells above 12% in the differential blood smear indicates exposure.

2. Tests to evaluate possible liver damage are described on p 75.

3. The urine may contain protein, red blood cells, or casts.

Prevention

Household products should not contain tetrachloroethane, and less toxic solvents should be substituted for tetrachloroethane in industrial processes whenever possible.

The exposure limit should never be exceeded. If a contaminated area must be entered, a gas mask with a canister approved for tetrachloroethane is safe for 30 minutes if the concentration does not go over 20,000 ppm (2%). For a concentration over 20,000 ppm, an airline hose mask or self-contained O_2 supply is necessary. Workers entering a high-concentration area must wear a rescue harness and lifeline attended by a responsible person outside the contaminated area.

If direct contact is unavoidable, aprons and gloves made of solvent-proof synthetics must be worn. Skin creams will not prevent penetration.

Alcohol ingestion increases the susceptibility to tetrachloroethane.

Treatment

Treatment is as described for carbon tetrachloride poisoning (see p 149).

Prognosis

Rapid progression of jaundice indicates a poor outcome. In some instances, mild symptoms will persist up to 3 months and then progress to acute yellow atrophy and death. Anuria may persist for as long as 2 weeks and still be followed by complete recovery.

ETHYLENE DICHLORIDE

Formula: CH_2ClCH_2Cl; bp: 83.5 °C; vapor pressure at 20 °C: 61 mm Hg.

Ethylene dichloride (1,2-dichloroethane) is used as a solvent in the rubber, plastic, and insecticide industries. It is sometimes used in rubber and plastic cement for hobby and household use. The fatal adult dose by ingestion is approximately 5 mL. The exposure limit in air is 10 ppm.

Ethylene dichloride depresses and injures almost all cells, but especially those of the central nervous system, liver, kidneys, and heart.

Postmortem evidences of injury include the following: edema of the brain with congestion of the intracranial vessels; edema, hemorrhage, and vascular congestion in the lungs, heart, and spleen; fatty degeneration in the liver; congestion, edema, and tubular injury in the kidneys.

Clinical Findings

The principal manifestations of poisoning with ethylene dichloride are coma, pulmonary edema, and renal injury.

A. Acute Poisoning: (From inhalation, skin absorption, or ingestion.) Initial symptoms are cyanosis, fall of blood pressure, vomiting, diarrhea, cardiovascular collapse, and coma. If exposure is severe, these progress rapidly to pulmonary edema and respiratory difficulty. If the effects are not immediately fatal, the patient may have a temporary symptom-free interval followed by jaundice and oliguria or anuria.

B. Chronic Poisoning: (From inhalation or skin absorption.)

Weight loss, low blood pressure, jaundice, oliguria, or anemia may occur after repeated minimal exposure.

C. Laboratory Findings: The urine may show red blood cells, protein, and casts. Liver function impairment may be revealed by appropriate tests (see p 75). Nitrogen retention due to renal injury is indicated by an increase in nonprotein nitrogen, urea, or creatinine.

Prevention

Maintain the concentration of ethylene dichloride in air below 50 ppm at all times. Ethylene dichloride should not be used as a plastic cement unless atmospheric levels are controlled.

Treatment

Treat as for methyl bromide poisoning (see p 151).

Prognosis

Survival for 48 hours usually implies complete recovery, although deaths have occurred up to 5 days after exposure.

ETHYLENE CHLOROHYDRIN

Formula: CH_2ClCH_2OH; bp: 128 °C; vapor pressure at 44 °C: 20 mm Hg.

Ethylene chlorohydrin is used to speed the germination of seeds and potatoes, as a cleaning solvent, and in chemical synthesis. Even in dangerous concentrations, it does not produce a warning odor or irritation of the nose or throat.

Deaths have occurred from exposure to liquid ethylene chlorohydrin in the open air, from skin absorption, or from exposure to vapors in warehouses. The exposure limit is 1 ppm. The fatal adult dose by ingestion or inhalation is 1–2 mL.

Ethylene chlorohydrin presumably irritates and damages cells after it is hydrolyzed to an acid (perhaps hydrochloric acid), producing pulmonary edema, vascular damage, direct inhibition of the cardiac muscle, central nervous system depression, and impairment of liver and kidney function.

Postmortem examination in fatal poisoning has revealed fatty infiltration of the liver, edema of the brain, congestion and edema of the lungs, dilatation of the heart with fatty degeneration of the myocardium, congestion of the spleen, and swelling and hyperemia of the kidneys with fat deposits and swollen epithelial cells in the tubules.

Clinical Findings

The principal manifestations in acute poisoning with ethylene chlorohydrin are respiratory and circulatory failure. Chronic poisoning does not occur.

Symptoms begin 1–4 hours after ingestion, inhalation, or skin absorption and include nausea and vomiting, headache, abdominal pain, excitability, dizziness, delirium, respiratory slowing, fall of blood pressure, twitching of muscles, cyanosis, and coma. Urine contains red cells, albumin, and casts. Death results from respiratory and circulatory failure.

Prevention

Ethylene chlorohydrin should never be used for cleaning in an open process. Exhaust ventilation in most open hoods is insufficient to prevent dangerous exposure.

Treatment of potatoes or seeds by ethylene chlorohydrin must be in an entirely closed space in which workers are not allowed until the space has been force-ventilated for 24 hours. The liquid must be sprayed into the fumigating chamber from a totally closed system to prevent any skin contact or inhalation of vapor. Transfer of the liquid from drums to the spraying system must be by means of an enclosed system and not by pouring.

Treatment of Acute Poisoning

A. Emergency Measures: Remove patient from further exposure to ethylene chlorohydrin vapor or liquid. Complete recovery must be ensured before the patient returns to work. Give artificial respiration if respiration is depressed. Give O_2 as soon as possible. Remove ingested ethylene chlorohydrin by thorough gastric lavage, using tap water. If gastric lavage cannot be accomplished immediately, use syrup of ipecac.

B. General Measures: Combat shock (see p 66) and treat pulmonary edema (see p 65). Administration of ethanol to suppress metabolism of ethylene chlorohydrin to toxic intermediates has been suggested.

Prognosis

Survival for 18 hours after poisoning has always been followed by complete recovery.

POLYCHLORINATED NAPHTHALENE & POLYCHLORINATED & POLYBROMINATED BIPHENYLS

Chloronaphthalenes, dichloronaphthalenes, polychlorinated naphthalene (Halowax), polybrominated biphenyl (PBB), and polychlorinated biphenyl (PCB, Arochlor) are used as high-temperature dielectrics for electric wires, electric motors, transformers, and other electrical equipment. They are also used as heat-exchange fluids, plasticizers, coatings, fillers, adhesives, paints, and inks and in duplicating papers. Depending on the amount of chlorination, the melting point for these compounds varies from 80 to 130 °C.

The exposure limit for these compounds is as follows (in mg/m³): chlorinated diphenyl oxide, 0.5; chlorodiphenyl (42% chlorine), 1; chlorodiphenyl (54% chlorine), 0.5; hexachloronaphthalene, 0.2; octachloronaphthalene, 0.1; tetrachloronaphthalene, 2; pentachloronaphthalene, 0.5; trichloronaphthalene, 5. At least 7 fatalities have been reported. It has been estimated that 40% of the US population has body fat levels of PCBs greater than 1 ppm, but the long-term effects of such levels have yet to be determined.

These compounds produce skin irritation and acute degeneration of the liver after prolonged exposure. Pathologic findings include acute necrosis of the liver, edema of the kidneys and heart, and, in some cases, necrosis of the adrenals.

Clinical Findings

The principal manifestations in chronic poisoning with chlorinated naphthalene and chlorinated diphenyl are chloracne and jaundice. Acute poisoning from single exposures has not been reported.

After exposure to vapors, the skin shows a pinhead to pea-sized papular, acnelike eruption consisting of straw-colored cysts formed by plugging of sebaceous glands. These progress to pustular eruptions. Symptoms and signs resulting from liver injury include drowsiness, indigestion, nausea, jaundice, liver enlargement, and weakness progressing to coma. Liver injury occurs at exposure levels of 1–2 mg/m³. Genetic injury has been reported in animal experiments. An increased incidence of cancer has occurred in some workers exposed to PCBs. Laboratory tests may reveal hypobilirubinemia, hyperbilirubinemia, or triglyceridemia. Tests to evaluate the extent of liver damage are described on p 75.

Prevention

Occurrence of acne in workers indicates inadequate control of fumes.

Treatment of Chronic Poisoning

Remove from further exposure. Treat liver damage (see p 77).

Prognosis

At least 50% of patients with liver damage from chlorinated naphthalenes or chlorinated biphenyls have died. If workers are removed from exposure at the onset of acne, recovery is likely. Because of the long-term stability of these compounds in human fat, there is increasing concern about their possible mutagenicity or carcinogenicity.

Letz G: The toxicology of PCBs. *West J Med* 1983;**138**:534.
Miller RW: Chemical and radiation hazards to children. *J Pediatr* 1982;**101**:495.

PHOSGENE

Phosgene ($COCl_2$) is a gas that liquefies at 8 °C. It is used in chemical synthesis and also results from the high-temperature decomposition of chlorinated hydrocarbons, especially carbon tetrachloride, chloroform, and methylene chloride. Thus, solvents, paint removers, and nonflammable dry cleaning fluids containing these substances will decompose to phosgene in the presence of fire or heat; deaths have occurred from such decomposition. The exposure limit for phosgene in air is 0.1 ppm.

Phosgene is hydrolyzed to hydrochloric acid in the body and thus irritates and damages cells.

Pathologic findings include extensive degenerative changes in the epithelium of the trachea, bronchi, and bronchioli and hemorrhagic edematous focal pneumonia.

Clinical Findings

The principal manifestations in acute poisoning with phosgene are respiratory and circulatory failure. Chronic poisoning does not occur.

A. Symptoms and Signs: After inhalation or skin absorption, symptoms and signs may begin any time up to 24 hours after exposure. These include a burning sensation in the throat, tightness in the chest, feeling of oppression, dyspnea, and cyanosis, with rapid progression to severe pulmonary edema and death from respiratory and circulatory failure.

B. Laboratory Findings: Radiologic examination of the chest shows diffuse opacities resulting from pulmonary edema.

Prevention

Paint removers and nonflammable dry cleaners should never be used in an enclosed space in the presence of fire or heaters of any kind.

Treatment

A. Emergency Measures: Remove patient from further exposure to phosgene or thermodecomposition products. Give artificial respiration if respiration is depressed. Give O_2 as soon as possible.

B. General Measures:

1. Give cortisone acetate, 1 mg/kg orally 1–3 times daily, or other steroid to reduce tissue response to injury.
2. Treat pulmonary edema (see p 65).

Prognosis

Survival for 48 hours has always been followed by complete recovery.

FLUOROCARBONS

The fluorocarbon (fluoroalkane) liquids and gases listed in Table 10–1 are used as refrigerants and aerosol propellants. They are either nonflammable or almost nonflammable, but at flame temperatures they decompose to fluorine, hydrofluoric acid, hydrochloric acid, and phosgene.

Laboratory experiments in animals have shown that, by usual exposure methods, these compounds are almost nontoxic. The only toxic effect from exposure is anesthesia, and this occurs at concentrations of 10% or more.

Recent experimental studies indicate that, in combination with asphyxia, at least some of these agents sensitize mice, rats, and dogs to fatal cardiac arrhythmias. The arrhythmias in mice include bradycardia, atrioventricular block, and ventricular T wave depression. These effects are not reversed by atropine.

Many fatalities have occurred in the USA as a result of the intentional inhalation of fluorocarbons obtained from aerosol cans. It has

Table 10–1. Fluorocarbons.

	Boiling Point (°C)	Exposure Limit (ppm)
Chlorodifluoromethane (Freon 22)	−40.8	1000
Chloropentafluoroethane	−39.1	1000
Chlorotrifluoromethane (Freon 13)	−81.1	
Dichlorodifluoromethane (Freon 12)	−29.8	1000
Dichlorofluoromethane (Freon 21)	− 9.0	10
1,1-Dichloro-1,2,2,2-tetrafluoroethane (Freon 114)	− 3.8	1000
Difluorodibromomethane (Freon 12B2)	24.5	100
1,1,1,2-Tetrachloro-2,2-difluoroethane (TCDFa)	91.67	500
1,1,2,2-Tetrachloro-1,2-difluoroethane (TCDF)	93	500
Trichlorofluoromethane (Freon 11)	23.7	1000
1,1,2-Trichloro-1,2,2-trifluoroethane (Freon 113)	45.8	1000
Trifluorobromoethane (Freon 13B1)		1000
Trifluorobromomethane	−58	1000

Table 10–2. Halogenated hydrocarbons.
(For treatment, see p 149.)

	Exposure Limit (ppm)	Fatal Dose (LD50 in mg/kg, LC in ppm)	Mucous Membrane, Skin, Lung, Cornea Irritation	Liver, Kidney Damage	CNS Effects	Carcinogen	Miscellaneous
Allyl bromide		30	+	+	+		
Allyl chloride	1	2000 ppm	+	+	+		
Benzoyl chloride			+	+	+		
Benzyl chloride	1	1230	+	+	+		
Bis(2-chlorethyl)sulfide		20	+	+			
Bis(2-chloroethoxy)methane	1?	65	+	+		+	
Bis(2-chloroisopropyl) ether	15	240	+	+		+	
Bis(chloromethyl) ether	0.001	210	+	+		+	
Bromoacetone		600*	+		+		
Bromodichloromethane		450	+	+	+	+	
Bromoform	0.5	400		+	+		
Butyl chloride		2670	+	+	+		
Carbon tetrabromide	0.1	1000		+	+		
Chloroacetaldehyde	1	23	+		+		
Chloroacetic acid		76	+		+		
Chlorobenzene	75	2900	+	+	+		
Chlorobromomethane	200	4300	+		+		
2-Chloro-1,3-butadiene	10	300	+	+	+	+	Cardiac.
Chlorobutane		2670	+		+		
Chlorodibromomethane		800	+	+	+	+	
2-Chloroethylvinyl ether		250	+				
Chloromethylmethyl ether	0	817	+	+		+	
3-Chloro-1,2-propanediol		152	+	+	+		
o-Chlorostyrene	50	5200	+	+			
o-Chlorotoluene	50	1600	+		+		
Dibromochloropropane	0.01	60	+	+	+		
Dibromoethane	0	117	+	+	+	+	
Dichloroacetic acid		2820	+				
Dichloroacetylene	0.1	19 ppm	+				
Dichlorobenzene (o- or p-)	50	500	+	+	+		
1,1-Dichloroethane	200	725			+		
1,1-Dichloroethylene	10	5750	+	+	+	+	
1,2-Dichloroethylene	200	770	+		+		
2,2'-Dichloroethyl ether	5	75	+		+		
2,3-Dichloro-1,4-naphthoquinone		1300	+	+	+		
Dichloropropane	75	860	+	+	+		Cardiac.

*mg/m^3.

†Tetrachloroethylene causes peripheral neuropathy, and vinyl chloride causes Raynaud's phenomenon and acroosteolysis.

Table 10–2 (cont'd). Halogenated hydrocarbons.
(For treatment, see p 149.)

	Exposure Limit (ppm)	Fatal Dose (LD50 in mg/kg, LC in ppm)	Mucous Membrane, Skin, Lung, Cornea Irritation	Liver, Kidney Damage	CNS Effects	Carcinogen	Miscellaneous
Dichloropropanol		90	+	+	+		
Dichloropropene	1	250	+	+			
1,1-Difluoroethylene	1	2000*					
Epichlorohydrin	2	90	+	+	+	+	
Ethyl bromide	200	2200 ppm	+	+	+		Cardiac.
Ethyl chloride	1000	13,000 ppm	+	+	+		Cardiac.
Hexachloroacetone		700	+	+			
Hexachlorobutadiene	0.02	87	+	+	+	+	
Hexachlorocyclopentadiene	0.1	1 ppm	+	+	+	+	
Hexachloroethane	10	4000	+	+	+		
Hexafluoroacetone	0.1	300		+			Testicular.
Pentachlorobenzene		2000	+			+	
Pentachloroethane		500	+	+	+		
Propylene chlorohydrin		220	+	+	+		Hemolysis.
sym-Tetrabromoethane	1	400	+	+	+		
Tetrachloroethylene†	50	4000	+	+	+		Cardiac.
Trichloroacetate		3320			+		
1,2,4-Trichlorobenzene	5	756	+	+	+		
Trichlorobenzoic acid		1600	+				
1,1,2-Trichloroethane	10	580	+	+	+		
1,2,3-Trichloropropane	50	320			+		
Vinyl bromide	5	250 ppm	+	+	+	+	
Vinyl chloride†	5	20,000 ppm		+	+	+	
Vinyl fluoride	1						

*mg/m^3.
†Tetrachloroethylene causes peripheral neuropathy, and vinyl chloride causes Raynaud's phenomenon and acroosteolysis.

also been suggested that the increase in mortality rates from asthma is a result of the use of fluorocarbon-propelled medications.

Pathologic findings have not been contributory.

Clinical Findings

Intentional exposure is produced by spraying the propellant into a plastic or paper bag and then inhaling deeply from the bag. Individuals who die as a result of the inhalation frequently show extreme physical activity—running or shouting or both—immediately prior to death. Difluorobromomethane causes central nervous system depression at lower concentrations than other fluorinated hydrocarbons. TCDF and TCDFa are respiratory irritants and central nervous system depressants and irritants. Dichlorofluoromethane has chronic effects like those of chloroform (see p 314). Fatal chemical pneumonia has occurred as a result of the delayed irritant effect of 1,1,2,3,3-pentafluoro-3-chloropropene.

Treatment

Death has been so rapid that no treatment has been possible.

RIOT CONTROL AGENTS
& PERSONAL PROTECTION DEVICES

Tear gas is 2-chloroacetophenone (1-phenyl-2-chloroethanone) (bp: 244 °C) in a hydrocarbon solvent with a fluorocarbon pressurizing agent for discharge as a fog from an aerosol container.

Tear gas guns contain 2-chloroacetophenone in a finely divided state with an explosive device to propel the charge several feet. Wadding of rubber, cardboard, or synthetic material is used to enclose the agent and increase the propelling force of the explosive.

Liquid riot control agents (Mace, Chemical Mace, Peacemaker, Streamer) contain 2-chloroacetophenone (1%) and one or more of a variety of solvents—including 1,1,1-trichloroethane (5%), a kerosenelike hydrocarbon (5%), or propylene glycol (50–90%)—to prolong and increase the effect on the skin and mucous membranes, plus a propellant fluorocarbon such as trichlorofluoromethane (see Table 10–1). Other forms of riot control agents may contain chloropicrin, bromobenzyl cyanide (BBC), and o-chlorobenzylmalononitrile. The exposure limits for substances used for riot control are as follows: 2-chloroacetophenone (CN), 0.05 ppm; o-chlorobenzylidene malononitrile (CS), 0.05 ppm; and chloropicrin, 0.1 ppm.

Clinical Findings

The principal manifestation of acute poisoning by riot control agents is irritation of the skin and mucous membranes.

Tear gas produces burning and irritation of the eyes with profuse tearing, irritation of the skin, laryngospasm, headache, and sometimes vomiting. If the duration of exposure is long, corneal burns, pigmentation, and second-degree burns of the skin may occur. Liquid riot control agents sprayed onto the eye can cause corneal perforation.

In addition to the effects of tear gas, tear gas guns can cause direct injury from the wadding or from direct deposition of 2-chloroacetophenone in the eyes or under the skin. These guns sometimes explode, causing severe hand injuries. Severe eye injury, corneal scarring, glaucoma, cataract, and hemorrhage have necessitated enucleation up to 15 years after the injury.

Liquid riot control agents (Mace, etc) have caused second-degree burns and hyperpigmentation of the skin, blurred vision, corneal scarring, skin sensitization, and hypertension.

Chloropicrin causes vomiting and choking, with the possibility of aspiration. Bromobenzyl cyanide is a nauseant and irritant. *o*-Chlorobenzylmalononitrile is a respiratory irritant that smells like pepper and causes uncontrollable sneezing.

Treatment

Emergency care personnel may need to wear protective equipment. Remove the victim's contaminated clothing, and wash exposed skin with soap and water. Irrigate eyes with water or normal saline solution (preferably sterile) for 15 minutes or longer. Injured eyes should be examined immediately by an ophthalmologist. Direct eye contact with riot control agents should be treated with 24-hour irrigation by means of a corneal contact irrigating device if the patient cannot be seen immediately by an ophthalmologist.

References

Wagoner JK: Toxicity of vinyl chloride and polyvinyl chloride: A critical review. *Environ Health Perspect* 1984;52:61.

11 | Alcohols & Glycols

METHANOL

Formula: CH_3OH; bp: 64.5 °C; vapor pressure at 20 °C: 94 mm Hg.

Methanol (methyl or wood alcohol) is used as an antifreeze, a paint remover, a solvent in shellac and varnish, in chemical synthesis, and as a denaturant in denatured alcohol. Preparations containing ethanol denatured with methanol and other chemicals appear to have greater toxicity than can be explained by their content of methanol and ethanol. For example, Solox (which contains approximately 5% methanol, 1% gasoline, 1% ethyl acetate, and 1% methylisobutylketone in ethanol) has caused severe hypoglycemia in addition to the usual findings from ethanol and methanol intoxication.

The fatal internal dose is 60–250 mL. The exposure limit is 200 ppm. More than 100 deaths in a single year have resulted from ingestion or inhalation of methanol, often as a substitute for ethanol.

The high oral or inhalation toxicity of methanol in comparison with that of ethanol has not been satisfactorily explained. Toxicity is probably due to metabolism of methanol to formic acid or formaldehyde, and formaldehyde has been shown to have selective injurious effects on retinal cells. Methanol is distributed in the body according to the water content of tissues.

Methanol is metabolized and excreted at a rate approximately one-fifth that of ethanol. After a single dose, excretion from the lungs and the kidneys may continue for at least 4 days. Severe acidosis is produced by the metabolic product, formic acid. The pH of the urine may reach 5.0.

Administration of ethanol reduces the toxic effects of methanol by blocking the metabolism of methanol to formaldehyde and formic acid; this allows the kidneys to excrete unchanged methanol.

In fatal cases, the liver, kidneys, and heart show parenchymatous degeneration. The lungs show desquamation of epithelium, emphysema, edema, congestion, and bronchial pneumonia. The brain may show edema, hyperemia, and petechiae. The eye shows degenerative changes in the retina and edema of the optic disk, and there may be optic nerve atrophy. The corneal epithelium may show degenerative changes.

Clinical Findings

The principal manifestations of methanol poisoning are visual disturbances and acidosis.

A. Acute Poisoning: (From ingestion, inhalation, or skin absorption.)

1. Mild–Fatigue, headache, nausea, and, after a latent period, temporary blurring of vision.

2. Moderate–Severe headache, dizziness, nausea and vomiting, and depression of the central nervous system. Vision may fail temporarily or permanently after 2–6 days.

3. Severe–The above symptoms progress to rapid, shallow respiration from acidosis; cyanosis; coma; fall of blood pressure; dilatation of the pupils; and hyperemia of the optic disk, with blurring of the margin. About 25% of those with severe poisoning (blood bicarbonate level < 20 meq/L) die of respiratory failure.

B. Chronic Poisoning: (From inhalation.) Visual impairment may be the first sign of poisoning; this begins with mild blurring of vision and progresses to contraction of visual fields and sometimes complete blindness.

C. Laboratory Findings: Severe acidosis is indicated by a blood bicarbonate level below 15 meq/L. A blood methanol level above 50 mg/dL is an indication for hemodialysis.

Prevention

Poison labels should be placed on all methanol containers. Workers should be instructed in the dangers of methanol ingestion. Spirit duplicators should be used only with adequate exhaust ventilation.

Treatment

A. Acute Poisoning:

1. **Emergency measures**–If ingestion of methanol is discovered within 2 hours, give syrup of ipecac (see p 21). Lavage thoroughly with 2–4 L of tap water with sodium bicarbonate (20 g/L) added.

2. **Antidote**–Give ethanol, 50% (100 proof), 1.5 mL/kg orally initially, diluted to not more than 5% solution, followed by 0.5–1 mL/kg every 2 hours orally or intravenously for 4 days in order to reduce metabolism of methanol and to allow time for its excretion. The blood ethanol level should be in the range 1–1.5 mg/mL.

3. **General measures**–

a. Combat acidosis by administration of sodium bicarbonate (see p 49).

b. Give up to 4 L of fluids daily orally or intravenously to maintain adequate urine output.

c. Extracorporeal dialysis should be used when symptoms progress rapidly and do not respond to administration of ethanol or alkalinizing agents or if the blood methanol level is above 50 mg/dL. Extracorporeal dialysis is at least 4 times as effective as peritoneal dialysis in removing methanol.

d. Maintain adequate nutrition by giving small meals at regular 3- to 4-hour intervals.

e. Maintain body warmth.

f. Treat coma (see p 52).

4. Special problems–Control delirium by use of pentobarbital sodium, 100 mg every 6–12 hours, or give diazepam, 10 mg slowly intravenously. Avoid respiratory depression.

B. Chronic Poisoning: Remove from exposure.

Prognosis

In acute methanol poisoning, particularly when it is unrecognized, 25–50% of victims do not recover. Visual impairment is not likely to show much improvement after 1 week.

Sejersted OM et al: Formate concentrations in plasma in patients poisoned with methanol. *Acta Med Scand* 1983;**213**:105.

ETHANOL

Formula: C_2H_5OH; bp: 78 °C; vapor pressure: 44 mm Hg at 20 °C.

Ethanol (ethyl or grain alcohol) is used as a solvent, an antiseptic, a chemical intermediate, and a beverage. For many commercial uses, ethanol is denatured. The following formulas are most common in pharmaceutical and household preparations: formulas 1 and 3A contain 5% methanol; formula 23A contains 10% acetone; formula 23H contains acetone and 1.5% methylisobutylketone; formula 39C contains 1% diethyl phthalate; formula 40 contains 1.25 mL of tertiary butyl alcohol and 0.25 g of brucine sulfate in each liter. The strength of alcoholic beverages is ordinarily given in vol%, indicating volumes of alcohol in 100 volumes of the beverage, or in proof spirits, in which the proof number is twice the concentration in vol%. Thus, 100 proof is 50 vol%. The usual concentration of ethanol in beverages is as follows: beer, 3%; wine, 10%; fortified wine, 20%; distilled spirits, 40%. Fermented beverages may contain more complex alcohols, which are more toxic.

The fatal dose for an average adult is 300–400 mL of pure ethanol (600–800 mL of 100 proof whiskey) if consumed in less than 1 hour, while serious symptoms have been produced in children by 1 mL/kg of denatured alcohol containing 5% methanol. The exposure limit is 1000 ppm. Chronic users have a greater tolerance for ethanol.

Ethanol, being a small, hydrophilic molecule, is rapidly absorbed from the gastrointestinal tract or alveoli and is distributed according to the water content of tissues. It is oxidized by way of acetaldehyde to CO_2 and water at a rate of 100–110 mg/kg/h. The ethanol metabolizing system saturates at a plasma ethanol level of 1 mg/mL. The volume of distribution (V_d) for ethanol is 0.6 L/kg (see p 90).

Ethanol depresses the central nervous system irregularly in descending order from cortex to medulla, depending on the amount ingested. The range between a dose that produces anesthesia and one that impairs vital functions is small. Thus, an amount that produces stupor is dangerously close to a fatal dose. Effects are potentiated by concomitant ingestion of barbiturates and other depressant drugs.

The pathologic findings in acute fatalities from ethanol include edema of the brain and hyperemia and edema of the gastrointestinal tract. Postmortem findings in patients dying after chronic ingestion of large amounts of ethanol include degenerative changes in the liver, kidneys, and brain; atrophic gastritis; and cirrhosis of the liver.

Interactions

Ethanol enhances the effects of coumarin anticoagulants, antihistamines, hypnotics, sedatives, tranquilizers, insulin, monoamine oxidase inhibitors, and antidepressants. Disulfiramlike intolerance to ethanol may occur from sulfonylureas, thiocarbamates, metronidazole, tolazoline, furazolidone, chloramphenicol, and quinacrine.

Clinical Findings

The principal manifestation of ethanol poisoning is central nervous system depression.

A. Acute Poisoning: (From ingestion.)

1. Mild (blood ethanol 0.05–0.15%; 0.5–1.5 mg/mL)–Decreased inhibitions, slight visual impairment, slight muscular incoordination, and slowing of reaction time. Approximately 25% of individuals in this group are clinically intoxicated.

2. Moderate (blood ethanol 0.15–0.3%; 1.5–3 mg/mL)–Definite visual impairment, sensory loss, muscular incoordination, slowing of reaction time, and slurring of speech. From 50 to 95% of individuals in this group are clinically intoxicated.

3. Severe (blood ethanol 0.3–0.5%; 3–5 mg/mL)–Marked muscular incoordination, blurred or double vision, approaching stupor. Severe hypoglycemia sometimes occurs, with hypothermia, conjugate deviation of the eyes, extensor rigidity of the extremities, unilateral or bilateral Babinski's sign, convulsions, and trismus. Children are especially susceptible. Fatalities begin to occur in this range.

4. Coma (blood ethanol above 0.5%; 5 mg/mL)–Unconsciousness, slowed respiration, decreased reflexes, and complete loss of sensations. Deaths are frequent in this range.

B. Chronic Poisoning: (From ingestion.) See Table 11–1.

1. General–Weight loss.

2. Gastrointestinal–Cirrhosis of the liver and gastroenteritis with anorexia and diarrhea.

3. Nervous system–

a. Polyneuritis with pain, and motor and sensory loss in the extremities.

b. Optic atrophy.

c. Mental deterioration with memory loss, tremor, impaired judgment, and loss or impairment of other abilities.

d. Ethanol withdrawal syndrome or acute alcoholic mania (delirium tremens) usually follows abstinence after a prolonged bout of steady drinking. Symptoms include uncontrollable fear; sleeplessness; tremors; restlessness progressing to visual, auditory, or gustatory hallucinations; and delirium. Exaggerated reflexes, tachycardia, and sometimes convulsions can occur. The most severe form of alcoholic withdrawal is delirium tremens.

e. Acute alcoholic psychosis (Korsakoff's syndrome) is characterized by severe mental impairment, suggestibility, disorientation, and impairment of memory.

Table 11–1. Chronic toxicity of ethanol.

Psychoneurologic syndromes	**Hematologic syndromes (cont'd)**
Acute alcoholism	Hemolytic anemia, thrombocytopenia
Intoxication, excitement, coma	Defective granulocyte mobilization
Withdrawal syndromes	**Neuromuscular syndromes**
Hallucinosis, convulsions, delirium	Peripheral polyneuropathy
tremens	Acute and chronic alcoholic myopathy
Nutritional syndromes	**Cardiovascular syndromes**
Wernicke-Korsakoff syndrome,	Alcoholic cardiomyopathy
pellagra (thiamine deficiency)	**Metabolic syndromes**
Gastrointestinal syndromes	Lactic acidosis, hypoglycemia, hypo-
Acute and chronic gastritis, malab-	magnesemia, hypouricemia, hyper-
sorption syndrome, fatty liver,	lipidemia
cirrhosis, acute and chronic pan-	**Pulmonary syndromes**
creatitis	Pulmonary aspiration, respiratory in-
Hematologic syndromes	fections. Lung volumes, airway re-
Anemia due to acute or chronic blood	sistance, diffusion, gas exchange
loss	all adversely affected.
Cytoplasmic vacuolization of eryth-	**Conditions aggravated by alcohol**
roid precursors	Traumatic encephalopathy, epilepsy,
Megaloblastic marrow alterations (in-	Hodgkin's disease, porphyria, pep-
hibition of folate metabolism) with	tic ulcer
anemia	**Drugs that contraindicate concomitant**
Sideroblastic bone marrow abnormal-	**use of alcohol**
ities	Disulfiram, sedatives, hypnotics, tran-
Stomatocytic erythrocyte changes	quilizers, phenformin.

f. In alcoholism of many years' duration, acute myopathy occasionally occurs after a period of unusually high alcohol intake. Symptoms are aching and tender muscles associated with muscular edema and degeneration of muscle fibers. The symptoms of pathologic change in the heart muscle are palpitation, extrasystoles, tachycardia, or other arrhythmias. The disease may progress to irreversible myocardial fibrosis and then to circulatory failure.

C. Laboratory Findings:

1. Most laboratories report blood ethanol levels that are 10–20% lower than serum or plasma ethanol levels. Blood ethanol levels (Table 11–2) correlate well with clinical findings except in chronic ethanol abusers, in whom levels are higher (see Acute Poisoning, above). Blood levels above 0.05–0.15% (0.5–1.5 mg/mL) are legal evidence of intoxication in many jurisdictions. Ethanol concentration in expired air can also be used to indicate blood level.

2. In chronic alcoholism, liver function should be evaluated by appropriate tests (see p 75).

3. Urinalysis may be positive for reducing sugar, acetone, or diacetic acid. Urine ethanol levels correlate well with blood ethanol levels.

4. Blood glucose levels should be determined after ingestion of ethanol-containing substances, especially in children.

5. Cardiomyopathy is indicated by electrocardiographic changes, including arrhythmias, extrasystoles from diverse foci, and deformed T waves.

6. Elevation of serum amylase indicates pancreatitis.

Prevention

Alcoholics Anonymous (see listing in local phone book) may be able to assist those patients who genuinely desire help.

Table 11–2. Blood ethanol levels after intake of alcoholic beverages.

Beverage (% Ethanol)	Amount Ingested (mL)	Peak Blood Level in a 60-kg Person (mg/mL)*
Beer (3%)	500	0.46
Wine (10%)	250	0.77
Distilled spirits (40%)	50	0.62

*The blood ethanol level falls at a rate of approximately 0.185 mg/mL/h. To calculate the expected blood ethanol level at any other body weight, use the following formula:

$$\left[\frac{60 \text{ kg}}{\text{Subject's weight in kg}} \right] \times \begin{array}{c} \text{Expected level} \\ \text{from table} \end{array} = \begin{array}{c} \text{Expected level} \\ \text{in subject} \end{array}$$

Disulfiram (Antabuse) administration induces sensitivity to ethanol and may be helpful in training the patient to avoid ethanol.

Treatment

A. Acute Poisoning:

1. Emergency measures–Remove unabsorbed ethanol by gastric lavage with tap water or by emesis (see p 21).

2. General measures for treatment of coma–

a. Maintain adequate airway. Give artificial respiration if necessary.

b. Maintain normal body temperature.

c. Give 2 g of sodium bicarbonate in 250 mL of water every 2 hours to maintain neutral or slightly alkaline urine.

d. Avoid administration of excessive fluids.

e. Avoid depressant drugs.

f. In the presence of hypoglycemia, administer 5–10% glucose intravenously plus thiamine, 100 mg intramuscularly.

g. Hemodialysis is indicated if the blood ethanol level is above 5 mg/mL.

B. Chronic Poisoning:

1. Emergency measures–

a. In acute alcoholic mania, give diazepam, 10 mg slowly intravenously initially, followed by 5 mg intravenously every 5–10 minutes until mania is controlled. Then give 5–10 mg orally every 1–8 hours as necessary.

b. Avoid physical restraint; maintain calm, quiet, and uniform surroundings.

2. General measures–

a. In patients with a history of seizures, give 500 mg of phenytoin and repeat in 4–6 hours. Phenytoin, 300 mg daily, is then continued.

b. Give high-vitamin, high-protein diet plus thiamine, 100 mg 3 times daily; pyridoxine, 100 mg/d; folic acid, 5 mg 3 times daily; ascorbic acid, 500 mg twice daily.

c. Give oral fluids to 4 L/d. Give 1–2 L of 5% dextrose in saline intravenously if patient is unable to take fluids orally.

Prognosis

In acute, uncomplicated alcoholism, survival for 24 hours is ordinarily followed by recovery.

In alcoholic psychosis, survival is likely but complete recovery is rare. In the presence of mental deterioration, complete withdrawal from ethanol may be followed only by minimal improvement.

Alcohol as a risk factor for injuries–United States. *MMWR* 1983;**32**:61.

Council on Scientific Affairs: Fetal effects of maternal alcohol use. *JAMA* 1983;**249**:2517.

O'Neill S et al: Survival after high blood alcohol levels. *Arch Intern Med* 1984;**144**:641.

Rosett HL, Weiner L: Alcohol and pregnancy: A clinical perspective. *Annu Rev Med* 1985;**36**:73.

Selbst SM et al: Mouthwash poisoning: Report of a fatal case. *Clin Pediatr* 1985;**24**:162.

West J et al: Alcoholism. *Ann Intern Med* 1984;**100**:405.

ETHYLENE GLYCOL & DIETHYLENE GLYCOL

These agents are heavy liquids with sweetish, acrid tastes. Their vapor pressures at room temperature are negligible. **Formula** (ethylene glycol): CH_2OHCH_2OH; bp: 198 °C. **Formula** (diethylene glycol): $HOCH_2CH_2OCH_2CH_2OH$; bp: 245 °C.

The fatal dose of ethylene glycol is approximately 100 g; of diethylene glycol, 15–100 g. Up to 60 deaths in a single year have been reported from ethylene glycol or diethylene glycol. The exposure limit for particulate ethylene glycol is 10 mg/m^3; for vapor, it is 50 ppm.

Ethylene glycol and its esters are distributed with body water, and some are metabolized to oxalic acid, which is thought to play a role in some of the toxic effects. The ethers of ethylene glycol, as well as diethylene glycol and its esters and ethers (none of which appear to be metabolized to oxalic acid), produce brain and kidney damage by unknown mechanisms. Many of these glycols produce profound acidosis.

The pathologic findings are congestion and edema of the brain, focal hemorrhagic necrosis of the renal cortex, and hydropic degeneration of the liver and kidneys. Calcium oxalate crystals may be found in the brain, spinal cord, and kidneys.

Clinical Findings

The principal manifestations of acute poisoning with these agents are anuria and narcosis.

A. Acute Poisoning: (From ingestion.) The initial symptoms in massive dosage (> 100 mL in a single dose) are those of alcohol intoxication. These symptoms soon progress to vomiting, cyanosis, headache, tachypnea, tachycardia, hypotension, pulmonary edema, muscle tenderness, stupor, anuria, prostration, and unconsciousness with convulsions. Hypoglycemia may occur. Death may occur within a few hours from respiratory failure or within the first 24 hours from pulmonary edema. Patients who have prolonged coma or convulsions may have irreversible brain damage. Hypocalcemic tetany as a result of calcium precipitation may follow ethylene glycol poisoning. Massive doses of these glycols may cause intravascular hemolysis.

Table 11–3. Alcohols and glycols. (For treatment, see p 177.)

	Exposure Limit (ppm)	Fatal Dose (LD50) (mg/kg)	Irritation	CNS Effects	Bone Marrow Damage	Kidney, Liver Damage	Miscellaneous
Allyl alcohol	2	64	+	+	+	+	Skin burns
Amyl alcohol	100	200	+	+	+		Headache
2-Butoxy ethanol	25	320	+	+	+	+	Hemolysis
Butyl alcohol	50	790	+	+		+	
Butyl carbitol		2000	+	+		+	
Carbitol	200*	3620	+	+		+	
Cyclohexanol	50	1300	+	+	+	+	Tremor
Decanol	50	2000	+	+		+	
Diacetone alcohol	50	4000	+	+		+	Anemia
Dipropylene glycol		14,000	+			+	
Dipropylene glycol methyl ether	100	4900	+			+	
2-Ethoxy ethanol	5	1400	+	+		+	Hemolysis
2-Ethoxy ethyl acetate	5	1910	+	+		+	
Ethyl octynol		400		+			
Furfuryl alcohol	10	40	+	+			
Glycerin		7750					
Hexylene glycol	25	3800	+	+			
Isopropoxyethanol	25	500	+		+		
2-Methoxy ethanol	5	890	+	+	+	+	Hemolysis
2-Methoxy ethyl acetate	5	1250	+	+	+	+	Hematuria
1-Methoxy-2-propanol	100	3000+		+		+	
Methylcyclohexanol	50	2000	+	+		+	
Methylisobutylcarbinol	25	2600	+	+			
Octanol	50	2000	+	+		+	
Polypropylene glycol		419		+			Cardiac
Propylene glycol		100/d		+			Convulsions
Propynol	1	0.07	+	+			
Tetrahydrofurfuryl alcohol		2300	+	+			

*mg/m^3.

If the ingestion of small amounts (15–30 mL) is repeated daily or if the patient recovers from acute poisoning, oliguria may begin in 24–72 hours and progress rapidly to anuria and uremia.

B. Chronic Poisoning: (From inhalation.) Continued exposure to the vapors from a process utilizing ethylene glycol is reported to induce unconsciousness, nystagmus, and lymphocytosis.

C. Laboratory Findings: The urine may contain calcium oxalate crystals, albumin, red blood cells, and casts. The blood pH or glucose level may be reduced. Methemoglobinemia may occur. Hypocalcemia and hyperkalemia may be present. The serum ethylene glycol level is diagnostic.

Treatment
A. Acute Poisoning:
1. Emergency measures–Remove ingested glycols by gastric lavage or emesis (see pp 21–28).

2. Antidote–

a. Give ethanol as in the treatment of methanol poisoning (see p 169) to prevent metabolism of ingested ethylene glycol to oxalate.

b. Give calcium gluconate, 10 mL of 10% solution diluted in 1 L of 5% glucose, intravenously as necessary to maintain normal serum calcium levels. Calcium administration may cause anuria due to precipitation of calcium oxalate in the kidney.

3. General measures–

a. Give artificial respiration with O_2 if respiration is depressed.

b. In the absence of renal impairment, force fluids to 4 L or more daily to increase excretion of the glycol.

c. Use dialysis.

d. Avoid stimulants.

e. For hypoglycemia, give 5% dextrose intravenously.

f. Control convulsions with diazepam, 0.1 mg/kg slowly intravenously.

4. Special problems–Treat pulmonary edema (see p 65), uremia (see p 72), shock (see p 66), acidosis (see p 49), and methemoglobinemia (see p 77).

B. Chronic Poisoning: Remove from exposure.

Prognosis
Complete recovery of renal function may follow 2 weeks of complete anuria. Cerebral damage may, however, be permanent.

Brown CG et al: Ethylene glycol poisoning. *Ann Emerg Med* 1983;**12**:501.
Jacobsen D, Ostby N, Bredesen JE: Studies on ethylene glycol poisoning. *Acta Med Scand* 1982;**212**:11.
Parry MF, Wallach R: Ethylene glycol poisoning. *Am J Med* 1974;**57**:143.

ISOPROPYL & n-PROPYL ALCOHOL

Formula (isopropyl alcohol [isopropanol]): $(CH_3)_2CHOH$; bp: 82.5 °C; vapor pressure at 23.8 °C: 40 mm Hg. **Formula** (n-propyl alcohol): $CH_3(CH_2)_2OH$; bp: 97–98 °C.

Isopropyl alcohol is used as rubbing alcohol, after-shave lotion, and window cleaner. n-Propyl alcohol is used in industry. These alcohols are about twice as toxic as ethanol; the fatal dose by ingestion is 250 mL. The exposure limit is 200 ppm for n-propyl alcohol and 400 ppm for isopropyl alcohol.

About 15% of an ingested dose of isopropyl alcohol is metabolized to acetone.

Pathologic findings after fatalities from isopropyl alcohol include hemorrhagic tracheobronchitis, bronchopneumonia, and hemorrhagic pulmonary edema. Pulmonary damage may occur as a result of pulmonary excretion of the alcohol.

Clinical Findings

The principal manifestation of acute isopropyl or n-propyl alcohol poisoning is central nervous system depression.

A. Symptoms and Signs: (From inhalation, ingestion, or skin absorption.) Symptoms are similar to ethanol intoxication, with more marked and more persistent nausea, vomiting, abdominal pain, hematemesis, refractory narcosis, areflexia, depressed respirations, and oliguria followed by diuresis. Deep coma has resulted from sponging with isopropyl alcohol. Generalized tenderness, induration, and edema of muscles may occur. Vapor exposure causes eye irritation. Prolonged contact with the skin can cause corrosion.

B. Laboratory Findings:
1. Elevated blood urea nitrogen.
2. Elevated SGOT.
3. Melena.
4. Fall in hemoglobin level as a result of hemolysis.
5. Acetonuria, acetonemia, and hypoglycemia.

Treatment of Acute Poisoning

A. Emergency Measures:
1. In respiratory depression, give O_2 by artificial respiration.
2. Give activated charcoal. Gastric lavage with protected airway (see p 24) is useful even if delayed. Do not attempt emesis if respiration is depressed.
3. Maintain blood pressure (see p 66).
4. Give glucose intravenously and correct electrolyte imbalance and dehydration (see p 49).

B. Special Measures:
1. In severe poisoning, hemodialysis can be lifesaving.
2. Treat renal failure (see p 72).

Prognosis

Symptoms persist 2–4 times as long as after ethanol ingestion. Patients who survive 48–72 hours ordinarily recover completely.

Lacouture PG et al: Acute isopropyl alcohol intoxication. *Am J Med* 1983;**75**:680.

Rosansky SJ: Isopropyl alcohol poisoning treated with hemodialysis: Kinetics of isopropyl alcohol and acetone removal. *J Toxicol Clin Toxicol* 1982;**19**:265.

12 | Esters, Aldehydes, Ketones, & Ethers

TRIORTHOCRESYL PHOSPHATE

Tricresyl phosphate, $(CH_3C_6H_4)_3PO_4$, exists in 3 isomeric forms: o-, m-, and p-. Only the o-form (triorthocresyl phosphate, TOCP) is of toxicologic importance; it is a liquid that fumes appreciably at 100 °C.

Triorthocresyl phosphate is used in lubricants, in fireproofers, and as a plasticizer in plastic coatings. Fatty foods stored in plastics containing free triorthocresyl phosphate will become contaminated.

The fatal dose by ingestion is estimated to be 1 g/kg, but the toxic dose is 6 mg/kg. Food contaminated to the extent of 0.4% has caused serious poisoning. The exposure limit is 0.1 mg/m³.

Demyelinization of nerves is the most prominent finding. Degenerative changes are also found in the muscles, anterior horn cells, and pyramidal tracts. As a result of these changes, a flaccid paralysis develops that affects the more distal muscles of the legs and arms.

Triorthocresyl phosphate inhibits nonspecific cholinesterase but not acetylcholinesterase. The relationship between this inhibition and the nerve demyelinization is unknown.

Clinical Findings

The principal manifestation of triorthocresyl phosphate poisoning is muscular paralysis.

A. Acute Poisoning: (From ingestion, inhalation, or skin absorption.) Symptoms begin 1–30 days after exposure and include weakness of the distal muscles progressing to foot drop, wrist drop, and loss of plantar reflex. Laryngeal, ocular, and respiratory muscles are affected in severe poisoning. Death is from respiratory paralysis.

B. Chronic Poisoning: The above symptoms may be produced by cumulative exposure over several months.

Prevention

Foods should never be stored in plastic containers containing unreacted triorthocresyl phosphate. Containers sold for food purposes are safe.

Processes utilizing triorthocresyl phosphate at high temperatures must be totally enclosed to avoid contamination of workroom air.

Treatment

A. Acute Poisoning:

1. Emergency measures–Remove ingested poison by gastric lavage or emesis (see pp 21–28). Give artificial respiration as needed.

2. General measures–If respiratory depression or weakness of respiratory muscles occurs, give artificial respiration with O_2. Assisted respiration may be necessary for several weeks.

B. Chronic Poisoning: Treat as for acute poisoning.

Prognosis

In paralysis from triorthocresyl phosphate, recovery may be gradual over a period of 1 year. Complete recovery may never occur.

FORMALDEHYDE

Formaldehyde (HCHO) is a gas that is ordinarily available as a 40% solution (formalin) for use as a disinfectant, an antiseptic, a deodorant, a tissue fixative, or an embalming fluid. The polymerized form, trioxymethylene (paraformaldehyde), can be decomposed by heat to formaldehyde for fumigating purposes. The fatal dose of formalin is 60–90 mL. The exposure limit for formaldehyde is 2 ppm (NIOSH). The American Society of Heating, Refrigeration and Air Conditioning Engineers has set a ceiling limit for formaldehyde of 0.12 mg/m^3 for indoor air. Polymers of formaldehyde are used to give paper and cloth wet strength and as adhesives in particle board and plywood. These polymers sometimes contain free formaldehyde. They decompose slowly, with the liberation of formaldehyde over a period of years. Air concentrations of formaldehyde ranging up to 1.9 ppm have been found in mobile homes with extensive use of particle board, plywood, and urea-formaldehyde insulation.

Although formaldehyde is a normal metabolite in humans, in high concentrations it can react chemically with most substances in cells and thus depress all cellular functions and lead to death of the cells. At least part of the toxic effect appears to be the result of conversion of formaldehyde to formic acid. Formaldehyde in very high concentrations is a carcinogen in animals, probably as a result of its capacity to irritate.

Pathologic findings from the ingestion of formaldehyde are necrosis and shrinking of the mucous membranes. Degenerative changes may be found in the liver, kidneys, heart, and brain.

Table 12—1. Aldehydes, ketones, ethers, and esters.
(For treatment, see p 186.)

	Exposure Limit (ppm)	LD50 (mg/kg) or LC (ppm)	Irritation	CNS Effects	Liver and Kidney Damage	Carcinogen	Miscellaneous and Remarks
Aldehydes							
Acetal		4570		+			
Acrolein	0.1	7	+	+			
Benzaldehyde		1000		+			Convulsions.
Crotonaldehyde	2	6	+				Sensitizer.
2-Furaldehyde	2	126	+		+		Pulmonary edema.
Glutaraldehyde	0.2	2380	+	+			
Malonaldehyde		632	+				Mutagen.
n-Valeraldehyde	50	310 ppm	+				
Ketones							
Acetone	750	5340	+	+			Hypoglycemia.
Acetophenone		900	+	+			
Acetyl butyrolactone	5		+				
Benzoquinone	0.1	130	+	+	+	+	
Butanone-2	200	3400	+	+			Neuropathy.
2-Butanone peroxide	0.2	472	+		+	+	
Cyclohexanone	25	1000	+	+			
Diethyl ketone	200	2000	+	+			Neuropathy?
Dihydroxyacetone		1000	+	+			Sensitizer.
Diisobutyl ketone	25	1416	+	+			
Dipropyl ketone	50	3730	+	+			
Ethyl amyl ketone	25	3000 ppm	+	+			
Ethyl butyl ketone	50	2760	+	+			
Hexanone-2	5	914	+	+			Neuropathy.
Isophorone	5	2330	+	+	+		
Ketene	0.5	1300	+				Like phosgene.
Mesityl oxide	15	1000	+	+			
Methylamyl ketone	50	3200	+	+			
Methylcyclohexanone	50	1000		+			
Methylisobutylketone	50	2080	+	+			
4-Methyl-pentanone-2	100	2080	+	+			Neuropathy.
Methyl propyl ketone	200	2000 ppm	+	+			
1,4-Naphthoquinone		190	+			+	Sensitizer, anemia.
Ninhydrin		250	+				
Pentanone-2	200	3730	+	+			
Ethers							
Allyl glycidyl ether	5	390	+	+			
Benzoyl peroxide	5*	250	+		+	+	Sensitizer.
n-Butyl glycidyl ether	25	1520	+	+			
Diglycidyl ether	0.1	170	+	+	+	+	Anemia.

*mg/m³.

Table 12—1 (cont'd). Aldehydes, ketones, ethers, and esters.
(For treatment, see p 186.)

	Exposure Limit (ppm)	LD50 (mg/kg) or LC (ppm)	Irritation	CNS Effects	Liver and Kidney Damage	Carcinogen	Miscellaneous and Remarks
Ethers (cont'd)							
Dioxane	25	2000	+	+	+	+	
Ethylene oxide	1	270	+	+	+	+	
Glycidol	25	450	+	+			
Isopropyl ether	250	800	+	+			
Isopropyl glycidyl ether	50	15,000 ppm	+	+			
Methylal	1000	3000	+	+	+		
Phenyl ether	1	4000	+		+		Nausea.
Phenyl glycidyl ether	1	14,000	+	+			
β-Propiolactone	0?	50	+			+	
Propylene oxide	20	1740 ppm	+	+		+	
Tetrahydrofuran	200	3000	+	+	+		
Trimellitic anhydride	0.005	2210	+	+			Lung damage.
Vinyl cyclohexene dioxide	10	620	+			+	
Esters							
Amyl acetate	100	4950	+	+	+		Anesthetic effect.
Butyl acetate	150	3200	+	+			
Butyl acrylate	10	3730	+		+	+	Sensitizer.
Butyl lactate	5	200	+				
Dibutylphosphate	1	3200	+				See p 199.
Diethylphthallate	5*	500	+				
Dioctylphthallate	5*	30,000	+				Teratogen.
Ethyl acetate	400	4930	+	+	+		Sensitizer.
Ethyl acrylate	5	420	+	+	+		Heart damage.
Ethyl formate	100	330	+	+			Like formic acid.
Ethyl methacrylate		5440	+	+			
Ethyl silicate	10	1000	+	+			Acid corrosive.
Hexyl acetate	50	4000 ppm	+	+			
Hydroxyethylacrylate		650	+				
Hydroxypropylacrylate	0.5	250	+				Sensitizer.
Methyl acetate	200	3700	+	+			Like methanol.
Methyl acrylate	10	280	+	+			
Methyl formate	100	1620	+	+			Formic acid.
Methyl methacrylate monomer	100	5000	+	+			Burning Plexiglas is similar.
Methylmethane sulfonate		125	+			+	
Propyl acetate	200	6630	+	+			
Triallylphosphate		71				+	

*mg/m^3.

Table 12–1 (cont'd). Aldehydes, ketones, ethers, and esters.
(For treatment, see p 186.)

	Exposure Limit (ppm)	LD50 (mg/kg) or LC (ppm)	Irritation	CNS Effects	Liver and Kidney Damage	Carcinogen	Miscellaneous and Remarks
Esters (cont'd)							
Tributylphosphate	0.2	3000	+				
Triethylphosphate		500	+				
Trimethylphosphate		840	+				
Trimethylphosphite	2	2890	+	+			Eye damage.
Triphenylphosphate	3*	3000	+	+			Like triortho-cresyl phosphate.
Tris(2,3-dibromopropyl) phosphate		1010				+	Sensitizer.
Vinyl acetate	10	1550 ppm	+				

*mg/m³.

Clinical Findings

The principal manifestations of formaldehyde poisoning are collapse and anuria.

A. Acute Poisoning: Ingestion causes immediate and severe abdominal pain followed by collapse, loss of consciousness, and anuria. There may be vomiting and diarrhea. Death is from circulatory failure. Exposure to formaldehyde in air causes respiratory tract and eye irritation. Such reactions can occur in some individuals at concentrations well below 1 ppm. Laryngeal edema and skin sensitivity reactions with urticarial swelling can also occur at these low concentrations.

B. Skin Manifestations: Clothing and papers containing free formaldehyde cause sensitivity dermatitis in some individuals.

C. Laboratory Findings: The urine may contain protein, casts, or red blood cells.

Treatment of Acute Poisoning

A. Emergency Measures:

1. Dilute, inactivate, or adsorb ingested formaldehyde by giving milk, activated charcoal, or tap water. Do not use gastric lavage or emetics. Any organic material will inactivate formaldehyde.

2. Treat shock (see p 66).

B. Special Problems: Treat anuria (see p 72). Esophageal stricture may occur.

Prognosis

Patients who survive for 48 hours will probably recover.

Acheson ED et al: Formaldehyde in the British chemical industry. *Lancet* 1984;**1**:611.

Coldiron VR et al: Occupational exposure to formaldehyde in a medical center autopsy service. *J Occup Med* 1983;**25**:544.

Halperin WE et al: Nasal cancer in a worker exposed to formaldehyde. *JAMA* 1983;**249**:510.

Hanrahan LP et al: Formaldehyde vapor in mobile homes: A cross-sectional survey of concentrations and irritant effects. *Am J Public Health* 1984;**74**:1026.

L'Abbe KA, Hoey JR: Review of the health effects of urea-formaldehyde foam insulation. *Environ Res* 1984;**35**:246.

Starr TB, Gibson JE: The mechanistic toxicology of formaldehyde and its implications for quantitative risk estimation. *Annu Rev Pharmacol Toxicol* 1985;**25**:745.

ACETALDEHYDE, METALDEHYDE, PARALDEHYDE

Metaldehyde—a tasteless, water-insoluble solid—and paraldehyde (bp: 124 °C)—a water-soluble (1:8) liquid with a burning taste and smell—are polymers of acetaldehyde (bp: 20 °C), a highly volatile, irritating, water-miscible liquid. In the presence of acids, paraldehyde decomposes readily and metaldehyde slowly to acetaldehyde. In the presence of moisture, paraldehyde slowly decomposes to acetaldehyde and acetic acid. Deaths have occurred from administration of decomposed paraldehyde; it should be stored in small, well-filled bottles in the dark at a temperature of 25 °C or lower and tested for acidity before administration. It should not be administered if the container has been opened for more than 24 hours. Paraldehyde is used as a hypnotic, metaldehyde as snail bait, and acetaldehyde as a reagent in chemical synthesis. Deaths have occurred from ingestion of 3 g (100 mg/kg) of metaldehyde. Amounts over 400 mg/kg are rapidly fatal.

The exposure limit for acetaldehyde is 100 ppm. Levels for paraldehyde and metaldehyde have not been established.

Paraldehyde and metaldehyde presumably are decomposed slowly to acetaldehyde in the body. In the case of paraldehyde, the rate apparently does not exceed the rate of acetaldehyde oxidation, so that acetaldehyde does not accumulate. With metaldehyde, however, the rate of decomposition to acetaldehyde may exceed the rate of oxidation of acetaldehyde, since persons who have died of metaldehyde poisoning have shown symptoms suggestive of acetaldehyde poisoning.

Acetaldehyde, a highly reactive chemical, is irritating and depressive to all cells. Metaldehyde apparently acts only after decomposition to acetaldehyde. Paraldehyde produces depression of the central nervous system without slowing of respiration.

Pathologic findings in deaths from acetaldehyde poisoning are pulmonary irritation and edema. After paraldehyde or metaldehyde poisoning, findings are not characteristic.

Clinical Findings

The principal manifestations of poisoning with these agents are irritation and coma.

A. Acute Poisoning:

1. Acetaldehyde–Exposure to the vapors causes severe irritation of mucous membranes, reddening of the skin, coughing, pulmonary edema, and narcosis. Ingestion causes nausea and vomiting, diarrhea, narcosis, and respiratory failure.

2. Paraldehyde–Ingestion ordinarily induces sleep without depression of respiration, although deaths occasionally occur from respiratory and circulatory failure after doses of 10 mL or more.

3. Metaldehyde–Ingestion of less than 50 mg/kg causes nausea, retching, severe vomiting, abdominal pain, temperature elevation, muscular rigidity, and hyperventilation. Ingestion of more than 100 mg/kg causes hyperreflexia, convulsions, and coma. Death from respiratory failure can occur up to 48 hours after ingestion. Liver and kidney injury also occurs.

B. Chronic Poisoning:

1. Acetaldehyde–Repeated exposure to the vapors causes dermatitis and conjunctivitis.

2. Paraldehyde–Chronic medicinal use of paraldehyde produces mental deterioration and delirium tremens.

3. Metaldehyde–Amounts less than necessary to produce acute poisoning are without effect.

C. Laboratory Findings:

1. The blood glucose level may be depressed.

2. The blood methemoglobin level may be raised.

3. Liver or kidney function impairment may be revealed by appropriate tests (see p 75). The serum transaminase level may be elevated.

4. Serum creatine kinase elevation indicates muscle damage from convulsions.

5. Blood acetaldehyde levels above 0.5 mg/dL are toxic.

Treatment (For Aldehydes, Ketones, Ethers, & Esters.)

A. Acute Poisoning From Fume Exposure:

1. Emergency measures–

a. Remove from exposure.

b. Maintain airway and respiration.

c. Give O_2 by inhalation.

2. General measures–Treat pulmonary edema (see p 65).

B. Acute Poisoning From Ingestion:

1. Emergency measures–

a. Remove poison by gastric lavage or emesis (see pp 21–28). Activated charcoal is useful. For metaldehyde, gastric lavage with 2–5% sodium bicarbonate solution will reduce conversion to acetaldehyde. Follow with saline catharsis. Gastric lavage and catharsis are effective up to 12–24 hours after poisoning, since metaldehyde is slowly absorbed and is also excreted into the gastrointestinal tract.

b. Maintain airway and respiration. Give O_2 if respiration is depressed.

2. Antidote–In metaldehyde poisoning in which convulsions cannot be controlled, cautious trial of D-penicillamine, N-acetylcysteine, ascorbic acid, or thiamine has been suggested on the basis that they lower blood acetaldehyde levels. Cautious trial of naloxone has also been suggested, since naloxone blocks the effect of salsolinol, a condensation product of acetaldehyde and dopamine that may contribute to convulsions.

3. General measures–

a. Treat coma (see p 52).

b. Treat hypoxia (see p 57).

c. Treat pulmonary edema (see p 65).

d. Give glucose intravenously for hypoglycemia.

e. Treat methemoglobinemia (see p 78).

f. Treat convulsions with diazepam, 0.1 mg/kg slowly intravenously. Do not use paraldehyde. Barbiturates and anticonvulsants such as phenytoin should not be given, since these inhibit acetaldehyde metabolism.

g. Treat renal failure (see p 72) or hepatic failure (see p 77).

h. In metaldehyde poisoning, maintain alkaline urine and treat acidosis by administering sodium bicarbonate or other alkalinizing agents (see p 49).

C. Chronic Poisoning From Fume Exposure: Remove from further exposure.

D. Chronic Poisoning From Paraldehyde Ingestion:

1. Remove from further exposure.

2. Treat mental symptoms.

Prognosis

Patients who survive for 48 hours after acute poisoning are likely to recover. Complete recovery after chronic poisoning from paraldehyde is not likely. Mental deficits after metaldehyde poisoning may persist for a year or more.

Booze TF et al: Metaldehyde toxicity: A review. *Vet Hum Toxicol* 1985;**27**:11.

Gooch WM III et al: Generalized arterial and venous thrombosis following intra-arterial paraldehyde. *Clin Toxicol* 1979;**15**:39.

Longstreth WT, Pierson DJ: Metaldehyde poisoning from slug bait ingestion. *West J Med* 1982;**137**:134.

References

Antti-Poika M: Prognosis of symptoms in patients with diagnosed chronic organic solvent intoxication. *Int Arch Occup Environ Health* 1982;**51**:81.

Babbich H: Butylated hydroxytoluene (BHT): A review. *Environ Res* 1982;**29**:1.

Beauchamp RO Jr et al: A critical review of the literature on acrolein toxicity. *CRC Crit Rev Toxicol* 1985;**14**:309.

Benson WG: Exposure to glutaraldehyde. *J Soc Occup Med* 1984;**34**:63.

Hemminki K et al: Spontaneous abortion in hospital staff engaged in sterilizing instruments with chemical agents. *Br Med J* 1982;**285**:1461.

Jedryckowski W: Styrene and methyl methacrylate in the industrial environment as a risk factor of chronic obstructive lung disease. *Int Arch Occup Environ Health* 1982;**51**:151.

Kluwe WM et al: Conference on phthallates. *Environ Health Perspect* 1982;**45**:1.

Kopelman PG, Kalfayan PY: Severe metabolic acidosis after ingestion of butanone. *Br Med J* 1983;**286**:21.

Landrigan PJ et al: Ethylene oxide: An overview of toxicologic and epidemiologic research. *Am J Ind Med* 1984;**6**:103.

McGrath KG et al: Four-year evaluation of workers exposed to trimellitic anhydride. *J Occup Med* 1984;**26**:671.

National Institute of Occupational Safety and Health: Ethylene oxide. *Current Intelligence Bulletin* 1981;**35**:1.

National Institute of Occupational Safety and Health: Glycol ethers. *Current Intelligence Bulletin* 1983;**39**:1.

Nethercott JR et al: Tetraethylene glycol diacrylate: A cause of delayed cutaneous irritant reactions and allergic contact dermatitis. *J Occup Med* 1984;**26**:513.

Seppäläinen AM, Rajaniemi R: Local neutrotoxicity of methyl methacrylate among dental technicians. *Am J Ind Med* 1984;**5**:471.

Smith RL: Toxic effects of glycol ethers. *Environ Health Perspect* 1984;**57**:1.

Zeiss CR et al: Syndromes in workers exposed to trimellitic anhydride. *Ann Intern Med* 1983;**98**:8.

Hydrocarbons | 13

PETROLEUM DISTILLATES: KEROSENE, SOLVENT DISTILLATE, & GASOLINE

Kerosene, mineral seal oil, diesel oil: bp: 150–300 °C. Solvent distillate (Stoddard solvent): bp: 100–150 °C. Gasoline, naphtha, petroleum ether, mineral spirits (benzine), paint thinner, petroleum spirit, ligroin: bp: 20–100 °C. The vapor pressure of distillates whose boiling point is above 100 °C is negligible at 25 °C. Lubricating oils, mineral seal oil, and petrolatum are nontoxic by ingestion unless aspiration occurs.

All the petroleum distillates are liquids. They contain mostly branched-chain or straight-chain aliphatic hydrocarbons and are used as fuels and solvents.

Petroleum distillates have far greater toxic effects when they are aspirated into the tracheobronchial tree than when they are merely ingested: ingestion of 500–1000 mL may produce only minor symptoms, but aspiration of as little as 1 mL can result in overwhelming chemical pneumonitis. The exposure limit for nonaromatic petroleum distillates (petroleum naphtha) is 500 ppm; for gasoline, 300 ppm; for mineral oil mist, 5 mg/m³; and for rubber solvent naphtha, 400 ppm. The presence of benzene increases the toxicity (see p 192). The exposure limit for Stoddard solvent, which contains aromatic hydrocarbons (benzene and derivatives), is 100 ppm. The exposure limit for ligroin, which contains aromatic hydrocarbons other than benzene, is 300 ppm. Pesticides, camphor, metals, or halogenated compounds dissolved in petroleum distillates also increase the toxicity.

Petroleum distillates are fat solvents and alter the function of nerves to produce depression, coma, and sometimes convulsions. The effects on liver, kidneys, and bone marrow may be caused by contaminants such as benzene.

Petroleum distillates with boiling points above 150 °C have little toxicity when they are absorbed after ingestion. Direct aspiration of these substances into the lungs during ingestion appears to be the principal cause of the pulmonary irritation. Because these petroleum hydrocarbons have a low surface tension and low viscosity, small quantities will spread over a large surface area, such as the lung.

Table 13–1. Hydrocarbons. (For treatment, see p 191.)

	Exposure Limit (ppm)	LD50 (mg/kg) or LC (ppm)	Irritation	Kidney and Liver Damage	Bone Marrow Damage	CNS Effects	Myocardial Sensitizer	Carcinogen
Acenaphthene			+	+				
Acetylene	2500					+	+	
Benzo(α)pyrene	0?	1000						+
Biphenyl	0.2	2180	+			+		
Butadiene-1,3	10		+	+	+	+		
Butane	800	658				+		
p-tert-Butyltoluene	10	900	+			+		
Chrysene	0?							+
Cumene	50	1400	+	+		+		
Cyclohexane†	300	813	+	+		+		
Cyclohexene†	300		+	+		+		
Cyclopentadiene	75	250 ppm	+	+		+		
Cyclopentane‡	600	110,000	+			+		
Decahydronaphthalene	50	4200	+			+		
Dicyclopentadiene	5	350	+	+		+		
Divinyl benzene	10	4100	+			+		
Ethane	500					+		
Ethylbenzene	100	5000	+			+		
Ethylidene norbornene	5	730 ppm	+	+	+			
Fluoranthrene	0?	2000						+
Heptane	400		+			+	+	
n-Hexane‡	50	1400 ppm	+		+	+	+	
Hexanes (branched)	500	1400	+			+	+	
Indene	10	800+ ppm	+	+				
Mesityl oxide	15	1000				+		
Methane	1000					+		
Methylacetylene	1000					+		
Methylcyclohexane	400	4000	+	+		+		
Nonane	200	3200 ppm	+			+		
Octane	300		+			+		
Paraffin wax	2							+
Pentane	600		+			+		
Petroleum gas	1000					+		
Propadiene	1000		+			+		
Propane	1000	50,000 ppm				+		
Styrene	50	316	+			+		
Terphenyls	0.5	1900	+	+				
Tetrahydronaphthalene	50	2860	+			+		
Trimethylbenzene	25	2400 ppm	+		+			
Vinyltoluene	50	4000	+			+		

*mg/m³.
†May contain benzene.
‡Peripheral neuropathy.

Pathologic findings in acute poisoning include pulmonary edema, bronchial pneumonia, and gastrointestinal irritation. Degenerative changes in the liver and kidneys and hypoplasia of the bone marrow occur after prolonged inhalation of high concentrations.

Clinical Findings

The principal manifestations of poisoning with these agents are pulmonary irritation and central nervous system depression.

A. Acute Poisoning: (From inhalation or ingestion.) Nausea and vomiting; cough; and pulmonary irritation progressing to pulmonary edema, bloody sputum, and bronchial pneumonia with fever and cough. Pneumothorax and emphysema may complicate recovery. If a large amount (> 1 mL/kg) is ingested and retained, symptoms of central nervous system depression and irritation occur and include weakness, dizziness, slow and shallow respiration, unconsciousness, and convulsions. Ventricular fibrillation can occur rarely after ingestion or inhalation. Petroleum distillates are irritating to skin.

B. Chronic Poisoning: (From inhalation.) Dizziness, weakness, weight loss, anemia, nervousness, pains in the limbs, peripheral numbness, and paresthesias.

C. Laboratory Findings:
1. The red blood cell count may be reduced.
2. The bone marrow may show hypoplasia.
3. The urine may contain protein and red cells.

Treatment

A. Acute Poisoning:

1. Emergency measures–Only hydrocarbons that are solvents for a toxic agent or are themselves toxic need be evacuated; most hydrocarbons are not toxic per se. Extreme care must be used to prevent aspiration. Gastric lavage with a cuffed endotracheal tube in place to prevent further aspiration should be done within 15 minutes. In the absence of depression or convulsions or impaired gag reflex, emesis can also be induced using syrup of ipecac without increasing the hazard of aspiration.

2. General measures–Give artificial respiration with O_2 if respiration is depressed.

3. Special problems–Treat bacterial aspiration pneumonia with organism-specific chemotherapy. Treat pulmonary edema (see p 65).

B. Chronic Poisoning: Treat as for acute poisoning.

Prognosis

After the first 24 hours, the extent of pulmonary involvement indicates severity. Infiltration of more than 30% of the lungs requires 2–4 weeks for resolution. Long-term pulmonary effects are not seen.

Banner W Jr, Walson PD: Systemic toxicity following gasoline aspiration. *Am J Emerg Med* 1983;**1**:292.

Saulsbury FT, Chobanian MC, Wilson WG: Child abuse: Parenteral hydrocarbon administration. *Pediatrics* 1984;**73**:719.

Voigts A, Kaufman CE Jr: Acidosis and other metabolic abnormalities associated with paint sniffing. *South Med J* 1983;**76**:443.

AROMATIC HYDROCARBONS:
BENZENE, XYLENE, TOLUENE

Benzene: liquid; bp: 80 °C; vapor pressure at 26 °C: 100 mm Hg; exposure limit: 1 ppm. **Xylene:** commercial preparation a mixture of *o-*, *m-*, *p-*; bp: 140 °C; vapor pressure at 28 °C: 10 mm Hg; exposure limit: 100 ppm. **Toluene:** liquid; bp: 110 °C; vapor pressure at 31 °C: 40 mm Hg; exposure limit: 100 ppm. Coal tar naphtha is a mixture of benzene, toluene, xylene, and other aromatic hydrocarbons.

These compounds are commonly used as solvents in rubber and plastic cement. Toluene is the usual ingredient in the cement used for glue sniffing. In experimental animals, the toxicities of benzene, toluene, and the 3 xylenes are similar either by injection or by inhalation, and the lethal quantity ranges from 2 to 5 g/kg; benzene is the most toxic. The toxic level of benzene in humans is around 0.2 g/kg, and for toluene and xylene it is 0.5–1 g/kg. In practice, the low vapor pressure of xylene reduces the inhalation hazard from this substance.

In large amounts, these compounds depress the central nervous system; repeated exposure to small amounts of benzene or toluene depresses the bone marrow.

In acute fatalities, the postmortem findings include petechial hemorrhages, noncoagulated blood, and congestion of all organs.

In fatalities from chronic exposure to benzene or toluene, the findings include severe bone marrow aplasia; anemia; necrosis or fatty degeneration of the heart, liver, and adrenals; and hemorrhages.

Clinical Findings

The principal manifestation of acute poisoning is coma. Anemia occurs after chronic exposure to benzene or toluene.

A. Acute Poisoning:

1. Inhalation or ingestion–Symptoms from mild exposure are dizziness, weakness, euphoria, headache, nausea and vomiting, tightness in the chest, and staggering. If exposure is more severe, symptoms progress to visual blurring, tremors, shallow and rapid respiration, and ventricular irregularities including fibrillation, paralysis, unconsciousness, and convulsions. Violent excitement or delirium may precede unconsciousness. Kidney or liver damage may occur.

2. Skin contact–Irritation, scaling, and cracking.

B. Chronic Poisoning: (From inhalation.) Symptoms include headache, loss of appetite, drowsiness, nervousness, and pallor. Anemia, petechiae, and abnormal bleeding occur after exposure to benzene or toluene. The anemia may progress to complete aplasia of the bone marrow, especially after benzene poisoning. Continued repeated inhalation of toluene to the point of euphoria has caused irreversible encephalopathy with ataxia, tremulousness, emotional lability, and diffuse cerebral atrophy. The incidence of leukemia in workers chronically exposed to benzene is 5–10 times that in nonexposed populations.

C. Laboratory Findings in Benzene Exposure:

1. The red blood cell count may be diminished to 20% of normal.

2. The white blood cell count may be diminished to 5–10% of normal. The differential count shows that the greatest decrease is in polymorphonuclear leukocytes.

3. The thrombocytes may be reduced to 10–50% of normal.

4. The tourniquet test (Rumpel-Leede) is positive.

5. The bone marrow may appear normal, hypoplastic, or hyperplastic.

Prevention

Adequate ventilation must always be supplied in workrooms where benzene is being used. The benzene concentration in air should be checked frequently. Where high vapor concentrations are unavoidable, forced air masks should be used. A lifeline attended by a responsible person outside the contaminated enclosure is essential.

If skin contact is unavoidable, neoprene gloves must be worn.

Treatment

A. Emergency Measures: Remove patient from contaminated air and give artificial respiration with O_2. Remove ingested hydrocarbon by gastric lavage, being careful to avoid aspiration (see p 191).

B. General Measures:

1. Control excitement or convulsions with diazepam, 0.1 mg/kg slowly intravenously.

2. Keep at complete bed rest until respiration is normal.

3. *Do not give* epinephrine or ephedrine or related drugs. They may induce fatal ventricular fibrillation. Monitor ECG to detect ventricular abnormalities foreshadowing possible cardiac arrest.

C. Special Problems: Treat anemia by repeated blood transfusions. Treat respiratory or pulmonary problems as described on p 191. Treat kidney or liver damage (see pp 72 and 77).

Prognosis

In acute poisoning, death may occur up to 3 days after poisoning.

Rapid progression of symptoms and lack of response to removal of the hydrocarbon indicate a poor outcome.

In chronic poisoning from benzene, a steady decrease in the cellular elements of the blood or bone marrow indicates a poor outcome. If the cellular elements remain at a constant low level or rise gradually, recovery is likely. Patients have recovered after as much as a year of almost complete absence of formation of new blood elements.

Aksoy M: Benzene as a leukemogenic and carcinogenic agent. *Am J Ind Med* 1985;8:9.
Aksoy M: Malignancies due to occupational exposure to benzene. *Am J Ind Med* 1985;7:395.

NAPHTHALENE

Melting point: 80 °C; bp: 218 °C; vapor pressure at 80 °C: 9.8 mm Hg.

Naphthalene, obtained from coal tar, is used as a moth repellent and synthetic intermediate.

The fatal dose of ingested naphthalene is approximately 2 g. This chemical is most dangerous in children up to age 6, in whom absorption occurs rapidly. The exposure limit is 10 ppm.

Naphthalene causes hemolysis with subsequent blocking of renal tubules by precipitated hemoglobin. Hepatic necrosis has been reported. Hemolysis only occurs in individuals with a hereditary deficiency of glucose-6-phosphate dehydrogenase in the red cells (primarily black males), which results in a low level of reduced glutathione and increased susceptibility to hemolysis by metabolites of naphthalene.

Clinical Findings

The principal manifestations from naphthalene poisoning are hemolysis, jaundice, oliguria, and convulsions.

A. Acute Poisoning: (From ingestion or inhalation.)

1. Ingestion–Nausea and vomiting, diarrhea, oliguria, hematuria, anemia, jaundice, and pain on urination progressing to oliguria or anuria. In more serious poisoning, excitement, coma, and convulsions may occur.

2. Inhalation–Headache, mental confusion, and visual disturbances have been reported from exposure to boiling naphthalene.

B. Chronic Poisoning:

1. Repeated ingestion will cause the symptoms described for acute poisoning.

2. Local effects–Continued handling of naphthalene may pro-

duce a dermatitis characterized by itching, redness, scaling, weeping, and crusting of the skin. Eye contact causes corneal irritation and injury. Workers exposed to high levels of naphthalene fumes have developed lens opacity.

C. Laboratory Findings:

1. The red blood cell count may be 20–40% of normal. The white blood cell count may be increased. Hemolysis may be present.

2. Urine may contain hemoglobin, protein, and casts.

Prevention

Store naphthalene safely. Exhaust ventilation is necessary during work with naphthalene. Naphthalene workers should have periodic eye, blood, and urine examinations.

Treatment

A. Emergency Measures: Remove ingested naphthalene by gastric lavage or emesis (see pp 21–28). Treat convulsions (see p 51).

B. General Measures:

1. Alkalinize urine–Give sodium bicarbonate, 5 g orally every 4 hours or as necessary to maintain alkaline urine. Give fluids, up to 15 mL/kg/h, with furosemide, 1 mg/kg, to produce maximum diuresis and reduce injury to the kidney from hemoglobin products.

2. Give repeated small blood transfusions until hemoglobin is 60–80% of normal.

3. Hemodialysis or exchange transfusions should be used in the presence of severe central nervous system symptoms.

C. Special Problems: Treat anuria (see p 72).

Prognosis

Rapid progression to coma and convulsions indicates poor prognosis. Anuria may persist for 1–2 weeks with eventual complete recovery.

Local effects disappear 1–6 months after discontinuing exposure.

ATMOSPHERIC ORGANIC COMPOUNDS

Organic compounds are liberated into the air during combustion and by the evaporation of solvents. These substances range from methane (CH_4) through aldehydes such as formaldehyde (HCHO) and acrolein (CH_2=CHCHO) to branched-chain, unsaturated hydrocarbons or polycyclic aromatic hydrocarbons (PAH). Many of these substances take part in reactions involving nitrogen dioxide, ozone, and energy from sunlight. Some combine to form particles that contribute to reduced visibility.

The main source of organic compounds in the atmosphere is the automobile. An automobile without crankcase or exhaust controls wastes 10% of the supplied fuel into the atmosphere, or 18 g (0.04 lb) per mile at a fuel consumption of 1 gallon each 15 miles. Of this total, 60% is in the exhaust, 24% in crankcase blowby, and 15% in carburetor and fuel tank evaporation. Exhaust emissions from cars with catalytic converters should not exceed 100 ppm of hydrocarbons.

Diesel vehicles emit 2% of the supplied fuel to the atmosphere, or 12 grams per mile for a vehicle at 5 miles per gallon. Evaporative losses from diesel vehicles are low, since they use low-volatility fuel.

The national maximum for hydrocarbons in community air is 0.24 ppm of compounds other than methane. The atmosphere of metropolitan regions without controls contains 2 ppm of hydrocarbons 90% of the time and 5 ppm 20% of the time.

Large organic molecules contaminating the atmosphere as a result of human activities may contribute to the incidence of cancer.

Couri D, Milks M: Toxicity and metabolism of the neurotoxic hexacarbons n-hexane, 2-hexanone, and 2,5-hexanedione. *Annu Rev Pharmacol Toxicol* 1982;**22**:145.

Døssing M: Antipyrine clearance during occupational exposure to styrene. *Br J Ind Med* 1983;**40**:224.

Tenenbein M et al: Peripheral neuropathy following intentional inhalation of naphtha fumes. [n-Hexane.] *Can Med Assoc J* 1984;**131**:1077.

Corrosives | 14

OXALIC ACID

Formula: COOH–COOH; soluble in water; fumes appreciably when heated to 100 °C.

Oxalic acid and oxalates are used as bleaches and metal cleaners in industry and in household products. The leaves of garden rhubarb (*Rheum* species) contain a high concentration of oxalate.

The fatal dose by ingestion is estimated to be 5–15 g. The exposure limit for oxalic acid is 1 mg/m^3.

Oxalic acid is a corrosive acid. Oxalates combine with serum calcium to form insoluble calcium oxalate. The reduction in available calcium leads to violent muscular stimulation with convulsions and collapse.

In deaths following oxalic acid poisoning, calcium oxalate crystals are found in the renal tubules and in other tissues. The kidneys show cloudy swelling, hyaline degeneration, and sclerosis of the tubules. Corrosive changes may be found in the mouth, esophagus, and stomach. Cerebral edema also is a frequent finding.

Clinical Findings

The principal manifestation of oxalic acid poisoning is anuria.

A. Acute Poisoning: (From ingestion of oxalic acid.) Symptoms begin with local irritation and corrosion of the mouth, esophagus, and stomach, with pain and vomiting. These symptoms are followed shortly by muscular tremors, convulsions, weak pulse, and collapse. Death may occur within minutes. After apparent recovery or if oxalate is ingested, acute renal failure may occur from blocking of renal tubules by calcium oxalate.

B. Chronic Poisoning: (From skin contact or inhalation.) Prolonged skin contact may cause discoloration and gangrene by a local corrosive effect. Prolonged inhalation of fumes produced by boiling oxalic acid solutions leads to oxalic acid poisoning with renal impairment.

C. Laboratory Findings:

1. Calcium oxalate crystals, red blood cells, and protein are found in the urine.

2. Other clinical laboratory tests are noncontributory.

Prevention

Avoid prolonged skin contact. Avoid fumes from boiling oxalic acid.

Treatment

A. Acute Poisoning:

1. Emergency measures–Precipitate oxalate by giving calcium in any form orally, such as milk, lime water, chalk, calcium gluconate, calcium chloride, or calcium lactate. Do not use gastric lavage or emesis if tissue corrosion has occurred. Dissolve 10 g (2 teaspoons) of calcium lactate in (or add milk to) lavage or emesis fluids.

2. Antidote–Give 10% calcium gluconate or calcium chloride, 10 mL slowly intravenously, and repeat if symptoms persist.

3. General measures–

a. If renal function remains normal, give fluids to 4 L daily to prevent precipitation of calcium oxalate in the renal tubules.

b. Treat as for acid ingestion (see p 201).

B. Chronic Poisoning: Remove from further exposure.

Prognosis

If calcium antidotes can be given promptly, recovery is likely.

MISCELLANEOUS ACIDS & ACIDLIKE CORROSIVES

The acids and acidlike corrosives listed in Table 14–1 are used for cleaning metals and other products and in a variety of chemical reactions.

Ingestion of 1 mL of a corrosive acid has caused death. (Exposure limits are listed in Table 14–1.) Death may occur up to 1 month after exposure to corrosive fumes such as nitrogen oxide, as in silo gas poisoning.

Corrosive acids destroy tissues by direct chemical action. The tissue protein is converted to acid proteinate, which dissolves in the concentrated acid. Hemoglobin is converted to dark acid hematin and is precipitated. The intense stimulation by acid causes reflex loss of vascular tone.

The pathologic findings are those of corrosion and irritation. After ingestion, corrosive penetration of the esophagus and stomach are commonly found. The area of contact is stained brown or black except in the case of nitric and picric acids, which produce a yellow stain. Precipitated blood (coffee-grounds material) is frequently found in the stomach. The epithelium of the esophagus may desquamate in portions or as

Table 14—1. Acids and acidlike corrosives.
(For treatment, see p 201.)

Legend: 1. Mild irritation and reddening, cough. 2. Strong irritation and erythema, blistering. 3. Superficial destruction of skin or mucous membrane. 4. Complete destruction of skin or mucous membrane.	Exposure Limit (ppm)	Estimated Fatal Dose (g or mL)	Corrosive Effect	Pulmonary Effect
Acetic acid (glacial)	10	5	3	3
Acetic anhydride	5	5	3	3
Acetyl chloride	5	1	4	4
Acrylic acid	10	5	3	3
Amyltrichlorocyclane		1	4	
Benzalchloride		1	4	4
Benzotrichloride		1	4	4
Bromine	0.1	1	4	4
Calcium chloride		30	2	
Chlorine	1		4	4
Chlorine dioxide	0.1		4	4
Chloroacetylchloride	0.05	1	4	4
Chlorosulfonic acid		1	4	4
Dibutylphosphate	1	10	2	3
2,2-Dichloropropionic acid		10	2	2
Ethyl chlorocarbonate		1	4	
Formic acid	5	30	2	
Furoyl chloride		1	4	
Hydrazoic acid	10		2	2
Hydriodic acid	10	1	4	4
Hydrobromic acid	3	1	4	4
Hydrochloric acid	5	1	4	4
Hydrogen bromate	3	1	4	
Hydrogen iodate		1	4	
Lactic acid		1	4	
Maleic anhydride	0.25	10	2	
Methacrylic acid	20	10	3	1
Methyl silicate	1	1	4	2
Methyl trichlorosilane		1	4	4
Osmic acid	0.0002	1	4	4
Peracetic acid		1	4	
Perchloric acid		1	4	
Phenylmagnesium chloride		5	3	
Phosphoric acid	1*	1	4	
Phosphorus pentachloride	0.1	1	4	4
Phosphorus trichloride	0.2	1	4	
Phthallic anhydride	1	1	3	3
Propionic acid	10	30	2	
Sulfamic acid		5	3	
Sulfosalicylic acid		10	3	
Tartaric acid		30	1	
Thioglycolic acid	1	1	3	
Titanium tetrachloride		1	4	4
Trichloroacetic acid	1	1	4	4

*mg/m^3.

a whole. The eye shows denudation of the corneal epithelium and, in severe cases, edema and necrosis of the deeper tissues.

Clinical Findings

The principal manifestation of acid poisoning is corrosion.

A. Acute Poisoning:

1. Ingestion–Severe, burning pain in the mouth, pharynx, and abdomen followed by vomiting and diarrhea of dark precipitated blood. The blood pressure falls sharply. Brownish or yellowish stains may be found around or in the mouth. Asphyxia occurs from edema of the glottis.

After initial recovery, onset of fever indicates mediastinitis or peritonitis from perforation of the esophagus or the stomach. However, the patient may have a rigid abdomen without perforation. If the patient recovers from the immediate damage, scar formation is more likely to produce stricture of the pylorus than stricture of the esophagus.

2. Inhalation–Inhalation of acid fumes or irritating gases causes coughing, choking, and variable symptoms of headache, dizziness, and weakness followed after a 6- to 8-hour latent period by pulmonary edema with tightness in the chest, air hunger, dizziness, frothy sputum, and cyanosis. The accompanying physical findings are moist rales, low blood pressure, and high pulse pressure. Hemoptysis and shortness of breath may continue for several weeks after a single exposure to chlorine or other corrosive vapor.

3. Skin contact–Symptoms are severe pain and brownish or yellowish stains. Burns usually penetrate the full thickness of the skin, have sharply defined edges, and heal slowly with scar formation.

4. Eye contact–Conjunctival edema and corneal destruction occur from even dilute acids in the eyes. The symptoms are pain, tearing, and photophobia.

B. Chronic Poisoning: (From inhalation.) Long exposure to acid fumes may cause erosion of the teeth followed by jaw necrosis. Bronchial irritation with chronic cough and frequent attacks of bronchial pneumonia are common. Gastrointestinal disturbances are also noted.

C. Laboratory Findings: In acute poisoning, hemoconcentration may be indicated by a rise in red blood cell count and hematocrit.

D. X-Ray Findings: After inhalation of corrosives, diffuse mottling of the lung fields may be seen on x-rays.

Prevention

The exposure limit must always be observed (see Table 14–1). Water bubbler eye fountains and showers must be available where skin or eye contact with acids is possible.

Tight-fitting goggles, rubber aprons, and rubber gloves *must* be worn when handling acids. Employees must be drilled in the constant use of safety equipment.

Enclosed spaces containing corrosive gases should be thoroughly ventilated before being entered. Use of proper gas masks is advisable.

Treatment

A. Ingestion:

1. Emergency measures–

a. Do not use gastric lavage or emesis.

b. Dilute the acid–Ingested acid must be diluted within seconds by drinking quantities of water or milk. If vomiting is persistent, administer fluids repeatedly. Ingested acid must be diluted approximately 100-fold to render it harmless to tissues.

c. Relieve pain–Give morphine sulfate, 5–10 mg every 4 hours as necessary. Avoid central nervous system depression.

2. General measures–

a. Treat asphyxia from glottal edema by maintaining an adequate airway (see p 58).

b. Treat shock–Maintain normal blood pressure by transfusion and by the administration of 5% dextrose in saline (see p 66).

c. If symptoms are severe and perforation of the stomach or esophagus is suspected, give nothing by mouth until endoscopic examination has been done.

d. Maintain nutrition by giving carbohydrate or hyperalimentation fluid intravenously.

e. Give prednisolone, 2 mg/kg/d in divided doses for 10 days, to reduce esophageal stricture formation or, in inhalation poisoning, to reduce progression of fibrocystic and hyaline lung disease.

3. Special problems–Esophageal stricture may require dilation.

B. Eye Contact:

1. Emergency measures–Dilute the acid. Flood affected area with quantities of water in a shower or by means of a water bubbler eye fountain for at least 15 minutes (see p 28). The eyelids must be held apart during the washing.

2. Antidote–Do not use chemical antidotes. The heat liberated in the chemical reaction may actually increase injury.

3. General measures–Eye burns require the immediate attention of an ophthalmologist. If an ophthalmologist is not immediately available, wash the eyes and apply sterile bandages without any medication. Allay pain by the systemic administration of analgesics. Then take the patient to an ophthalmologist.

C. Skin Contact:

1. Emergency measures–Remove acid by flooding with water for at least 15 minutes. If the clothing is contaminated, a stream of water must be directed under the clothing while the clothes are being removed in order to remove the acid rapidly.

2. Antidote–Do not use chemical antidotes (see above).

3. General measures–Treat damaged areas as for thermal burns.

D. Inhalation:

1. Give artificial respiration.

2. Treat shock (see p 66).

3. Treat pulmonary edema (see p 65).

4. Treat bacterial pneumonia with organism-specific chemotherapy.

E. Chronic Poisoning: Remove from further exposure.

Prognosis

In one series, 32 of 105 persons who ingested acid died. Damage to the esophagus and stomach after ingestion may progress for 2–3 weeks. Death from peritonitis may occur as late as 1 month after ingestion. Approximately 95% of those who ingest acid and recover from immediate effects have persistent esophageal stricture.

Skin burns from acid are followed by extensive scarring. Skin grafting is required if a good cosmetic effect is desired. Corneal damage almost always results in blindness.

After inhalation of corrosive atmospheres, convalescence may be prolonged and frequent relapses may occur. Death may occur 30 days or more after exposure to such corrosive atmospheres as silo gas.

Gapany-Gapanavičius M et al: Chloramine-induced pneumonitis from mixing household cleaning agents. *Br Med J* 1982;**285:**1086.

Sellu DP: Obstructive jaundice caused by corrosive injury to the duodenum. *Br Med J* 1985;**290:**356.

Szerlip HM et al: Hyperchloremic metabolic acidosis after chlorine inhalation. *Am J Med* 1984;**77:**581.

Wason S et al: Phosphorus trichloride toxicity: Preliminary report. *Am J Med* 1984;**77:**1039.

NITROGEN OXIDES

The nitrogen oxides important in air contamination and in reactions that form atmospheric oxidants (see p 206) include nitric oxide (NO, colorless), nitrogen dioxide (NO_2, brown color), nitrogen trioxide (N_2O_3, colorless), nitric acid (HNO_3), and nitrogen pentoxide (N_2O_5, colorless). Nitrous oxide (N_2O, laughing gas, colorless) and nitrogen tetroxide (N_2O_4, colorless) do not occur in the atmosphere in significant amounts.

The nitrogen oxides are emitted into the atmosphere as a result of combustion of any nitrogen-containing substances. Thus, missile fuels, explosives, cigarettes, and agricultural wastes liberate nitrogen oxides. Nitrogen dioxide is also liberated during the rapid decomposition of plant material, as happens in silos. In an enclosed silo, the concentration of nitrogen dioxide may reach as high as 1500 ppm. In addition, combustion at high temperatures of nitrogen-free fuels in the presence of air oxidizes the nitrogen of the air to nitric oxide ($N_2 + O_2 = 2NO$). At 1800 °K, 1% of the reactants will be converted, and at 2675 °K, 5% of the reactants will be converted. Unmodified auto or diesel exhaust contains 1100 ppm of nitric oxide, producing an emission of 0.13 lb per gallon of fuel or 4 g per mile for a vehicle consuming 1 gallon of fuel each 15 miles. For 1977 and after, federal regulations limit all new automobiles to emission of 0.31 g of nitrogen oxides per mile. Cigarette smoke contains 200–650 ppm of nitrogen oxides, and pipe smoke contains 1100 ppm.

On reaching the air, nitric oxide oxidizes spontaneously to nitrogen dioxide, which gives smog its brown color. This reaction is slow if the concentration of nitric oxide is below 1 ppm, but it is speeded by the presence of other contaminants in the air, especially ozone. This color can be seen most clearly by looking into an air-polluted basin from above the temperature inversion boundary on any day with low wind velocity.

The exposure limit for industrial exposure to nitrogen dioxide is 3 ppm (NIOSH 1 ppm) and for submarines in the US Navy 0.5 ppm. The industrial exposure limit for nitric acid is 2 ppm. The exposure limit for nitric oxide is 25 ppm. The fatal dose of nitric acid is 1 mL. The national maximum annual average for nitrogen dioxide in community air has been set at 0.05 ppm. A concentration of 0.2 ppm was exceeded for a total of 487 hours in San Francisco in 1967 and for 2594 hours in the same year in Burbank, California.

Experimental studies in humans have used nitrogen dioxide, since it is reasonably stable and reproducible conditions can be established. The taste and odor of this compound can be detected at 1 ppm by experienced subjects. Chest discomfort occurs at a concentration of 15 ppm for 1 hour, the sensation becoming unpleasant at 25 ppm. After 1 minute at 50 ppm, subjects feel substernal pain. Longer exposure at this concentration has caused inflammatory changes in the lungs that ordinarily are reversible. Higher concentrations have been fatal.

Pathologic findings show that the effects on the lungs from inhaled silo gas (nitrogen dioxide) are typical of bronchiolitis fibrosa cystica. These effects include hemorrhage; fibrous stroma replacing the terminal bronchi, alveolar ducts, and sacs; hyaline membrane formation; and hyalinization of the basement membrane.

Exposure of rats to 0.5 ppm for 4 hours causes reversible degranulation of lung cells. Mice exposed continuously for 3 months to 0.5 ppm are more susceptible when exposed to pneumococci. Monkeys lose weight when exposed at this concentration, but other animals are not affected. Continuous exposure of rats to 2 ppm of nitrogen dioxide for 3 days caused epithelial hyperplasia in the terminal bronchioles, and exposure for more than 1 year caused thinning of the membrane lining the lungs. Intermittent exposure of rats to 4 ppm for a year caused no discernible permanent damage to the lungs.

Clinical Findings

The principal manifestation of nitrogen dioxide poisoning is dyspnea. For nitric acid, see p 200.

A. Acute Poisoning: (From inhalation.) Progressive weakness, dyspnea, cough, and cyanosis begin 1–3 weeks after single or repeated exposure to concentrations of 50–300 ppm. Concentrations above 300 ppm cause fulminating pulmonary edema or bronchopneumonia with onset within hours or days. Exposure to pure nitric oxide causes methemoglobinemia.

B. Laboratory Findings: Pulmonary function tests reveal reductions in inspiratory capacity and vital capacity and impaired diffusion capacity. These findings improve as the inflammatory process subsides, but some impairment of function may be permanent.

Prevention

Silos and other enclosed spaces in which decomposition of organic material can liberate nitrogen dioxide should be ventilated thoroughly before being entered.

Treatment

A. General Measures:

1. Give O_2 for dyspnea and cyanosis.

2. Give prednisone or prednisolone, 5 mg orally every 6 hours, to reduce pulmonary inflammatory reaction. After 1 month, gradually reduce dosage to zero over 1–2 months.

B. Special Problems:

1. Treat pulmonary edema (see p 65).

2. Treat bronchopneumonia with organism-specific chemotherapy.

Prognosis

Recovery from the acute phase requires 1–6 months. Emphysematous change persists depending on the severity of the original damage.

Silo-filler's disease in rural New York. *MMWR* 1982;**31**:389.

DIMETHYL SULFATE & DIETHYL SULFATE

Formula (dimethyl sulfate): $(CH_3)_2SO_4$; bp: 188 °C; vapor pressure at 76 °C: 15 mm Hg. **Formula** (diethyl sulfate): $(C_2H_5)_2SO_4$; bp: 209 °C; vapor pressure at 47 °C: 1 mm Hg.

Dimethyl sulfate is used in organic synthesis. The lethal dose is 1–5 g. The exposure limit is 0.1 ppm. Diethyl sulfate is also used in organic synthesis. The lethal dose is probably in excess of 10 g. No exposure limit has been established.

Dimethyl sulfate hydrolyzes in the presence of water to methanol and sulfuric acid. It is caustic to mucous membranes of the eyes, nose, throat, and lungs. Pulmonary edema is the usual cause of death. Diethyl sulfate hydrolyzes slowly in water to monoethyl sulfate and ethanol. Monoethyl sulfate is corrosive to mucous membranes.

Pathologic changes are those of extreme irritation. The eyes, nose, mouth, throat, lungs, liver, heart, and kidneys are affected.

Clinical Findings

The principal manifestation of acute dimethyl sulfate or diethyl sulfate poisoning is extreme irritation.

A. Symptoms and Signs: (From inhalation, skin absorption, or ingestion.) The immediate effects of vapor exposure are irritation and erythema of the eyes progressing to lacrimation, blepharospasm, and chemosis. Cough, hoarseness, and edema of the tongue, lips, larynx, and lungs occur later.

Ingestion or direct contact with mucous membranes causes corrosion equivalent to that from sulfuric acid. After absorption, pulmonary edema and injury to the liver and kidneys are the most prominent findings.

Diethyl sulfate is suspected of being a carcinogen after long exposure.

B. Laboratory Findings:

1. Hematocrit determination may reveal hemoconcentration. Hypoglycemia also occurs.

2. The urine may contain protein and red blood cells.

Prevention

If dimethyl sulfate or diethyl sulfate is spilled, the building must be evacuated and the agent decomposed by hosing with water or spraying with 5% sodium hydroxide (caustic soda).

Workers who enter contaminated areas must wear positive-pressure airline hose masks or self-contained breathing apparatus. Canister type gas masks are not safe.

Treatment of Acute Poisoning

A. Emergency Measures: Remove the patient to fresh air and wash skin or mucous membranes with copious amounts of water. Showers and bubbler eye fountains must be available where these agents are used. Washing should continue for at least 15 minutes. Treat skin corrosion the same as a burn. Observe exposed individuals for at least 24 hours for the development of symptoms.

B. General Measures:

1. Maintain adequate arterial O_2 saturation—if necessary, by artificial ventilation with 60–100% O_2.

2. Treat bronchospasm—

a. Give isoproterenol, 1:200, 0.5 mL in 3 mL of saline, by intermittent positive-pressure nebulizer for 15-minute periods every 2–4 hours. Cardiac arrhythmias may occur.

b. Give aminophylline, 250–500 mg in 50 mL of saline intravenously over 30 minutes every 6 hours as necessary. Cardiac arrhythmias and tachycardia may occur.

3. Administration of hydrocortisone, 300 mg in divided doses daily for 2 days, may be useful to limit pulmonary injury.

C. Special Problems: Treat pulmonary edema (see p 65).

Prognosis

The first 24 hours after poisoning constitute the most dangerous period. If pulmonary edema can be controlled, recovery is likely. Complete recovery from eye irritation may take up to 1 month.

ATMOSPHERIC OXIDANTS

Oxidants are atmospheric substances with an oxidizing power sufficiently great to liberate iodine from a solution of potassium iodide. One oxidant, ozone (O_3), accelerates the cracking of rubber, a property that can be used to measure the total exposure to ozone over a period of time. These oxidants make up the eye irritants in photochemical smog resulting from the action of sunlight on air containing nitrogen dioxide and certain organic compounds.

Sources

The reactions that initiate the formation of oxidants depend on the absorption of light energy. The amount of energy in a light quantum is given by the expression h (Planck's constant, with a value of 6.62×10^{-27} erg second) $\times \nu$ (frequency of the light). For this reason, the light in the ultraviolet spectrum is more important, since it has greater energy. The following reactions are considered to be important in the absorption of light energy (hv) and the production of monatomic oxygen ($\dot{O}$) and free organic radicals ($\dot{R}$):

$$NO_2 + hv = NO + \dot{O} \qquad\qquad RONO + hv = R\dot{O} + NO$$

$$RCHO + hv = \dot{R} + H\dot{C}O \qquad\qquad RONO + hv = \dot{R} + NO_2$$

$$RCO \cdot R + hv = \dot{R} + R\dot{C}O$$

Other reactions, including some or all of the following, occur in the dark:

$$\dot{O} + O_2 = O_3 \qquad\qquad CH_3O\dot{O} + O_2 = CH_3\dot{O} + O_3$$

$$O_3 + NO = O_2 + NO_2 \qquad\qquad CH_3\dot{O} + NO = CH_3ONO$$

$$\dot{O} + C_4H_8 = \dot{C}H_3 + C_3H_5O \qquad\qquad CH_3\dot{O} + O_2 = H_2CO + HO\dot{O}$$

$$\dot{C}H_3 + O_2 = CH_3O\dot{O} \qquad\qquad O_3 + 2NO_2 = N_2O_5 + O_2$$

The following reaction scheme from ethylene (C_2H_4) to peroxyacetylnitrate (PAN) has been suggested.

$$C_2H_4 + O_3 = C_2H_4O_3$$

$$2\,C_2H_4O_3 = HCHO + CH_3O + CH_3CO + O_3$$

$$CH_3CO + O_2 = CH_3CO_3$$

$$CH_3CO_3 + NO_2 = CH_3CO \cdot O \cdot ONO_2 \text{ (PAN)}$$

The concentration of ozone does not begin to rise until nitric oxide (NO) has been completely converted to nitrogen dioxide (NO_2). Although nitrogen dioxide alone contributes to the formation of a small amount of ozone, the levels found in urban atmospheres do not occur unless some of the carbon compounds indicated in the above schemes are present. These include aldehydes, ketones, and unsaturated hydrocarbons. The reactivity of these substances in atmospheres forms the basis for the restriction of their use in various solvents for paints, lacquers, and other finishes. Methane (CH_4), which makes up about half of the organic compounds in the atmosphere, does not react. Some of the reaction intermediates are possible contributors to eye irritation, but they are so unstable that analysis or experimental testing has not been possible. PAN has been tested in volunteers and found to be eye-irritating at concentrations of 0.5 ppm. This concentration is higher than that likely to occur in the atmosphere. A combination may be more irritating that the individual chemicals.

At the peak of oxidant concentration in the atmosphere (shortly after midday), ozone makes up more than 90% of the total. By nightfall, ozone falls to a low level but oxidants may still be present. The chemical makeup of all the dark-reaction oxidants has not as yet been defined. One compound has been identified as PAN (see above); its concentration during air pollution episodes is not known.

Ozone is also produced by electrical discharges such as lightning and by the effect of intense ultraviolet light. At an altitude of 75,000 ft, the concentration of ozone is raised to 16 ppm by the direct action of sunlight. Unless some means is used to decompose the ozone, the concentration inside pressurized aircraft flying between 30,000 and 40,000 ft reaches 0.3–0.4 ppm. Some ozone found at ground level is brought down to this level by atmospheric mixing, but this amount does not exceed 0.01–0.03 ppm except during lightning storms.

The national maximum 1-hour average for ozone in community air has been set at 0.12 ppm. In 1967, San Jose, California, exceeded 0.1 ppm for 272 hours; Burbank, California, for 1191 hours; and Pasadena, California, for 1245 hours. In the same year, a level of 0.05 ppm was exceeded for 1032 hours in San Jose, 2198 hours in Burbank, and 2243 hours in Pasadena, while San Francisco had 129 hours above 0.05 ppm and 25 hours above 0.1 ppm. The industrial exposure limit for ozone is 0.1 ppm.

Effects on Humans & Animals

The odor threshold for ozone in the most sensitive individuals is 0.01 ppm, but it is only recognized by all persons at 0.05 ppm. At a concentration of 0.1 ppm of ozone or oxidants, more than 5% of individuals will have symptoms of eye irritation. Mice exposed for 3 hours to this concentration plus a streptococcus had a statistically significant increase in the mortality rate as compared to mice exposed only to the streptococcus. Guinea pigs exposed to 0.1 ppm of ozone and tubercle bacilli continuously for 17 weeks also showed an increased mortality rate as compared to guinea pigs exposed only to tubercle bacilli.

Patients with obstructive lung diseases such as asthma or emphysema, when exposed to an ambient atmosphere containing 0.1–0.15 ppm of oxidants, showed increased breathing resistance, increased O_2 consumption, and decreased arterial O_2 concentration, as compared to the same patients exposed to charcoal-filtered air during episodes with outside air at 0.1–0.15 ppm of oxidants. Recovery from the effects of oxidant-containing ambient air required several days.

Experiments have shown that exposure to 0.2 ppm of ozone for 3 hours reduces visual acuity, increases peripheral vision, decreases night vision, and alters the balance of the muscles controlling the position of the eye.

Asthmatic patients report more attacks when the daily peak of oxidants goes over 0.25 ppm. A level of 0.3 ppm of ozone causes cough and some respiratory tract irritation after 30 minutes of exposure. This same concentration of PAN raised O_2 consumption during voluntary exercise. Progressively higher concentrations are more irritating; lung function is distinctly impaired at ozone concentrations of 0.6 ppm.

Mechanisms of Ozone Action

Ozone and other oxidants presumably produce their irritant action as a result of their chemical reactivity at the point of contact. These oxidants would be expected to react so rapidly on contact with any organic compounds that they could not be absorbed as such into the bloodstream. Thus, effects on tissues not directly exposed to ozone or oxidants are difficult to explain. Peroxidized fatty acids have been suggested as carriers of the energy. For example, subjects exposed to 1 ppm of ozone for 10 minutes showed a reduction in the ability of hemoglobin of the red blood cells to release O_2 in the tissues. The shape of red blood cells was altered by exposure of subjects to ozone at concentrations down to 0.2 ppm.

An effect of ozone similar to that of ionizing radiation has been suggested. Ionizing radiation appears to act on tissues by producing free radicals, and ozone could also have this effect. Substances that combine quickly with free radicals are effective as protective agents against both ionizing radiation and ozone. Both ozone and ionizing radiation cause chromosomal damage and age animals prematurely. On the other hand, in one series of experiments, exposure to ozone protected mice against simultaneous exposure to radiation.

Treatment

The use of activated charcoal adsorbers in rooms has been suggested as a means of lowering air contaminant concentrations.

Bates DV: Epidemiologic basis for photochemical oxidant standards. *Environ Health Perspect* 1984;52:125.

SULFUR OXIDES

The following sulfur oxides occur as atmosphere contaminants: sulfur dioxide (SO_2), sulfur trioxide (SO_3), sulfurous acid (H_2SO_3), and sulfuric acid (H_2SO_4). Sulfur monochloride (S_2Cl_2) and thionyl chloride ($SOCl_2$) are used in industrial processes. A number of salts of sulfur oxides are used as bleaches, oxidizers, reducing agents, and cleaning agents. Their estimated fatal doses and exposure limits (if established) are as follows: sodium acid sulfate ($NaHSO_4$), 10 g; sodium sulfite (Na_2SO_3), 10 g; sodium hydrosulfite (sodium sulfoxylate, $Na_2S_2O_4$), 30 g; sodium bisulfite (NaHSO$_3$), 10 g, 5 mg/m^3; sodium metabisulfite (Na$_2$S$_2$O$_5$), 10 g, 5 mg/m^3; sodium, potassium, or ammonium persulfate (Na$_2$S$_2$O$_8$, K$_2$S$_2$O$_8$, [NH$_4$]$_2$S$_2$O$_8$), 10 g, 0.5 mg/m^3; sodium thiosulfate (Na$_2$S$_2$O$_3$), 50 g. Sodium hydrosulfite releases sulfur dioxide on contact with acids. Persulfate salts release ozone and sulfuric acid on contact with water.

Sulfur dioxide reduces visibility by taking part in reactions between organic compounds and nitrogen oxides to form particulates. Oxidation to sulfur trioxide, which then combines with water to form small droplets of sulfuric acid, also reduces visibility.

Sulfur oxides come from fuel oil and coal combustion, from petroleum refining, and from the chemical and metallurgic industries.

The national maximum annual average for sulfur dioxide in community air is 0.03 ppm, and the maximum 24-hour average is 0.14 ppm. For industrial exposures, the exposure limit for sulfur dioxide is 2 ppm; for sulfur trioxide, 2 ppm; for sulfuric acid, 1 mg/m^3; for sulfurous acid, 10 ppm; for thionyl chloride, 1 ppm; and for sulfur monochloride, 1 ppm. The estimated fatal dose for sulfuric acid is 1 mL; for sulfurous acid, 10 mL.

Trained observers can recognize the presence of sulfur dioxide at a concentration of 0.3 ppm, but concentrations up to 1 ppm have little effect on lung function except for possible increase in respiratory rate. Increased resistance to breathing begins to occur at 1.6 ppm in normal individuals and possibly at 0.7 ppm in patients with respiratory disease. Concentrations in air pollution disasters such as occurred in Donora, Pennsylvania, and in London have ranged from 1 to 3 ppm. The eye irritation level is 10 ppm. Rats show decreased life span with accelerated aging and heart, lung, and kidney damage on uninterrupted exposure to 1 ppm.

Sulfites are potent sensitizers, and anaphylaxis can occur from exposure to residues in food or drugs.

Clinical Findings & Treatment

See pp 13 and 200–202.

Prevention

Persons sensitive to sulfites should be identified and warned to avoid foods that may contain residues. Physicians should not prescribe drugs containing sulfites for sensitive individuals.

Koepke JW: Dose-dependent bronchospasm from sulfites in isoetharine. *JAMA* 1984;**251**:2982.

Twarog FJ, Leung DY: Anaphylaxis to a component of isoetharine (sodium bisulfite). *JAMA* 1982;**248**:2030.

ALKALIES & PHOSPHATES
(Potassium Hydroxide, Sodium Hydroxide [Lye], Sodium Phosphates, Potassium Carbonate, & Sodium Carbonate)
(Table 14–2)

These agents are used in the manufacture of soaps and cleansers and in chemical synthesis. Urine sugar test tablets contain sodium hydroxide. Button batteries contain sodium hydroxide or potassium hydroxide.

The fatal doses of alkalies are listed in Table 14–2.

The alkalies combine with protein to form proteinates and with fats to form soaps, thus producing soft, necrotic, deeply penetrating areas on contact with tissues. The solubility of these products allows further penetration that may continue for several days.

Sodium and potassium hexametaphosphates, polyphosphates, tripolyphosphates, pyrophosphates, and other phosphates used as water softeners form complexes with calcium and, after ingestion, are capable of seriously reducing the serum level of ionic calcium. They have less corrosive effect on mucous membranes than sodium or potassium hydroxide. Hydrolysis of the polymeric phosphates can also produce acidosis.

Pathologic findings include gelatinous necrotic areas at the sites of contact.

Intense stimulation by alkalies causes reflex loss of vascular tone and cardiac inhibition.

Clinical Findings

The principal manifestation of poisoning with the alkalies is corrosion.

A. Acute Poisoning:

1. Ingestion of strong alkalies–Ingestion of alkali is followed by severe pain, vomiting, diarrhea, and collapse. The vomitus contains blood and desquamated mucosal lining. If death does not occur in the first 24 hours, the patient may improve for 2–4 days and then have a sudden onset of severe abdominal pain, boardlike abdominal rigidity, and rapid fall of blood pressure indicating delayed gastric or esophageal perforation. Button batteries can cause corrosive damage to the esophagus and upper gastrointestinal tract.

Even though the patient recovers from the immediate damage, esophageal stricture can occur weeks, months, or even years later to make swallowing difficult. Carcinoma is a risk in later life.

2. Ingestion of other alkalies–Ingestion of hexametaphosphate, tripolyphosphate, and other phosphates in the form of detergents or laxatives causes a shocklike state, fall of blood pressure, slow pulse,

Table 14—2. Alkali corrosives.

Legend: 1. Mild irritation and reddening. 2. Strong irritation and erythema, blistering. 3. Superficial destruction of skin or mucous membrane. 4. Complete destruction of skin or mucous membrane.	Exposure Limit (ppm)	Estimated Fatal Dose (g)	Corrosive Effect
2-Aminobutane		10	2
2-Aminopropane	5	10	2
Butylamine	5	20	3
Calcium carbide		15	3
Calcium hydroxide	5	30	2
Calcium oxide	2*	10	3
Cement (Portland)	10*	60	3
Cesium hydroxide	2*	15	2
Cyclohexylamine	10	30	2
2-N-Dibutylaminoethanol	2	30	2
Diethanolamine	3	20	2
Diethylamine	10	20	2
Diethylaminoethanol	10	20	2
Diethylene triamine	1	20	2
Diisopropylamine	5	20	2
Dimethylamine	10	10	3
Ethanolamine	3	50	2
Ethylamine	10	20	2
Ethylenediamine†	10	10	2
Isopropylamine	5	20	2
Lithium hydride	0.025*	5	4
Lithium hydroxide		5	4
Methylamine	10	50	1
Potassium carbonate		20	3
Potassium hydroxide	2*	5	4
Sodium carbonate		30	3
Sodium hydroxide	2*	5	4
Sodium phosphates		50	2
Sodium silicate		50	2
Tetrasodium pyrophosphate	5*	50	2
Triethanolamine		50	2
Triethylamine	10	20	2
Trimethylamine	10	20	2
Tris(hydroxymethyl)-aminomethane		50	1

*mg/m^3.
†Sensitizer.

cyanosis, coma, and sometimes tetany as a result of reduction in ionic calcium.

3. Eye contact–Eye contact with concentrated alkali causes conjunctival edema and corneal destruction. Dilute solutions of the amines shown in Table 14–2 can cause corneal damage.

4. **Skin contact**–Alkalies penetrate skin slowly. The extent of damage therefore depends on duration of contact.

5. Diethylaminoethanol and 2-N-dibutylaminoethanol inhibit cholinesterase (see p 115–116 for clinical findings).

B. Chronic Poisoning: (From skin contact.) A chronic dermatitis may follow repeated contact with alkalies.

C. Laboratory Findings: The red blood cell count and hematocrit are increased. Button batteries lodged in the esophagus or a Meckel's diverticulum can be seen on x-ray.

Prevention

Store corrosive alkalies safely. The manufacturer's "safety caps" on containers should not be replaced with regular caps. Water bubbler eye fountains and showers must be available where skin or eye contact with alkalies is possible. Tight-fitting goggles, rubber aprons, and rubber gloves *must* be worn when handling alkalies in concentrated solutions. Employees must be drilled in the constant use of safety equipment.

Treatment

A. Ingestion:

1. **Emergency measures**–Dilute the alkali by giving water or milk to drink immediately, and allow vomiting to occur. Avoid gastric lavage or emetics. These increase the possibility of perforation. Esophagoscopy is the only way to exclude the possibility of corrosion in the upper gastrointestinal tract; if corrosion is suspected, esophagoscopy should usually be performed within 24 hours.

2. **Antidote**–For hypocalcemia after phosphate ingestion, give calcium gluconate, 5 mL of 10% solution slowly intravenously, to restore ionic calcium to normal level.

3. **General measures**–Give nothing by mouth until esophagoscopy has been done. In children, give prednisolone orally or intramuscularly, 2 mg/kg/d in divided doses for 10 days. A broad-spectrum antibiotic and penicillin should be given to patients with fever or other signs indicating the possibility of perforation. After the acute injury has subsided, esophageal dilation can be done.

4. **Specific measures**–Button batteries lodged in the esophagus should be removed endoscopically or surgically. Batteries that have passed beyond the esophagus will ordinarily be expelled within 1–3 days; surgical intervention is unnecessary unless the battery lodges in a Meckel's diverticulum. Catharsis may speed passage of the battery through the intestinal tract.

B. Eye Contact:

1. **Emergency measures**–Wash eye for 15 minutes with running

water and then irrigate eye for 30–60 minutes with normal saline solution.

2. General measures–Apply sterile bandages, allay pain by systemic administration of analgesics, and take the patient to an ophthalmologist for evaluation of the injury.

C. Skin Contact: Wash with running water until skin is free of alkali as indicated by disappearance of soapiness.

D. Chronic Poisoning: Remove from further contact and treat dermatitis (see p 83).

Prognosis

Approximately 25% of those who ingest strong alkali die from the immediate effects. Damage to the esophagus and stomach after ingestion may progress for 2–3 weeks. Death from peritonitis may occur as late as 1 month after ingestion. Approximately 95% of those who ingest strong alkali and recover from the immediate effects have persistent esophageal stricture.

Button batteries that pass the esophagus usually travel through the gastrointestinal tract with little or no damage.

Corneal damage is almost always permanent. Corneal transplant may be useful.

Crain EF et al: Caustic ingestions. *Am J Dis Child* 1984;**138**:863.
Litovitz TL: Battery ingestions: Product accessibility and clinical course. *Pediatrics* 1985;**75**:469.
Litovitz TL: Button battery ingestions. *JAMA* 1983;**249**:2495.
Litovitz TL et al: Button battery ingestion: Assessment of therapeutic modalities and battery discharge state. *J Pediatr* 1984;**105**:868.

AMMONIA & AMMONIUM HYDROXIDE

Ammonia (NH_3) is a gas at ordinary temperatures. Ammonium hydroxide (NH_4OH) is a liquid containing 25–29% NH_3; vapor pressure at 27 °C: 500 mm Hg.

Ammonia is used in organic synthesis, as a refrigerant, and as a fertilizer. Ammonium hydroxide is used in organic synthesis and as a cleaner.

The exposure limit of ammonia is 25 ppm. The fatal dose of ammonium hydroxide by ingestion is about 30 mL (1 oz) of a 25% concentration.

Ammonia and ammonium hydroxide injure cells directly by alkaline caustic action and cause extremely painful irritation of all mucous membranes.

The pathologic findings in inhalation poisoning are pulmonary edema, pulmonary irritation, and pneumonia. After ingestion, the findings are the same as with alkalies (see p 211), although usually less severe.

Clinical Findings

The principal manifestation of acute poisoning with these compounds is extreme irritation.

A. Ingestion: Ingested ammonia causes severe pain in the mouth, chest, and abdomen, with cough, vomiting, and shocklike collapse. Gastric or esophageal perforation may occur later, with exacerbation of abdominal pain, fever, and abdominal rigidity. Lung irritation and pulmonary edema may appear rapidly or after a delay of 12–24 hours.

B. Inhalation: Ammonia fumes (1000 ppm) cause irritation of the eyes and upper respiratory tract, with cough, vomiting, conjunctival injection, and redness of the mucous membranes of the lips, mouth, nose, and pharynx. Higher concentrations cause swelling of the lips and conjunctiva, temporary blindness, restlessness, tightness in the chest, frothy sputum indicating pulmonary edema, cyanosis, and rapid, weak pulse.

C. Skin Contact: If skin contact is prolonged more than a few minutes, it causes severe burning pain and corrosive damage.

D. Eye Contact: Eye contact with concentrated ammonia causes immediate and severe pain followed by conjunctival edema and corneal clouding. Later, cataract formation and atrophy of the retina and iris may occur.

Prevention

Employees working in areas where ammonia is used must be trained in escape methods and in the use of safety equipment, including goggles, gas masks, showers, eye fountains, water hoses, exits, lifelines, and first-aid equipment. Ammonia equipment must be constantly inspected to prevent accidents. All valves should be labeled to prevent accidental opening.

If a contaminated area must be entered, a full-face airline mask or self-contained oxygen mask must be worn. Protective clothing is also necessary if the concentration is above 10,000 ppm.

Treatment

A. Emergency Measures:

1. Ingestion–Dilute ingested poison as described on p 213.

2. Eye contamination–Wash eyes in a water bubbler eye fountain for at least 15 minutes. Follow this by repeated irrigation with normal saline solution. The patient should be taken to an ophthalmologist for further treatment.

3. Inhalation–Remove patient from contaminated area and keep at bed rest.

4. Skin contamination–Wash skin for at least 15 minutes.

B. Antidote: Milk may be given by mouth, or water can be used externally.

C. General Measures: Treat as described on p 201.

D. Special Problems:

1. Treat pulmonary edema (see p 65).
2. Treat esophageal stricture (see p 201).

Prognosis

Patients who survive 48 hours are likely to recover. Eye contact is frequently followed by permanent blindness.

FLUORINE, HYDROGEN FLUORIDE, & DERIVATIVES

Fluorine, hydrogen fluoride, and many derivatives of fluorine are gases at ordinary temperatures. Sulfur pentafluoride is a liquid.

Fluorine is used in organic synthesis. Hydrogen fluoride (hydrofluoric acid) is useful in the petroleum and semiconductor industries and in etching glass. Cryolite (sodium aluminum fluoride) is used in aluminum reduction and many other industrial processes. Fluoride salts are used in the prevention of dental caries and in rodenticides. A 90-g tube of fluoride toothpaste contains 67 mg of fluoride. Methyl sulfonyl fluoride is used as a fumigant.

The exposure limits for fluorine and derivatives are as follows: fluorine, 1 ppm; hydrogen fluoride, 3 ppm; fluoride salts, 2.5 mg/m^3; boron trifluoride, 1 ppm; bromine pentafluoride, 0.1 ppm; carbonyl fluoride, 2 ppm; chlorine trifluoride, 0.1 ppm; nitrogen trifluoride, 10 ppm; oxygen difluoride, 0.05 ppm; perchloryl fluoride, 3 ppm; selenium hexafluoride, 0.05 ppm; sulfur hexafluoride, 1000 ppm; sulfur pentafluoride, 0.01 ppm; sulfur tetrafluoride, 0.1 ppm; sulfuryl fluoride, 5 ppm; tellurium hexafluoride, 0.02 ppm. The fatal dose of sodium fluoride is 5–10 mg of fluorine per kilogram, and toxic effects occur below 1 mg of fluorine per kilogram. The fatal plasma level of fluorine is 3 mg/L. Patients with osteoporosis tolerate up to 60 mg of sodium fluoride per day, but osteosclerosis may occur at a urinary excretion level of 10 mg of fluoride per day in workers exposed to fluoride. The fatal dose of fluorosilicates is about the same as for fluorides, but that of cryolite is much higher (above 10 g). The LD50 for methyl sulfonyl fluoride in experimental animals is 3.5 mg/kg.

Fluorine and fluorides act as direct cellular poisons by interfering with calcium metabolism and enzyme mechanisms. Fluorides form an insoluble precipitate with calcium and lower the plasma calcium level.

Fluorine, hydrogen fluoride (hydrofluoric acid), and most fluorine derivatives are corrosive to tissues.

Skin or mucous membrane contact with hydrogen fluoride produces deeply penetrating, necrotic ulcerations.

Neutral fluorides in 1–2% concentrations will cause inflammation and necrosis of mucous membranes. After death, rigor mortis sets in rapidly. Postmortem findings are cerebral hyperemia and edema, pulmonary edema, and degenerative changes in the liver and kidneys.

In fatalities caused by inhalation of hydrogen fluoride or fluorine, pulmonary edema and bronchial pneumonia are the most prominent findings.

In deaths following prolonged absorption of fluoride, the bone structure shows thickening with calcification in the ligamentous attachments. Bone marrow space is greatly reduced.

Clinical Findings

The principal manifestation of fluorine and fluoride poisoning is corrosion.

A. Acute Poisoning:

1. Inhalation–Inhalation of hydrogen fluoride, fluorine, and most fluorine derivatives causes coughing, choking, and chills lasting 1–2 hours after exposure. After an asymptomatic period of 1–2 days, fever, cough, tightness in the chest, rales, and cyanosis indicate pulmonary edema. These symptoms progress for 1–2 days and then regress slowly over a period of 10–30 days. Sulfuryl fluoride causes narcosis, convulsions, and pulmonary irritation. Nitrogen trifluoride causes methemoglobin formation. Bromine pentafluoride causes nephrosis and hepatitis. Sulfur hexafluoride (sulfur fluoride) is nearly nontoxic.

2. Ingestion–Ingestion of neutral fluorides such as sodium fluoride or sodium silicofluoride causes salivation, nausea and vomiting, diarrhea, and abdominal pain. Later, weakness, tremors, shallow respiration, carpopedal spasm, and convulsions occur. Death is by respiratory paralysis. If death does not occur immediately, jaundice and oliguria may appear. Experience with oral fluoride supplements used to prevent tooth decay has been reassuring; no adverse effects occur unless enormous amounts are ingested.

3. Contact–Skin or mucous membrane contact with hydrogen fluoride solution results in damage depending on the concentration. Concentrations above 60% result immediately in severe, extremely painful burns. Such burns are deep and heal slowly. Concentrations less than 50% may cause slight immediate irritation of the skin or none at all. The acid penetrates readily, however, and a deep-seated ulceration results if contact continues for more than a few minutes. A fatality has occurred from systemic poisoning following exposure of 2.5% of the body surface to hydrofluoric acid.

B. Chronic Poisoning: (From inhalation or ingestion.) Intake of more than 6 mg of fluorine per day results in fluorosis. Symptoms are weight loss, brittle bones, anemia, weakness, general ill health, stiffness of joints, and discoloration of the teeth when exposure occurs during tooth formation.

C. Laboratory Findings:

1. In acute poisoning from fluoride salts or skin exposure to hydrofluoric acid, serum calcium and serum magnesium are reduced.

2. In chronic exposure, x-ray evidence of osteosclerosis and calcification of ligaments is indicative of fluorosis.

3. In severe fluorosis, both red and white blood cell counts may be diminished.

4. Fluorine workers should have urine fluoride determinations at 6-month intervals.

Prevention

Hydrogen fluoride workers must be carefully instructed in the dangers of skin contact with hydrogen fluoride and in the necessity for immediate removal of even dilute solutions by prolonged washing. Showers and water bubbler eye fountains must be available where hydrogen fluoride is being used. Processes utilizing hydrogen fluoride must be totally enclosed. Workers should wear long rubber gauntlets, long rubber aprons, high rubber boots, and wide plastic face shields while handling hydrogen fluoride. Full safety suits that are checked daily for leaks may be necessary. Forced-air face masks should be worn if the air concentration of hydrogen fluoride is sufficiently high to cause nasal irritation. Tools and benches must be decontaminated immediately by washing with ammonia or lye solutions after hydrogen fluoride is spilled.

Treatment

A. Skin or Mucous Membrane Burns: Wash thoroughly under a stream of water for 15–60 minutes. Do not wait until symptoms appear before giving treatment. Coat the burn with a magnesium oxide–water paste containing 20% glycerin. Do not use oily ointments. Open all blisters; if hydrogen fluoride has penetrated under the fingernails, consider removing the nails using local anesthesia. Wash these areas for 15–30 minutes. The injection of 0.5 mL of 10% calcium gluconate with local anesthetic per square centimeter under the burn area is effective but painful and must be repeated; an alternative that is proving far more acceptable and effective is injection of 0.5–2 mL of 10% calcium gluconate or calcium chloride into the radial or ulnar artery. Treat systemic effects promptly (see below).

B. Eye Burns: Wash eyes with running water for 15 minutes (see p 28) and then irrigate the eye with normal saline for 30–60 minutes. Cover the eyes with sterile bandages, allay pain by giving systemic analgesics, and take the patient to an ophthalmologist for evaluation of injury. Do not use chemical antidotes.

C. Inhalation: Remove patient to fresh air. Keep at complete rest. Treat pulmonary edema (see p 65).

D. Ingestion of Hydrogen Fluoride: Treat as for acid ingestion (see p 201).

E. Ingestion of Neutral Fluorides:

1. Emergency measures–Give soluble calcium in any form: milk, calcium gluconate solution, or calcium lactate solution. For calcium salts, the concentration should be 10 g in 250 mL of water. Give calcium gluconate, 10 g, and magnesium sulfate, 30 g, in 200 mL of water orally to precipitate and remove fluoride from the intestine.

2. Antidote–Give calcium gluconate, 10 mL of 10% solution intravenously slowly; repeat until symptoms disappear. If serum magnesium level is low, give milk of magnesia, 10 mL every hour.

3. General measures–

a. Give milk and cream every 4 hours to relieve irritation of the esophagus and stomach.

b. Treat shock (see p 66).

c. Give maximum amounts of fluids either orally or intravenously.

F. Fluorosis: Remove from further exposure.

Prognosis

After ingestion of neutral fluoride, survival for 48 hours is followed by recovery. After inhalation, survival for 3–4 days is usually followed by recovery. Skin burns require 1–2 months to heal.

In fluorosis from chronic exposure, removal from exposure for a year or more may be necessary before joint stiffness begins to reverse.

The prognosis in burns of the esophagus or stomach from hydrofluoric acid is the same as in acid burns (see p 202).

Grandjean P et al: Mortality and cancer morbidity after heavy occupational fluoride exposure. *Am J Epidemiol* 1985;**121**:57.

Mayer TG et al: Fatal systemic fluorosis due to hydrofluoric acid burns. *Ann Emerg Med* 1985;**14**:149.

Trevino MA et al: Treatment of severe hydrofluoric acid exposures. *J Occup Med* 1983;**25**:861.

15 | Metallic Poisons

ANTIMONY & STIBINE

Antimony is used in alloys, type metal, foil, batteries, ceramics, textiles, safety matches, ant paste, and a number of chemicals, including tartar emetic (antimony potassium tartrate). Acid treatment of metals containing antimony releases the colorless gas stibine (SbH_3).

The exposure limit for antimony is 0.5 mg/m^3. The exposure limit for stibine is 0.1 ppm. The fatal dose of antimony compounds by ingestion is 100–200 mg. Fatalities from antimony poisoning are rare.

The mechanism of poisoning is similar to that of arsenic poisoning, presumably by inhibition of enzymes through combination with sulfhydryl ($-SH$) groups.

Antimony is strongly irritating to mucous membranes and to tissues. Stibine causes hemolysis and irritation of the central nervous system.

Pathologic findings include fatty degeneration of the liver and parenchymatous degeneration in the liver and other organs. The gastrointestinal tract shows marked congestion and edema.

Clinical Findings

The principal manifestations of antimony poisoning are gastrointestinal disturbances. Stibine causes hemolysis.

A. Acute Poisoning:

1. Ingestion–The symptoms are nausea, vomiting, and severe diarrhea with mucus and later with blood. Hemorrhagic nephritis and hepatitis may also occur.

2. Inhalation (of stibine)–Headache, nausea and vomiting, weakness, jaundice, hemolysis, anemia, weak pulse.

B. Chronic Poisoning: (From fume and dust exposure.) Itching skin pustules, bleeding gums, conjunctivitis, laryngitis, headache, weight loss, and anemia. Antimony is suspected of being a carcinogen.

C. Laboratory Findings:

1. The red blood cell count is diminished. Eosinophils may reach 25% of total white cells.

2. The urine contains hemoglobin and red cells.

Prevention

Adequate fume and dust control is necessary to prevent the exposure limit from being exceeded.

Treatment

A. Acute Poisoning:

1. Emergency measures–

a. Remove ingested antimony compounds by gastric lavage or emesis (see pp 21–28).

b. Remove patient from further exposure to stibine.

2. Antidote–Give dimercaprol (see p 84).

3. General measures–

a. Treat as for arsenic poisoning (see p 223).

b. Treat hemolysis from stibine (see p 80).

B. Chronic Poisoning: Remove from further exposure and give dimercaprol (see p 84).

Prognosis

If the patient survives for 48 hours, recovery is probable.

ARSENIC & ARSINE

Arsenic is used in ant poisons, insecticides, weed killers, paint, wallpaper, ceramics, and glass. The action of acids on metals in the presence of arsenic forms arsine gas. Alloys such as ferrosilicon may release arsine upon contact with water, since the ferrosilicon may be contaminated with arsenic.

The fatal dose of arsenic trioxide is about 120 mg. In the USA, the allowable food residue is limited by federal law to 1.4 mg/kg. The exposure limit for arsine is 0.05 ppm (NIOSH 0.002 mg/m³); for arsenic, arsenic acid, arsenates, arsenites, and other compounds of arsenic, it is 0.5 mg/m³ (NIOSH 0.002 mg/m³). Organic arsenicals, such as arsphenamine, acetarsone, methane arsonic acid, and dimethylarsinic (cacodylic) acid, release arsenic slowly and are therefore less likely to cause acute poisoning, although at least one fatality has occurred from the vaginal use of acetarsone suppositories. The fatal dose for these compounds is estimated at 0.1–0.5 g/kg.

Arsenic presumably causes toxicity by combining with sulfhydryl (–SH) enzymes and interfering with cellular metabolism.

If death occurs within a few hours, the stomach mucosa shows inflammation but other pathologic changes are absent. If death occurs more than a few hours after poisoning, pathologic examination shows inflammatory changes and partial desquamation of the intestinal mucosa. The capillaries of the gastrointestinal tract are distended, and ecchymoses may be found. In immediate deaths from arsine poisoning, intravascular hemolysis is found. If death is delayed for several days after poisoning with arsenic in any form, the liver and kidneys show degenerative changes.

Clinical Findings

The principal manifestations of arsenic poisoning are gastrointestinal disturbances. The principal manifestation of arsine poisoning is hemolysis.

A. Acute Poisoning:

1. Ingestion—After ingestion of overwhelming amounts of arsenic (10 times the MLD), initial symptoms are those of violent gastroenteritis: burning esophageal pain, vomiting, and copious watery or bloody diarrhea containing shreds of mucus. Later, the skin becomes cold and clammy, the blood pressure falls, and weakness is marked. Death is from circulatory failure. Convulsions and coma are the terminal signs. If death is not immediate, jaundice and oliguria or anuria appear after 1–3 days.

Doses approaching the MLD cause restlessness, nausea and vomiting, headache, dizziness, chills, cramps, irritability, and variable paralysis that may progress over a period of several weeks. Ventricular arrhythmias may occur.

2. Inhalation—Inhalation of arsenic dusts may cause acute pulmonary edema, restlessness, dyspnea, cyanosis, cough with foamy sputum, and rales.

3. Arsine—Exposure to arsine causes burning and stinging of the face and, after 3–4 hours, tightness of the chest, dysphagia, nausea and vomiting, diarrhea, and electrocardiographic abnormalities. Later, pulmonary edema, massive hemolysis, cyanosis, hemoglobinuria, renal failure, and liver damage can occur. The liver and spleen may be enlarged. At 10 ppm, arsine rapidly causes delirium, coma, and death.

B. Chronic Poisoning: (From ingestion or inhalation.) The following are affected variably:

1. Central nervous system—Polyneuritis, optic neuritis, anesthesias, paresthesias such as burning pains in the hands and feet.

2. Skin—Bronzing, alopecia, localized edema, dermatitis.

3. Gastrointestinal tract—Cirrhosis of the liver, nausea and vomiting, abdominal cramps, salivation.

4. General effects—Anemia and weight loss. Aplastic anemia has occurred.

5. Cardiovascular system and kidneys—Chronic nephritis, cardiac failure, dependent edema.

6. Tryparsamide administration has caused visual impairment and optic atrophy.

7. Melarsoprol has caused mild cardiac damage, hypertension, neuritis, colic, proteinuria, and rare fatalities.

8. Glycobiarsol has caused sensitivity reactions and hepatitis after oral administration.

9. Acetarsone (acetarsol) has caused sensitivity dermatitis, exfoliative dermatitis, jaundice, and angioneurotic edema.

10. Arsenic and its compounds are carcinogenic for skin, lungs, and liver and possibly other organ systems.

C. Laboratory Findings:

1. Acute poisoning–

a. The urine may contain red blood cells, protein, and casts.

b. Arsenic compounds may appear as bariumlike radiopaque material after ingestion.

c. In fatal arsenic poisoning, the blood level has ranged from 1 to 15 μg/mL.

d. After arsine inhalation, the urine contains hemoglobin and hemosiderin. The serum contains hemoglobin and methemalbumin.

2. Chronic poisoning–

a. Urinary excretion of arsenic at a rate above 100 μg/24 h or a blood arsenic level above 0.1 mg/L indicates exposure.

b. Renal or hepatic function may be impaired as shown by suitable tests (see pp 72 and 75).

c. Blood counts reveal neutrophilic leukopenia as well as anemia.

Prevention

Store arsenic safely. The exposure limit of arsine in air must be observed at all times. Acid treatment of metals or dilution of acid sludge must be done with adequate fume control.

Treatment

A. Acute Poisoning From Arsenic:

1. **Emergency measures**–Remove ingested arsenic by gastric lavage or emesis (see pp 21–28). Follow with a saline cathartic.

2. **Antidote**–Give dimercaprol (see p 84) for 2 days, then penicillamine (see p 87). Discontinue antidote when the urine arsenic level falls below 50 μg/24 h.

3. **General measures**–

a. Treat dehydration by giving 5% glucose in normal saline intravenously.

b. Treat shock (see p 66).

c. Treat pulmonary edema (see p 65).

d. Treat anuria (see p 72).

e. Treat liver damage (see p 77).

f. In severe poisoning, use hemodialysis after dimercaprol therapy to remove combined dimercaprol and arsenic.

B. Acute Poisoning From Arsine: Treat hemolytic reaction (see p 80). Exchange transfusions are useful to remove the hemoglobin-arsine complex. Dialysis is necessary during the period of hemoglobinuric renal failure. Antidotes appear to be useless.

C. Chronic Poisoning: Remove from further exposure and give dimercaprol (see p 84) or penicillamine (see p 87). Signs of arsenic intoxication disappear slowly.

Prognosis

In acute arsenic poisoning, survival for more than 1 week is usually followed by complete recovery. Complete recovery from chronic arsenic poisoning may require 6 months to 1 year.

Armstrong CW et al: Outbreak of fatal arsenic poisoning caused by contaminated drinking water. *Arch Environ Health* 1984;**39**:276.

Landrigan PJ: Arsenic: State of the art. *Am J Ind Med* 1981;**2**:5.

Landrigan PJ et al: Occupational exposure to arsine. *Scand J Work Environ Health* 1982;**8**:169.

Peters HA et al: Seasonal arsenic exposure from burning chromium-copper-arsenate-treated wood. *JAMA* 1984;**251**:2393.

Takahashi W et al: Urinary arsenic, chromium, and copper levels in workers exposed to arsenic-based wood preservatives. *Arch Environ Health* 1983;**38**:209.

BERYLLIUM

Beryllium is used in alloys for electrical and other equipment. It is present in some fluorophors used in cathode ray tubes but is no longer used in fluorophors in fluorescent lamps.

The fatal dose of beryllium is not known. The exposure limit in air for beryllium is 0.002 mg/m^3.

Between 1941 and 1966, 760 cases of berylliosis were recorded in a national registry (Massachusetts General Hospital, Boston). Between 1966 and 1973, 76 new cases were recorded. Beryllium appears to inhibit certain magnesium-activated enzymes. The relationship between this effect and the pathologic changes induced by beryllium is not understood.

Soluble beryllium salts are directly irritating to skin and mucous membranes and induce acute pneumonitis with pulmonary edema. At least some of the changes present in acute pneumonitis and chronic pulmonary granulomatosis develop as a result of hypersensitivity to the beryllium in the tissues.

At pathologic examination, granulomas consisting of monocytes, lymphocytes, and fibrous tissue are found at the site of beryllium localization. In deaths from acute pneumonitis, the lung alveoli are filled with mononuclear and plasma cells.

Clinical Findings

The principal manifestation of beryllium poisoning is dyspnea.

A. Acute Poisoning:

1. Inhalation–Acute pneumonitis, with chest pain, bronchial spasm, fever, dyspnea, cyanosis, cough, blood-tinged sputum, and nasal discharge. Right heart failure may occur as a result of increased pulmonary arterial resistance. Onset of symptoms occurs 2–5 weeks after an exposure of 1–20 days.

2. Skin contact–Cuts from beryllium-contaminated objects form deep ulcerations that are slow to heal. Acute dermatitis from contact with dust stimulates first- and second-degree burns.

3. Eye contact–Dust contamination causes acute conjunctivitis with corneal maculae and diffuse erythema.

B. Chronic Poisoning:

1. Inhalation–In chronic pulmonary granulomatosis (berylliosis), weight loss and marked dyspnea begin 3 months to 11 years after the first exposure. The disease may pursue a steady downhill course or may be marked by exacerbations and remissions. Right heart failure may occur as a result of increased pulmonary resistance. Fever is variable. The incidence of lung cancer is increased in workers exposed to beryllium.

2. Skin contact–Eczematous dermatitis with a maculopapular, erythematous, vesicular rash appears in a large percentage of workers exposed to beryllium dusts. In such patients, patch tests with dilute beryllium solutions show positive reactions.

C. Laboratory Findings: These are noncontributory.

D. X-Ray Findings:

1. Radiologic examination in acute pneumonitis reveals a diffuse increase in density of the lung fields.

2. In chronic pulmonary granulomatosis, radiologic examination reveals a "snowstorm" appearance of the lungs.

Prevention

Dusts and fumes from beryllium processes must be rigidly controlled. No beryllium is allowable in air.

Chest x-rays are not useful in controlling exposure or in case-finding. Positive radiologic findings may be seen in the absence of symptoms or may occur only at the onset of symptoms. Workers may be asymptomatic and have normal chest x-rays during exposure to beryllium, and yet they may develop symptoms and positive chest x-ray findings many years after discontinuing exposure.

Treatment

A. Acute Pneumonitis:

1. Emergency measures–

a. Complete bed rest is necessary.

b. If cyanosis is present, give 40–60% O_2 by mask or intratracheal tube as necessary to maintain arterial P_{O_2} above 60 mm Hg. Ventilatory assistance may be necessary.

2. Antidote–The administration of calcium edetate has been suggested (see p 85).

3. General measures–

a. Relieve bronchial spasm–Give epinephrine, 0.2 mg (0.2 mL of 1:1000 solution) subcutaneously, or aminophylline, 0.25 g intravenously every 6 hours.

b. Treat bronchial pneumonia–Give organism-specific chemotherapy.

c. For right heart failure–Digitalize.

d. Give prednisone or equivalent corticosteroid, 25–50 mg/d orally, to decrease the hypersensitivity reaction to beryllium. These hormones relieve symptoms for varying lengths of time but are not curative.

B. Chronic Granuloma of Lungs (Berylliosis): Moderate activity is allowable. Maintain arterial P_{O_2} above 60 mm Hg by intermittent O_2 administration—if necessary, by mechanical ventilation. Adequate oxygenation delays the onset of pulmonary hypertension and cor pulmonale.

C. Skin Granuloma and Ulcers: Excise beryllium-contaminated areas of skin surgically.

D. Beryllium Dermatitis or Conjunctivitis:

1. Remove from further exposure. Wash skin and eyes thoroughly (see pp 28–29).

2. Apply local anesthetic ointment to control pain.

Prognosis

Recovery from acute pneumonitis requires 2–6 months. Deaths have been rare. Approximately 2% of patients with chronic pulmonary granulomatosis from beryllium (berylliosis) die. Adrenocortical hormones appear to improve symptoms without appreciably affecting the outcome of the disease.

Cotes JE et al: A long-term follow-up of workers exposed to beryllium. *Br J Ind Med* 1983;**40**:13.

CADMIUM

Cadmium is used for plating metals and in the manufacture of bearing alloys and silver solders. Cadmium plating is soluble in acid foods such as fruit juices and vinegar. When products containing cadmium are heated above its melting point (321 °C), cadmium fumes are released.

The fatal dose by ingestion is not known. Ingestion of as little as 10 mg will cause marked symptoms. At least 10 fatalities have occurred after exposure to cadmium fumes. The exposure limit for cadmium dusts or cadmium oxide fumes is 0.05 mg/m^3 (NIOSH 0.04 mg/m^3). Cadmium is damaging to all cells of the body.

The pathologic findings in cases of fatal cadmium ingestion are severe gastrointestinal inflammation and liver and kidney damage. In fatal acute poisoning from the inhalation of cadmium fumes, pathologic examination reveals inflammation of the pulmonary epithelium and pulmonary edema. Pathologic examination in fatalities following prolonged exposure to cadmium fumes reveals emphysema.

Clinical Findings

A. Acute Poisoning:

1. Ingestion–Nausea and vomiting, diarrhea, headache, muscular aches, salivation, abdominal pain, shock, liver damage, and renal failure.

2. Inhalation of cadmium fumes causes a metallic taste in the mouth, shortness of breath, pain in the chest, cough with foamy or bloody sputum, weakness, and pains in the legs. Chest examination reveals bubbling rales. Urine formation may be diminished later. Progression of the disease is indicated by onset of fever and by development of signs of lung consolidation.

B. Chronic Poisoning: (From inhalation.) Loss of sense of smell, cough, dyspnea, weight loss, anemia, irritability, and yellow-stained teeth. The liver and kidneys may be damaged. The incidence of carcinoma of the prostate is increased in workers exposed to cadmium.

C. Laboratory Findings:

1. Hematuria and proteinuria are present.

2. The red and white blood cell counts are low. The erythrocyte sedimentation rate may be elevated.

3. After ingestion or chronic inhalation, hepatic cell function may be impaired as shown by appropriate tests (see p 75).

D. X-Ray Findings: After inhalation, early chest x-rays show a diffuse increase in lung density; later findings are those of bronchial pneumonia.

Prevention

The exposure limit for cadmium fumes must always be observed. Acid foods should never be stored or prepared in cadmium-plated cooking utensils.

Treatment

A. Inhalation:

1. Remove patient from further exposure.

2. Treat pulmonary edema (see p 65).

3. Calcium disodium edetate (see p 85) given intravenously or intramuscularly appears to be effective. Give 25 mg/kg twice daily for 1 week and repeat if necessary after a 2-day interval. Do not give dimercaprol.

B. Ingestion:

1. Allay gastrointestinal irritation–Give milk or beaten eggs every 4 hours.

2. Catharsis–Remove unabsorbed cadmium by catharsis with Fleet's Phospho-Soda, 30–60 mL diluted 1:4 in water.

3. Give calcium disodium edetate (see p 85) if symptoms persist. Do not give dimercaprol.

4. Treat liver damage (see p 77).

5. Treat renal failure (see p 72).

Prognosis

Symptoms from cadmium ingestion usually last no more than 24 hours. In fume inhalation, the mortality rate has been approximately 15%. Survival for more than 4 days is followed by recovery, but complete recovery may take 6 months.

Engvall J, Perk J: Prevalence of hypertension among cadmium-exposed workers. *Arch Environ Health* 1985;**40**:185.

Friberg L: Cadmium. *Annu Rev Public Health* 1983;**4**:367.

National Institute of Occupational Safety and Health: Cadmium. *Current Intelligence Bulletin* 1984;**42**:1.

CHROMIUM

Chromium is used in chemical synthesis, steel-making, electroplating, and leather tanning and as a radiator anti-rust.

The fatal dose of a soluble chromate such as potassium chromate, potassium bichromate, or chromic acid is approximately 5 g. The toxicity of chromium compounds depends on the valence state of the metal. The exposure limit for metal dust and chromium salts of valence 2 or 3 is 0.5 mg/m^3. Most soluble and insoluble compounds of valence 6, including chromic acid, chromates, bichromates, zinc chromate, lead chromate, and chromite ore, have an exposure limit of 0.05 mg/m^3. The exposure limit for tertiary butyl chromate is 0.1 mg/m^3, and that for chromyl chloride is 0.025 ppm or 0.15 mg/m^3. Up to 20% of chromium workers develop dermatitis.

Chromium and chromates are irritating and destructive to all cells of the body. In fatalities from acute poisoning, hemorrhagic nephritis is found.

Clinical Findings

The principal manifestation of chromium poisoning is irritation or corrosion.

A. Acute Poisoning: (From ingestion.) Dizziness, intense thirst, abdominal pain, vomiting, shock, and oliguria or anuria. Death is from uremia.

B. Chronic Poisoning: (From inhalation or skin contact.) Repeated skin contact leads to incapacitating eczematous dermatitis with edema, and ulceration that heals slowly. Breathing chromium fumes over long periods causes painless ulceration, bleeding, and perforation of the nasal septum accompanied by a foul nasal discharge. Conjunctivitis, lacrimation, and acute hepatitis with jaundice have also been observed. Findings in acute hepatitis include nausea and vomiting, loss of appetite, and an enlarged, tender liver.

The incidence of lung cancer is increased up to 15 times normal in workers exposed to dusty chromite, chromic oxide, and chromium ores. All compounds in which chromium has a valence of 6 are considered to be carcinogens.

C. Laboratory Findings:

1. Proteinuria and hematuria are present.

2. Hepatic cell function impairment may be revealed by appropriate tests (see p 75).

Prevention

The exposure limit must always be observed. Chromic mist, fumes, and dust must be controlled. Chromate solutions must not come in contact with the skin.

Treatment

A. Acute Poisoning:

1. Emergency measures–Remove swallowed chromate by gastric lavage or emesis (see pp 21–28).

2. Antidote–Use of dimercaprol has been suggested on the basis of findings in animals (see p 84).

3. General measures–If oliguria or anuria is present, carefully maintain fluid and electrolyte balance (see p 72).

B. Chronic Poisoning:

1. Treat weeping dermatitis with 1% aluminum acetate wet dressings. Avoid further exposure to chromate.

2. Treat liver damage by giving high-carbohydrate, high-protein, high-vitamin diet.

Prognosis

In acute poisoning, rapid progression to anuria indicates a poor outcome. Dermatitis and liver damage will respond when the patient is removed from further exposure.

Ellis EN et al: Effects of hemodialysis and dimercaprol in acute dichromate poisoning. *J Toxicol Clin Toxicol* 1982;**19**:249.

Franchini I et al: Mortality experience among chrome plating workers. *Scand J Work Environ Health* 1983;**9**:247.

LEAD

Lead is used in type metal, storage batteries, industrial paint, solder, electric cable covering, pottery glaze, rubber, toys, gasoline (tetraethyl lead), and brass alloys. Other sources include plastic beads or jewelry coated with lead to give a pearl appearance; illicit whiskey; home-glazed pottery; leaded glass; the dust in shooting galleries; ashes and fumes from burning old painted wood, newspapers, magazines, and battery cases; and artists' paint pigments. The amount of lead in a sample of ash resulting from burning black-ink newsprint was less than 5 mg/kg, and that in a sample of ash from burned colored-ink newsprint (comics) was 57.7 mg/kg.

The amount of lead in economic circulation or that has been lost from use is enormous. From 1720 to 1979, 54,867,900 tons of lead were added to the supply in the USA. In 1979, 731,000 tons of lead were added to the supply in the USA by importation and mine production. In the same year, 187,000 tons of lead were used in gasoline additives, down from 253,000 tons used in 1970. In total, more than 7 million tons of lead have been used in gasoline additives in the USA. Much of the lead from gasoline additives and paints is still distributed on the earth's surface. House dust may have 7500 mg of lead per kilogram, compared to an average of 15 mg/kg in the earth's crust. Undisturbed surface soils in urban areas usually contain more than 500 mg of lead per kilogram in the top centimeter.

The fatal dose of absorbed lead has been estimated to be 0.5 g. Accumulation and toxicity occur if more than 0.5 mg/d is absorbed. The half-life of lead in bone is 32 years, and the half-life of lead in the kidney is 7 years. The exposure limit for lead and lead arsenate in air is 0.15 mg/m^3. The average level of lead in community air should not exceed 1.5 μg/m^3 per calendar quarter. The exposure limit for lead in food is 2.56 mg/kg. The exposure limit for tetraethyl or tetramethyl lead is 0.07 mg of lead per cubic meter.

Since 1972, 3,350,000 children between ages 1 and 5 years have been screened for blood lead levels. Of these, 6.6% had a blood lead level in the toxic range. In the past, as many as 200 deaths per year were due to lead encephalopathy; most were in children who lived in homes built before 1940 and resulted from exposure to lead-based paints.

The most serious toxic effects result from effects of lead on the brain and peripheral nervous system. The brain and liver lead levels may be 5–10 times the blood level. The lead in these tissues is only slowly removable by deleading agents. Since only uncombined lead is removed effectively by deleading agents, the increased excretion of lead brought about by such agents is only temporary. The deleading agent only becomes effective again when further lead has been released from combination.

Erythrocyte δ-aminolevulinic acid dehydratase, an enzyme important in hemoglobin synthesis, is one of the most sensitive indicators of the effect of lead. The free erythrocyte protoporphyrin level is an even more sensitive indicator of lead toxicity. Free erythrocyte protoporphyrin levels above 25–50 μg/dL are considered abnormal; however, because free erythrocyte protoporphyrin levels are also high in iron deficiency states, they cannot be used alone to diagnose lead poisoning. The activity of erythrocyte δ-aminolevulinic acid dehydratase is partially inhibited at blood lead levels of 10 μg/dL. Half of all individuals had blood lead levels greater than this in 1980. In 1976, the mean blood lead level was 15.8 μg/dL.

In acute poisoning, pathologic findings include inflammation of the gastrointestinal mucosa and renal tubular degeneration. In chronic lead poisoning, cerebral edema and degeneration of nerve and muscle cells occur. There may be cellular infiltration around capillaries and arterioles. The liver and kidneys show intranuclear inclusion bodies.

Clinical Findings
(Table 15–1)

Any symptoms suggestive of incipient encephalopathy should be considered an emergency. A rapid presumptive diagnosis can be based on the presence of the following: blood lead level above 50–80 μg/dL; free erythrocyte protoporphyrin above 200–250 μg/dL; and the appearance of radiopaque material on a plain film of the abdomen and radiopaque lead lines in the wrists and knees. Any positive finding in addition to suggestive symptoms may be sufficient indication to start therapy. Any child who has minor symptoms of poisoning can develop acute encephalopathy suddenly if the blood lead level is above 80 μg/dL.

To determine abnormal lead exposure, give calcium disodium edetate, 25 mg/kg as a single intramuscular injection or intravenously over $1\frac{1}{2}$ hours as a 0.5% solution in 5% dextrose in water. Collect all urine for 24 hours if kidney function is normal or for 3–4 days in renal insufficiency. Compare the urine lead level after calcium disodium edetate with prior urine lead levels.

The principal manifestations of lead poisoning are gastrointestinal or central nervous system disturbances and anemia.

Table 15–1. Symptoms and signs in the diagnosis of lead poisoning.

	Suggestive	Incipient Intoxication	More Advanced or Definite Plumbism
General appearance	Patient feels restive, moody, easily excited, "flustered."	Pallor, lead line, jaundice.	Lead line, jaundice, emaciation, "premature aging," weight loss, lethargy.
Digestive system	Persistent metallic taste, slight loss of appetite, slight constipation.	Metallic taste, definite loss of appetite, slight abdominal colic, constipation.	Nausea and vomiting, marked abdominal pain, rigid abdomen, marked constipation, blood in stool.
Nervous system	Patient is irritable and uncooperative.	Slight headache, insomnia, slight dizziness, palpitation, increased irritability, increased reflexes.	Persistent headaches, ataxia, confusion. Marked reflex changes, tremor, fibrillary twitching, neuritis, visual disturbances, encephalitis (hallucinations, convulsions, coma), paralysis.
Miscellaneous changes	None.	Muscle soreness, easy fatigability, hypotension.	General weakness, joint pains, hypertension, bone density.
Urine examination	Urine excretion of lead greater than 0.08 mg/d.	Trace of protein, few granular casts.	Increase in protein and casts. Coproporphyrinuria, hematuria, glycosuria, aminoaciduria, oliguria.
Blood changes	Polycythemia or anemia, polychromatophilia, increased platelets, percentage of reticulocytes about doubled.	Increase in reticulocytes. From 50 to 100 stippled cells per 100,000 erythrocytes. Blood lead over 60 μg/dL. Decrease in hemoglobin. Decrease in total number of red blood cells below 4 million. Increase in all forms of basophilic cells. Increase in percentage of mononuclears. Anisocytosis and poikilocytosis. Nucleated red cells present in peripheral circulation. Decreased platelets.	

A. Acute Poisoning: (From ingestion or injection of soluble or rapidly absorbed compounds of lead.) Metallic taste, abdominal pain, vomiting, diarrhea, black stools, oliguria, collapse, and coma.

B. Chronic Poisoning: (From ingestion, skin absorption, or inhalation of particulate or organic lead.) The diagnosis should be considered in any walking or crawling child with any of the symptoms given below who lives in or visits a house built before 1940.

1. Early–Loss of appetite, weight loss, constipation, apathy or irritability, occasional vomiting, fatigue, headache, weakness, metallic taste, lead line on gums, loss of recently developed skills, and anemia.

2. More advanced–Intermittent vomiting; irritability; nervousness; incoordination; vague pains in arms, legs, joints, and abdomen; sensory disturbances of extremities; paralysis of extensor muscles of

arms and legs with wrist and foot drop; disturbance of menstrual cycle; and abortion.

3. Severe–Persistent vomiting, ataxia, periods of stupor or lethargy, encephalopathy (with visual disturbances), elevated blood pressure, papilledema, cranial nerve paralysis, delirium, convulsions, and coma. Severe symptoms occur most frequently in lead poisoning in children or in adults exposed to tetraethyl lead.

4. Exposure to tetraethyl lead or tetramethyl lead causes insomnia, disturbing dreams, emotional instability, hyperactivity, convulsions, and even toxic psychosis. The organic form of lead localizes in neural tissue.

C. Laboratory Findings: The following findings are suggestive of lead poisoning (Table 15–1).

1. Blood–Hemoglobin below 13 g/dL of blood. A blood lead level above 5 μg/dL indicates exposure to lead, and one above 25 μg/dL suggests the need for a search for the source of lead and its elimination. The risk of encephalopathy is great at blood lead levels over 80 μg/dL; a level of 100 μg/dL should be considered an emergency, although much higher levels have been found in asymptomatic individuals.

Free erythrocyte protoporphyrin is a sensitive test of lead toxicity (as well as of iron deficiency), and erythrocyte porphyrin fluorescence can be measured directly on diluted whole blood as a screening test.

2. Urine–

a. Urinary lead excretion greater than 0.08 mg/d or urine coproporphyrin above 0.15 mg/24 h. A urine coproporphyrin level above 0.8 mg/L occurs only in symptomatic poisoning in adults. A urine δ-aminolevulinic acid level above 6 mg/L indicates that some lead effects have occurred. A level above 19 mg/L is associated with symptoms of lead poisoning. Glycosuria, hematuria, and proteinuria also occur.

b. Urinary excretion of more than 1 μg of lead per milligram of calcium edetate after intramuscular administration of calcium edetate at 25 mg/kg but not exceeding 1 g total.

3. Spinal fluid–Lumbar puncture should be avoided unless necessary for diagnosis. Spinal fluid examination reveals elevated protein, pleocytosis, and increased spinal fluid pressure in approximately one-third of children with lead poisoning.

D. X-Ray Findings: X-ray evidence of transverse bands of increased density at the ends of growing bones is present in chronic poisoning in children and is most likely at ages 2–5 years. Multiple bands represent repeated episodes of poisoning. A film of the abdomen reveals opaque particles, especially in the rectosigmoid area, if paint or other lead products have been ingested recently. Cerebral edema is evident on CT scans.

Prevention

Lead-containing paint should not be used indoors. Painters and lead workers must change clothing and bathe before eating. Effective dust-control filter masks should be worn when sanding or wire-brushing lead-containing paint. Lead-containing paint should only be burned with adequate fume control, since lead-containing fumes are emitted. Precautions must be taken to keep lead in air below the exposure limit. Children must not be allowed to play with lead toys.

Treatment

It may be necessary to start treatment as soon as blood and urine samples are obtained for lead analysis.

A. Emergency Measures: Remove ingested soluble lead compounds by gastric lavage with dilute magnesium sulfate or sodium sulfate solution or by emesis (see pp 21–28). Treat cerebral edema with mannitol and prednisolone or other corticosteroid (see below).

B. Antidotes: Dimercaprol and calcium disodium edetate, and later penicillamine, should be given to all patients with clinical symptoms of lead poisoning and should be considered for asymptomatic patients with blood lead levels over 80–100 μg/dL or free erythrocyte protoporphyrin levels over 250–300 μg/dL of whole blood.

1. Urine flow–Initiate urine flow first. Give 10% dextrose in water intravenously, 10–20 mL/kg body weight over a period of 1–2 hours. If urine flow does not start, give mannitol, 20% solution, 5–10 mL/kg body weight intravenously over 20 minutes. Fluid must be limited to requirements, and catheterization may be necessary in coma. Daily urine output should be 350–500 mL/m^2/24 h. Excessive fluids further increase cerebral edema.

2. Use in children–Give dimercaprol, 4 mg/kg intramuscularly every 4 hours for 30 doses. Beginning 4 hours later, give calcium disodium edetate at a separate injection site, 12.5 mg/kg intramuscularly every 4 hours as 20% solution, with 0.5% procaine added, for a total of 30 doses. If significant improvement has not occurred by the fourth day, increase the number of injections by 10 for each drug. In patients without encephalopathy who respond well, dimercaprol can be discontinued after the third or fourth day and edetate reduced to 50 mg/kg/24 h for the remainder of the 5-day course of injections. Two to 3 weeks after the first course, if the blood lead level is still above 80 μg/dL, give a second course of 30 injections each of both drugs. Courses of calcium disodium edetate should not exceed 500 mg/kg, with at least 1 week between courses.

For follow-up care, place the child in a protected environment to make certain that further ingestion of lead does not occur; give penicillamine (Cuprimine) orally, 30 mg/kg daily in 2 doses, for 3–6 months or until blood lead level falls below 60 μg/dL. The maximum dose is

500 mg/d. Give penicillamine on an empty stomach 90 minutes before meals.

3. Use in adults–Adults with acute encephalopathy should be given dimercaprol and calcium disodium edetate in the same way as for children. For other symptomatic adults, the course of dimercaprol and calcium disodium edetate can be shortened or calcium disodium edetate only can be given in a dosage of 50 mg/kg intravenously as 0.5% solution in 5% dextrose in water or normal saline by infusion over not less than 8 hours for not more than 5 days. Follow with penicillamine, 500–750 mg/d orally for 1–2 months or until urine lead level drops below 0.3 mg/24 h.

C. General Measures in Acute Encephalopathy:

1. For cerebral edema, give mannitol, 20% solution, 5 mL/kg by intravenous injection at a rate not to exceed 1 mL/min. Give prednisolone, 1–2 mg/kg intravenously or intramuscularly, or other corticosteroid in equivalent doses, every 4 hours.

2. Do not use catharsis or enemas in the presence of severe symptoms.

3. Control convulsions with cautious administration of phenobarbital, hydantoin anticonvulsants, or diazepam. Associated depression of respiration may increase cerebral edema and can be hazardous in the acute stage.

4. Reduce fever with cooling blanket.

5. Maintain urine output at 350–500 mL/m²/24 h by giving 10% dextrose in water parenterally. Avoid administration of sodium-containing fluids.

6. Withhold oral fluid, food, and medication for at least 3 days.

D. Special Problems:

1. In the presence of impaired renal function, dialysis is mandatory.

2. Wrist drop and foot drop may be corrected by splinting and passive exercise until function returns.

3. Toxicity from tetraethyl lead and tetramethyl lead does not respond to chelation therapy. Give barbiturates or diazepam to control hyperactivity.

Prognosis

Until recently, the mortality rate in patients with lead encephalopathy was about 25%. About half of those who survived had permanent mental deterioration. The effect of calcium disodium edetate on the prognosis in lead encephalopathy has not been determined as yet.

Complete recovery from other forms of lead poisoning takes up to 1 year.

Annest JL et al: Chronological trend in blood lead levels between 1976 and 1980. *N Engl J Med* 1983;**308:**1373.

Baker EL et al: Occupational lead neurotoxicity: A behavioural and electrophysiological evaluation. *Br J Ind Med* 1984;**41:**352.

Bellinger DC, Needleman HL: Lead and relationship between maternal and child intelligence. *J Pediatr* 1983;**102:**523.

Beritić T: Lead neuropathy. *CRC Crit Rev Toxicol* 1984;**12:**149.

Berwick BM, Komaroff AL: Cost effectiveness of lead screening. *N Engl J Med* 1982;**306:**1392.

Bose A et al: Azarćon por empacho: Another cause of lead toxicity. *Pediatrics* 1983;**72:**106.

Charney E et al: Childhood lead poisoning: A controlled trial of the effect of dust control measures on blood lead levels. *N Engl J Med* 1983;**309:**1089.

Coulihan JL et al: Gasoline sniffing and lead toxicity in Navajo adolescents. *Pediatrics* 1983;**71:**113.

Farfel MR: Reducing lead exposure in children. *Annu Rev Public Health* 1985;**6:**333.

Folk remedy-associated lead poisoning in Hmong children—Minnesota. *MMWR* 1983;**32:**555.

Hryhorczuk DO et al: Elimination kinetics of blood lead in workers with chronic lead intoxication. *Am J Ind Med* 1985;**8:**33.

Jeyaratnam J et al: Neurophysiological studies on workers exposed to lead. *Br J Ind Med* 1985;**42:**173.

Lead poisoning-associated deaths from Asian-Indian folk remedies—Florida. *MMWR* 1984;**33:**638.

Lilis R: Long-term occupational lead exposure, chronic nephropathy, and renal cancer. *Am J Ind Med* 1981;**2:**293.

Maracek J: Low-level lead exposure in childhood influences neuropsychological performance. *Arch Environ Health* 1983;**38:**355.

Markowitz ME, Rosen JF: Assessment of lead stores in children: Validation of an 8-hour CaNa$_2$EDTA provocative test. *J Pediatr* 1984;**104:**337.

Needleman HL, Landrigan PJ: The health effects of low level exposure to lead. *Annu Rev Public Health* 1982;**2:**277.

Piomelli S et al: Management of childhood lead poisoning. *J Pediatr* 1984;**105:**523.

Results of blood lead determinations among workers potentially exposed to lead—United States. *MMWR* 1983;**32:**216.

Ross CA: Gasoline sniffing and lead encephalopathy. *Can Med Assoc J* 1982;**127:**1195.

MANGANESE

Manganese is used in the manufacture of steel and dry cell batteries. Manganese dietary supplements are sometimes available. Their toxicity is unknown.

The exposure limits for manganese and manganese compounds are as follows: dust, 5 mg/m^3; fumes, 1 mg/m^3; tetroxide, 1 mg/m^3; manganese cyclopentadienyl tricarbonyl, 0.1 mg/m^3; methyl manganese cyclopentadienyl tricarbonyl, 0.2 mg/m^3. Manganese cyclopentadienyl tricarbonyl and methyl manganese cyclopentadienyl tricarbonyl are used as anti-knock additives in gasoline. These substances are readily absorbed through the skin.

The toxic amount from inhalation is not known. Fatalities are rare.

The mechanism of manganese poisoning is not known. Inhalation of manganese fumes or dusts produces progressive deterioration in the central nervous system. Large oral doses of manganese compounds are without systemic effect in experimental animals.

The findings in one death suspected to be from ingesting manganese-contaminated drinking water were atrophy and disappearance of cells of the globus pallidus. Experimental animals show inflammatory changes in both gray and white matter.

Clinical Findings

The principal manifestations of poisoning with these compounds are central nervous system disturbances.

A. Acute Poisoning: (From ingestion, inhalation, or skin absorption.) Single exposure to the manganese cyclopentadienyl tricarbonyls causes edema, bleeding, hypotension, nerve atrophy, renal damage, hyperactivity, convulsions, and coma.

B. Chronic Poisoning: (From ingestion or inhalation.)

1. Ingestion–Drinking manganese-contaminated well water caused lethargy, edema, and symptoms of extrapyramidal tract lesions in one outbreak. Chronic poisoning from ingesting manganese in other forms has not been reported.

2. Inhalation–Inhalation of manganese dusts causes acute bronchitis, nasopharyngitis, pneumonia, headache, itching, numbness of the extremities, impairment of libido, sleep disturbances, dermatitis, and liver enlargement. Later, there are gradually progressive signs that simulate parkinsonism. These include weakness in the legs, increased muscle tone, hand tremor, slurred speech, muscle cramps, spastic gait, fixed facial expression, and mental deterioration.

3. Chronic exposure to the manganese cyclopentadienyl tricarbonyls causes effects like those of tetraethyl lead (see p 233).

C. Laboratory Findings:

1. Hepatic cell function may be impaired as shown by appropriate tests (see p 75).

2. Increased hemoglobin and red blood cell count; decrease in monocytes.

3. Cerebrospinal fluid may contain traces of globulin.

Prevention

Workers should change clothing and bathe on leaving work. Quarterly physical examinations of all exposed workers will aid in the discovery of early changes.

Batteries must not be buried near water supplies.

Treatment of Chronic Poisoning

A. Immediate Measures: Remove from further exposure.

B. Antidote: Calcium edetate is effective in removing manganese but has no permanent effect on symptomatic patients in the late stages of manganism.

C. General Measures: Oral levodopa, beginning with 0.1 g 3–5 times a day and gradually increasing to a total daily dose of 8 g/d, or D,L-5-hydroxytryptophan, up to 3 g daily, is reported to be effective against some central nervous system symptoms.

Prognosis

While liver damage and respiratory system damage from manganese are reported to improve with administration of calcium disodium edetate, this antidote has no effect on the symptoms of central nervous system deterioration. If exposure is discontinued when central nervous system symptoms first appear, recovery is possible.

Bencko V: Manganese: A review of occupational and environmental toxicology. *J Hyg Epidemiol Microbiol Immunol* 1984;**28**:139.

Chandra SV et al: An exploratory study of manganese in welders. *Clin Toxicol* 1981;**18**:407.

Taylor PA, Price JDE: Acute manganese intoxication and pancreatitis in a patient treated with contaminated dialysate. *Can Med Assoc J* 1982;**126**:503.

MERCURY

Mercury is a liquid. Air saturated with mercury at 20 °C contains about 15 mg/m^3. At 40 °C, saturated air contains 68 mg/m^3.

Mercury and its salts are used in the manufacture of thermometers, felt, paints, explosives, lamps, electrical apparatus, and batteries. The diethyl and dimethyl mercury compounds are used in treating seeds. Mercurous chloride (calomel) and organic mercurials were formerly used medicinally.

The fatal dose of mercuric salts such as mercuric chloride (corrosive sublimate) is 1 g. Ingested metallic mercury is ordinarily not toxic, since it is not absorbed. However, metallic mercury retained in the lung or injected intravenously can produce toxicity, although often it does not. Mercury vapor is in the monatomic state and is lipophilic. It is transferred to brain cells, where it is oxidized to Hg^{2+} to produce toxic effects. Inhaled mercury vapor causes acute pneumonitis. Mercurous chloride, ammoniated mercury, mercury protoiodide, and organic antiseptic mercurials such as acetomeroctol, merbromin, mercocresol, nitromersol, phenylmercuric salts and esters, and thimerosal (Merthiolate) are not likely to cause acute poisoning because they are poorly absorbed. The single fatal dose of these compounds is 2–4 times the fatal dose of soluble inorganic mercury salts. The mercurial diuretics (mersalyl, meralluride, mercurophylline, mercumatilin, mercaptomerin, chlormerodrin, and merethoxylline) are almost as toxic as mercuric chloride in experimental animals when mercury content is compared. The exposure limit for mercury or mercury compounds is 0.05 mg/m^3 as mercury. Alkyl mercury compounds such as methyl mercury chloride, methyl mercury cyanide, methyl mercury hydroxide, methyl mercury pentachlorophenate, methyl mercury toluene sulfonate, ethyl mercury chloride (Ceresan), ethyl mercury phosphate, and ethyl mercury toluene sulfonate are more toxic than mercuric chloride, and the exposure limit is 0.01 mg of mercury per cubic meter. Other organic mercury compounds, such as hydroxymercuriphenol and cyanomethyl-mercuri-guanidine, are as toxic as an equivalent amount of mercury in mercuric chloride.

Environmental contamination from industrial discharge of organic mercury compounds has resulted in organic mercurial poisoning from eating fish from the discharge area (Minamata disease) and in teratogenesis. Seed grains treated with organic mercury fungicides have caused poisoning when used as food. The concentration of alkyl mercury compounds (methyl mercury) in food should not exceed 0.5 mg/kg; for foods at this level, intake should be limited to not more than 0.5 kg per week.

Mercury depresses cellular enzymatic mechanisms by combining with sulfhydryl (−SH) groups; for this reason, soluble mercuric salts are toxic to all cells. The high concentrations attained during renal excretion lead to specific damage to renal glomeruli and tubules.

In fatalities from mercury poisoning, the pathologic findings are acute tubular and glomerular degeneration or hemorrhagic glomerular nephritis. The mucosa of the gastrointestinal tract shows inflammation, congestion, coagulation, and corrosion.

Clinical Findings

The principal manifestations of mercury salt poisoning are gastrointestinal, hepatic, and renal damage.

A. Acute Poisoning:

1. Ingestion–Ingestion of mercuric salts causes metallic taste, thirst, severe abdominal pain, vomiting, and bloody diarrhea. Diarrhea of mucus shreds and blood may continue for several weeks. One day to 2 weeks after ingestion, urine output diminishes or stops. Death is from uremia. Esophageal, gastric, or intestinal stenosis may occur after mercuric chloride ingestion.

2. Inhalation–Inhalation of a high concentration of mercury vapor can cause almost immediate dyspnea, cough, fever, nausea and vomiting, diarrhea, stomatitis, salivation, and metallic taste. The symptoms may resolve or may progress to necrotizing bronchiolitis, pneumonitis, pulmonary edema, and pneumothorax. This syndrome is often fatal in children. Acidosis and renal damage with renal failure may occur. Inhaling volatile organic mercurials in high concentrations causes metallic taste, dizziness, clumsiness, slurred speech, diarrhea, and sometimes fatal convulsions.

3. Alkyl mercury compounds are concentrated in the central nervous system, with ataxia, chorea, athetosis, tremors, and convulsions. Damage tends to be permanent.

B. Chronic Poisoning:

1. Injection or ingestion–Injection of organic mercurial compounds or ingestion of insoluble or poorly dissociated mercuric salts— including mercurous chloride and organic mercurial compounds—over a prolonged period causes urticaria progressing to weeping dermatitis, stomatitis, salivation, diarrhea, anemia, leukopenia, liver damage, and renal damage progressing to acute renal failure with anuria. Injection of organic mercurial diuretics has caused depression or irregularities of cardiac function and anaphylaxis. In children, repeated administration of calomel in "teething powders" caused a syndrome known as erythredema polyneuropathy (acrodynia, or "pink disease"). Symptoms are photophobia, anorexia, restlessness, stomatitis, pains in the arms and legs, pink palms, oliguria, and severe diarrhea. The symptoms may persist for weeks or months.

2. Inhalation or skin contact–Inhalation of mercury vapor, dusts, or organic vapors or skin absorption of mercury or mercury compounds over a long period causes mercurialism. Findings are extremely variable and include tremors, salivation, stomatitis, loosening of the teeth, blue line on the gums, pain and numbness in the extremities, nephritis, diarrhea, anxiety, headache, weight loss, anorexia, mental depression, insomnia, irritability, instability, hallucinations, and evidence of mental deterioration.

C. Laboratory Findings:

1. The lowest blood concentration of methyl mercury associated with identifiable symptoms is 0.2 μg/mL. A tentative blood standard for methyl mercury or other organic mercury derivatives has been set: these should not exceed 0.1 μg/mL. Neuromuscular toxicity occurs at blood levels of inorganic mercury below 0.1 μg/mL.

2. Urinary excretion of more than 0.3 mg of mercury per 24 hours indicates the possibility of mercury poisoning. An average urinary mercury excretion rate above 0.1 mg/24 h in a group of mercury workers indicates the need for corrective measures for the work situation. An individual who shows over 0.2 mg/24 h in urine should be removed from

further exposure if the urinary excretion of mercury goes above 0.05 mg/24 h. The county or state health department will make arrangements for mercury analyses.

3. Proteinuria and hematuria (may be absent in chronic poisoning).

Prevention

The exposure limit must be observed at all times; frequent air sampling is necessary.

Floors in rooms where mercury is used must be impervious and free from cracks. Spilled mercury should be picked up immediately by water pump suction or by a wet sweeping compound. After handling mercury or mercury compounds, the skin must be thoroughly cleaned.

The administration of mercury in any form to children should be avoided. Ammoniated mercury should be replaced by less hazardous agents.

Treatment

A. Acute Poisoning:

1. Emergency measures–Remove ingested poison by gastric lavage with tap water or by emesis and catharsis (see pp 21–28).

2. Antidote–Give dimercaprol (see p 84). Hemodialysis will speed the removal of the mercury-dimercaprol complex. Penicillamine is also effective (see p 87). Neither penicillamine nor dimercaprol is effective against the neurologic effects of alkyl mercury compounds. A chelating agent should be continued until the urine mercury level falls below 50 μg/24 h.

3. General measures–

a. Treat anuria (see p 72) and shock (see p 66).

b. Treat stenotic lesions of the gastrointestinal tract after appropriate endoscopy. It has been suggested that neostigmine, 15–22.5 mg, and atropine, 2–3 mg daily in divided doses, will increase muscle strength in late stages of alkyl mercury poisoning.

B. Chronic Poisoning: Remove from further exposure. Give dimercaprol (see p 84). Treat oliguria (see p 72). Maintain nutrition by intravenous or oral feedings.

Prognosis

In acute and chronic poisoning, recovery is likely if dimercaprol treatment is given for at least 1 week. Recovery from mental deterioration caused by chronic mercury poisoning may never be complete. Brain damage from alkyl mercury compounds is more likely to be permanent. Improvement requires 1–2 years.

Adams CR et al: Mercury intoxication simulating amyotrophic lateral sclerosis. *JAMA* 1983;**250**:642.

Clark JA et al: Mercury poisoning from merbromin therapy of omphalocele. *Clin Pediatr* 1982;**21**:445.

Clarkson TW: Mercury. *Annu Rev Public Health* 1983;**4**:375.

El Hassani SB: The many faces of methyl mercury poisoning. *J Toxicol Clin Toxicol* 1982;**19**:875.

Fawer RF et al: Measurement of hand tremor induced by industrial exposure to metallic mercury. *Br J Ind Med* 1983;**40**:204.

Hryhorczuk DO et al: Treatment of mercury intoxication in a dentist with N-acetyl-d,1-penicillamine. *J Toxicol Clin Toxicol* 1982;**19**:401.

Jaffe KM et al: Survival after acute mercury vapor poisoning. *Am J Dis Child* 1983;**137**:749.

Lund ME et al: Treatment of acute methyl mercury ingestion by hemodialysis with N-acetylcysteine (Mucomyst) infusion and 2,3-dimercaptopropane sulfonate. *J Toxicol Clin Toxicol* 1984;**22**:31.

Roels H et al: Surveillance of workers exposed to mercury vapor. *Am J Ind Med* 1985;**7**:45.

Rohyans JA et al: Mercury toxicity following Merthiolate ear irrigations. *Pediatrics* 1984;**73**:311.

Stack P et al: Mercuric chloride poisoning in a 23-month-old child. *Br Med J* 1983;**287**:1513.

Tamachiro H et al: Causes of death in Minamata disease: Analysis of death certificates. *Int Arch Occup Environ Health* 1984;**54**:135.

NICKEL CARBONYL

Nickel carbonyl is formed by passing carbon monoxide over finely divided metallic nickel. Nickel carbonyl is a liquid that boils at 43 °C. It is important in the Mond process for refining nickel. It is also used in petroleum refining.

The exposure limit for nickel carbonyl is 0.05 ppm. Inhaled nickel carbonyl decomposes to metallic nickel, which deposits on the epithelium of the lung. This finely divided nickel is rapidly absorbed and damages the lung and brain. Postmortem examination in deaths caused by nickel carbonyl inhalation reveals edema and hyperemia of the lungs and brain. Areas of necrosis and hemorrhage are found in the brain and lungs.

Clinical Findings

The principal manifestation of nickel carbonyl poisoning is dyspnea.

A. Acute Poisoning: Inhalation of nickel carbonyl immediately causes cough, dizziness, headache, and malaise, which ordinarily can be relieved by removal to fresh air. Progressive dyspnea, cough, cyanosis, fever, rapid pulse, and nausea and vomiting may follow in 12–36 hours, and death from respiratory failure within 4–12 days.

B. Chronic Poisoning: Workers exposed to nickel carbonyl have a high incidence of lung cancer. Some workers develop dermatitis.

Prevention

The exposure limit for nickel carbonyl must always be observed. No person with chronic pulmonary disease should work where nickel carbonyl exposure can occur. Contaminated atmospheres can only be entered by using an airline face mask.

Treatment

A. Acute Poisoning:

1. Emergency measures–Treat cyanosis and dyspnea by giving 100% O_2 by mask. If pulmonary edema is present, treat as described on p 65.

2. Antidote–Give dimercaprol (see p 84). The administration of sodium diethyldithiocarbamate, 50–100 mg/kg/d orally or intramuscularly, has also been suggested.

3. General measures–After any exposure, keep the patient at absolute bed rest for the first 4 days after poisoning, even if asymptomatic. Thereafter, keep at bed rest until cyanosis is relieved.

B. Chronic Poisoning: Remove from further exposure.

Prognosis

Survival for more than 14 days is followed by recovery. Cyanosis and dyspnea are indices of the severity of poisoning.

Brown S, Sunderman FW Jr: *Nickel Toxicology*. Academic Press, 1981.
Sunderman FW: Chelation therapy in nickel poisoning. *Ann Clin Lab Sci* 1981;**11**:1.

PHOSPHORUS, PHOSPHINE, & PHOSPHIDES

Phosphorus exists in 2 forms: a red, granular, nonabsorbed, and nonpoisonous form; and a yellow, waxy, water-insoluble and fat-soluble, highly poisonous form that will burn on contact with air. Red phosphorus is sometimes contaminated with yellow phosphorus. The striking surface of a safety match contains 50% red phosphorus. Yellow phosphorus is used in rodent and insect poisons, fireworks, and fertilizer manufacture. The action of water or acids on metals will liberate phosphine if phosphorus is present as a contaminant. Phosphine may also be present in acetylene. Phosphides, which are used as rat poisons, release phosphine on contact with water. Phosphorus sesquisulfide (tetraphosphorus trisulfide) has low toxicity. The heads of 20 large wooden matches contain 220 mg.

Table 15—2. Uncommon poisons.

	Exposure Limit (ppm)	Effects	Treatment
Bacillus subtilis enzymes	0.00006*	Irritant, sensitizer.	Remove from exposure.
Bismuth telluride	10*	Granulomatous pulmonary lesions.	Remove from exposure.
Bismuth telluride with selenium	5	Granulomatous pulmonary lesions.	Remove from exposure.
Carbon dioxide gas	5000	3%—dyspnea and headache. 10%—visual disturbances, tinnitus, tremor, and loss of consciousness in 1 minute.	Give artificial respiration.
Cerium fumes		Pulmonary fibrosis, emphysema.	Remove from exposure.
Cobalt dust and fumes	0.05*	Inhalation causes shortness of breath, lung densities, dermatitis with hyperemia and vesiculation. Ingestion causes hypotension, pericardial effusion, polycythemia, congestive failure, pain, vomiting, nerve deafness, convulsions, enlargement of the thyroid.	Give calcium disodium edetate (see p 85).
Copper fumes or copper powder	0.2* 1*	Metal fume fever, sneezing, nausea. Renal damage may occur.	Give calcium disodium edetate (see p 85).
Epoxy hardeners (catalyst)		Consist of amines, organic acids or acid anhydrides, or polyamines. These cause irritation, sensitivity reactions, and corrosion of skin or mucous membranes after prolonged contact. Vapor hazard possible.	Remove ingested hardener by gastric lavage or emesis. Remove skin contamination by gentle scrubbing with soap and water. Avoid use of organic solvents, which may increase penetration.
Epoxy monomer (unpolymerized resin)		Skin irritant and sensitizer.	Remove by scrubbing gently with soap and water.
Epoxy resin (polymerized)		Inert, but may decompose at high temperature with release of irritating products, causing pulmonary edema.	Treat pulmonary edema.

*mg/m^3.

Table 15—2 (cont'd). Uncommon poisons.

	Exposure Limit (ppm)	Effects	Treatment
Ferrovanadium	1*	Irritation of the eyes and respiratory tract, bronchitis, pneumonitis.	Remove from exposure.
Fluorocarbon polymer fumes (Teflon)		Malaise; weakness; numbness and tingling in arms, fingers; pain in throat; and some difficulty in breathing. (From high-temperature decomposition of solid or aerosol Teflon or other fluorinated hydrocarbons.)	Remove from exposure.
Germanium compounds	0.6*	Bronchitis; pneumonitis; liver, kidney damage; hemolysis.	Remove from exposure.
Germanium tetrahydride	0.2	Like arsine.	See p 223.
Hafnium	0.5*	Salts are irritants and can cause liver damage.	Remove from exposure.
Indium	0.1*	Pulmonary damage.	Remove from exposure.
Iron, dicyclopentadienyl	10*	No effect?	
Iron dust, iron oxide fumes, iron salt fumes	10* 5* 1*	Conjunctivitis, choroiditis, and retinitis.	
Iron pentacarbonyl	0.01	Dizziness, headache, vomiting, coma.	
Magnesium metal		Skin implants cause necrosis, gangrene, subcutaneous emphysema.	Remove implant surgically.
Magnesium oxide fumes	10*	Fever.	Remove from exposure.
Molybdenum	5*	Possible irritation, CNS effects, liver and kidney damage.	Remove from exposure.
Molybdenum salts and fumes	5*	Irritation, weight loss, ataxia in animals.	Remove from exposure.
Nickel, nickel compounds	1 0.1*	Skin sensitization with itching dermatitis. Asthma occurs. Lung cancer.	Remove from exposure.
Platinum metal, platinum salts	1* 0.002*	Irritant, sensitizer, dermatitis, asthma.	Remove from exposure.
Polyurethane polymer		High temperature decomposition releases carbon monoxide.	See p 262.

*mg/m^3.

Table 15–2 (cont'd). Uncommon poisons.

	Exposure Limit (ppm)	Effects	Treatment
Polyvinyl chloride polymers		High-temperature decomposition releases hydrochloric acid, carbon monoxide, and phosgene.	See p 201.
Rhodium salts, rhodium fumes	0.01* 1*	Irritant and possible sensitizer.	Remove from exposure.
Selenate and selenium compounds orally		Damages liver, kidneys, gastrointestinal tract, heart, lungs. Death has occurred from therapeutic use.	Treat symptomatically. Both calcium edetate and dimercaprol have been shown to increase toxicity in experimental animals.
Selenium fumes	0.2*	Garlic breath, gastrointestinal upset, nervousness.	
Selenium hexafluoride, hydrogen selenide	0.05	Pneumonitis, pulmonary edema, bronchial pneumonia.	
Selenium oxide fumes	0.2*	Severe irritation, bronchospasm, difficulty in breathing, chills, fever, headaches, pneumonitis with consolidation clearing after 1–4 weeks.	
Silane	5	Irritant.	Remove from exposure.
Solder, rosin core pyrolysis products	0.1* (as HCHO)	Eye, bronchial, and pulmonary irritation.	Remove from exposure.
Tantalum	5*	Irritant.	Remove from exposure.
Tellurium fumes	0.1*	Garlic odor of breath, metallic taste, nausea, loss of appetite, liver injury.	Treat symptomatically.
Tributyl tin	0.1*	Severe irritation to necrosis.	Remove from exposure and treat symptomatically.
Triethyl tin	0.1*	Brain damage that may be permanent.	
Triphenyl tin	0.1*	Liver damage.	
Tungsten, insoluble salts and metal	5*	Pulmonary fibrosis.	Remove from exposure.
Tungsten, soluble salts	1*		
Uranium salts	0.2*	Pulmonary irritation, severe kidney degeneration, and cancers from radiation effects.	Give calcium disodium edetate (see p 85).

*mg/m^3.

Table 15–2 (cont'd). Uncommon poisons.

	Exposure Limit (ppm)	Effects	Treatment
Vanadium fumes, vanadium dust	0.05* 0.5*	Rhinorrhea, sneezing, sore chest, wheezing, dyspnea, weakness, bronchitis, pneumonitis.	Give ascorbic acid, 1 g/d. Calcium edetate may be useful (see p 85).
Welding fumes	5*	Irritation, pulmonary damage.	Remove from exposure.
Yttrium salts	1*	Pulmonary irritation.	Remove from exposure.
Zirconium oxide and salts	5*	Granulomas from skin application. Possible pneumonitis.	Remove from exposure.

*mg/m^3.

The fatal dose of yellow phosphorus or phosphides is approximately 1 mg/kg. The exposure limit for yellow phosphorus is 0.1 mg/m^3; for phosphine, 0.3 ppm; and for phenyl phosphine, 0.05 ppm.

Phosphorus causes tissue destruction, with disturbances in carbohydrate, fat, and protein metabolism in the liver. Deposition of glycogen in the liver is inhibited; deposition of fat is increased.

Chronic absorption of phosphorus increases bone formation under the epiphyseal cartilage and impairs blood circulation in bone by bone formation in haversian and marrow canals. These changes lead to necrosis and sequestration of bone; they occur most frequently in the mandible.

The pathologic findings in yellow phosphorus poisoning are jaundice, fatty degeneration and necrosis of the liver and kidneys, and hemorrhages, congestion, and erosion of the gastrointestinal tract. Pathologic findings from phosphine inhalation are pulmonary hyperemia and edema and focal myocardial necrosis. Zinc phosphide ingestion causes both fatty degeneration and necrosis of the liver and pulmonary hyperemia and edema.

Clinical Findings

The principal manifestations of poisoning with these compounds are jaundice and collapse.

A. Acute Poisoning:

1. Ingestion–Ingestion of yellow phosphorus is followed within 1–2 hours by nausea and vomiting, diarrhea, cardiac arrhythmias, and a garlic odor of breath and excreta. The breath and excreta may appear to smoke. Death in coma or cardiac arrest may occur in the first 24–48 hours, or symptoms may improve for 1 or 2 days and then return, with nausea and vomiting, diarrhea, liver tenderness and enlargement, jaun-

dice, prostration, fall of blood pressure, oliguria, hypocalcemic tetany, hypoglycemia, and multiple petechial hemorrhages. Onset of Cheyne-Stokes respiration followed by convulsions, coma, and death may occur up to 3 weeks after poisoning. Phosphide ingestion causes jaundice, liver tenderness and enlargement, and pulmonary edema with dyspnea and cyanosis. Death may occur up to a week after poisoning.

2. Skin contact–Yellow phosphorus allowed to dry on the skin will ignite and cause second- to third-degree burns surrounded by blisters. These burns heal slowly.

3. Inhalation–Inhalation of phosphorus is followed after 1–3 days by the symptoms of acute phosphorus poisoning. Phosphine or phosphide inhalation causes nausea and vomiting, fatigue, cough, jaundice, paresthesias, ataxia, intention tremor, diplopia, fall of blood pressure, dyspnea, pulmonary edema, collapse, cardiac arrhythmias, convulsions, and coma. Death usually occurs within 4 days; it may be delayed 1–2 weeks. Renal damage and leukopenia may appear after several days. Exposure to phenyl phosphine at 0.6 ppm causes hypersensitivity to sound and touch and hyperemia of the skin. Exposure at levels above 2 ppm causes hematologic effects, with decrease in red blood cell count, dermatitis, and nerve and testicular degeneration.

B. Chronic Poisoning: (From ingestion or inhalation of yellow phosphorus, phosphine, or phosphides.) The first symptom is toothache, followed by swelling of the jaw and then necrosis of the mandible (phossy jaw). Other findings are weakness, weight loss, loss of appetite, anemia, and spontaneous fractures.

C. Laboratory Findings:

1. Impairment of liver function is shown by appropriate tests (see p 75).

2. Blood urea nitrogen and bilirubin are increased. Acidosis may occur.

3. Hematuria and proteinuria may be present.

Prevention

The exposure limit for phosphorus, phosphine, and phosphides in the air must be observed at all times. Special clothing, to be changed daily, should be provided for phosphorus workers. Workers must bathe on leaving work and must be educated in the hazards of phosphorus exposure. Safety showers and eye fountains must be provided where yellow phosphorus is being used. Dental examination should be made frequently, depending on exposure.

Treatment

A. Acute Poisoning:

1. Emergency measures–Remove poison by gastric lavage with 5–10 L of tap water. If a gastric tube is not immediately available, induce emesis. Remove phosphorus contamination from the skin or eyes by copious irrigation with tap water for at least 15 minutes.

2. General measures–Treat pulmonary edema (see p 65). Treat shock (see p 66). Give 10% calcium gluconate, 10 mL intravenously, to maintain serum calcium. Give 1–4 L of 5% glucose in water or 10% invert sugar (Travert) in water intravenously daily until a high-carbohydrate diet can be given by mouth. Treat hepatic failure (see p 77).

B. Chronic Poisoning: Remove from further exposure. Treat jaw necrosis by surgical excision of sequestered bone.

Prognosis

In poisoning from ingestion of phosphorus, the mortality rate is about 50%. In phosphine inhalation, survival for 4 days is ordinarily followed by recovery.

Konjoyan TR: White phosphorus burns: Case report and literature review. *Milit Med* 1983;**148**:881.

McCarron MM et al: Acute yellow phosphorus poisoning from pesticide pastes. *Clin Toxicol* 1981;**18**:693.

Singh S et al: Aluminum phosphide ingestion. *Br Med J* 1985;**290**:1110.

Wilson R et al: Acute phosphine poisoning aboard a grain freighter. *JAMA* 1980;**244**:148.

ZINC FUMES & METAL FUME FEVER

Zinc fumes are produced in welding, metal cutting, and smelting zinc alloys or galvanized iron. Zinc fumes are most often responsible for metal fume fever, but other metal fumes, including magnesium oxide fumes, will also cause the disease. Soluble zinc salts, such as zinc chloride, are used in smoke generators.

The exposure limit for zinc oxide fumes is 5 mg/m^3; for zinc chloride fumes, 1 mg/m^3; and for magnesium oxide fumes, 10 mg/m^3. No fatalities from breathing zinc oxide or zinc chloride fumes have been reported in recent years.

Fumes from zinc or soluble zinc salts irritate the lungs. Other physiologic changes are not known.

The pathologic findings in fatalities from zinc chloride or zinc fume inhalation are pulmonary edema and damage to the respiratory tract.

Clinical Findings

The principal manifestations of acute zinc fume or other metal fume poisoning are muscular aches and fever. Chronic poisoning does not occur.

Inhalation of zinc oxide or other metal oxide fumes causes fever, chills, nausea and vomiting, muscular aches, and weakness. Inhaling fumes of soluble zinc salts such as zinc chloride may cause pulmonary edema with cyanosis and dyspnea.

Prevention

Zinc chloride smoke generators should not be operated in such a way that workers will be exposed. Fumes from melting zinc must be controlled by proper air exhaust.

Treatment of Acute Poisoning

A. Specific Measures: Treat pulmonary edema (see p 65). Give prednisone, 25–50 mg orally daily, or other corticosteroid, to reduce tissue response to inhaled metal fumes. Decrease dosage as the patient improves.

B. Other measures: Treat metal fume fever by bed rest and give aspirin for fever and pain.

Prognosis

In zinc fume fever, recovery occurs in 24–48 hours. In pulmonary edema from zinc chloride fumes, the mortality rate has been 10–40%.

Armstrong CW et al: An outbreak of metal fume fever. *J Occup Med* 1983;**25**:886.

References

Bencko V: Nickel: A review of its occupational and environmental toxicity. *Z Gesamte Hyg* 1984;**30**:259.

Demayo A et al: Effects of copper on humans, laboratory and farm animals, terrestrial plants, and aquatic life. *Crit Rev Environ Control* 1982;**12**:183.

Demedts M et al: Cobalt lung in diamond polishers. *Am Rev Respir Dis* 1984;**130**:130.

Greaves IA et al: Respiratory effects of two types of solder flux used in the electronics industry. *J Occup Med* 1984;**26**:81.

Kizer KW et al: Health effects of silicon tetrachloride. *J Occup Med* 1984;**26**:33.

Kruger GL et al: The health effects of aluminum compounds in mammals. *CRC Crit Rev Toxicol* 1984;**13**:1.

Nechay BR: Mechanisms of action of vanadium. *Annu Rev Pharmacol Toxicol* 1984;**24**:501.

Rey C et al: Methyl tin intoxication in six men: Toxicologic and clinical aspects. *Vet Hum Toxicol* 1984;**26**:121.

Selenium intoxication—New York. *MMWR* 1984;**33**:157.

Cyanides, Sulfides, & Carbon Monoxide | 16

HYDROGEN CYANIDE & DERIVATIVES:
ACRYLONITRILE, CYANAMIDE, CYANOGEN CHLORIDE, CYANIDES, NITROPRUSSIDES, & CYANOGENETIC GLYCOSIDES
(Table 16–1)

Hydrogen cyanide (HCN) is used as a fumigant and in chemical synthesis. Acrylonitrile is used in the production of synthetic rubber. Cyanamide is used as a fertilizer and as a source of hydrogen cyanide. Cyanogen chloride is used in chemical synthesis. Cyanide salts are used in metal cleaning, hardening, and refining and in the recovery of gold from ores. Nitroprussides are used in chemical synthesis and as hypotensive agents. The seeds of apple, cherry, peach, apricot, plum, jetberry bush, and toyon contain cyanogenetic glycosides such as amygdalin that release cyanide on digestion. The fatal dose of these seeds varies from 5 to 25 seeds for a small child. They are only dangerous if the seed capsule is broken.

Natural oil of bitter almonds contains 4% hydrogen cyanide, and artificial oil of bitter almonds contains mandelonitrile. Some species of the lima bean *(Phaseolus lunatus)* contain 300 mg of HCN per 100 g of bean. American white lima beans contain 10 mg of HCN per 100 g of bean. The dried root of cassava *(Manihot utilissima,* tapioca) may contain 245 mg of HCN per 100 g of root. Hydrolysis and leaching can reduce the amount of HCN to 1 mg per 100 g. When raw plant material containing cyanogenetic glycoside is ingested, enzymes in the plant material release HCN. In the absence of enzymes in ingested material, bacterial enzymes in the intestine release HCN. One man was poisoned after eating about 48 apricot kernels that had been roasted at 300 °F for 10 minutes. Laetrile, claimed to be a cancer cure, is reported to be made from apricot kernels and contains a cyanide-releasing substance. It has caused fatal cyanide poisoning.

Cyanide apparently poisons by inhibiting the cytochrome oxidase

Table 16–1. Hydrogen cyanide and derivatives.

	Formula	Boiling Point (°C)	Exposure Limit (ppm)	LD50 (mg/kg) or LC (ppm)	Cyanide-releasing	Remarks
Acetone cyanohydrin	CH₃C(OH)CN·CH₃	82		15	+	
Acetonitrile	CH₃CN	81.6	40	120	+	Irritant.
Acrylonitrile	CH₂=CHCN	78.5	0	35	+	Bullae. Carcinogen.
Benzonitrile	C₆H₅CN	190.7		180	0	
Benzylcyanide	C₆H₅CH₂CN	234		32	+	Irritant.
Bromobenzylcyanide	C₆H₅CH₂BrCN	Solid		3500*	+	Irritant.
n-Butyronitrile	CH₃CH₂CH₂CN	118		10	+	
Cyanamide	HN=C=NH	Solid		1000	0	
Cyanide salts	CN⁻	Solid	2*	2	+*	
Cyanoacetic acid	N≡CCH₂COOH	108	5*	2000	0	
Cyanogen	N≡C–C≡N	Gas	10	13	+	
Cyanogen chloride	ClC≡N	61	0.3	13	+	
Ferricyanide	Fe(CN)₆³⁻	Solid		1600	0	
Ferrocyanide	Fe(CN)₆⁴⁻	Solid		1600	0	
Fumaronitrile	NCCHCHCN	186		50	+	
Hydrogen cyanide	HCN	26.5	10	0.5		
Malononitrile	N≡CCH₂C≡N	Solid	3	6	+	
Mandelonitrile	C₆H₅CH(OH)CN	Liquid		6	+	
Methyl acrylonitrile	CH₂=C(CH₃)CN	90	1		+	Carcinogen.
Methyl 2-cyanoacrylate	CH₂:C(CN)COOCH₃	Liquid	2			Irritant.
Methyl isocyanate	CH₃NCO	39	0.02	2 ppm		Irritant, sensitizer.
Nitroprusside (see p 391)	Fe(CN)₅(NO)²⁻	Solid		10	+ (?)	Releases nitrite.
m-Phthalodinitrile	C₆H₄(CN)₂	Solid	5*		0	Irritant.
Propionitrile	C₂H₅CN	97		40	+	
o-Tolunitrile	CH₃C₆H₄CN	204		600	0	
Trichloroacetonitrile	CCl₃CN	84.6		200	+	Extreme irritation.

*mg/m³.

system for O_2 utilization in cells. Other enzyme systems are also inhibited, but to a lesser degree.

Cyanide first causes a marked increase in respiration by affecting chemoreceptors in the carotid body and respiratory center and then paralyzes all cells. Pathologic findings in fatal cases are not characteristic. The odor of bitter almonds may be noticeable at autopsy; however, the ability to perceive this odor is genetically determined, and some humans do not possess it. Ingestion of potassium cyanide or sodium cyanide causes congestion and corrosion of the gastric mucosa.

Clinical Findings

The principal manifestations of poisoning with these compounds are rapid respiration, blood pressure fall, convulsions, and coma.

A. Acute Poisoning:

1. Cyanide, cyanogen chloride, acetonitrile, and other cyanide-releasing substances–Ingestion or inhalation of large amounts of these compounds (10 times the MLD) causes immediate unconsciousness, convulsions, and death within 1–15 minutes. Ingestion, inhalation, or absorption through the skin of an amount near the MLD causes dizziness, rapid respiration, vomiting, flushing, headache, drowsiness, drop in blood pressure, rapid pulse, and unconsciousness. Death in convulsions occurs within 4 hours with all cyanide derivatives except sodium nitroprusside, which may cause death as late as 12 hours after ingestion.

2. Acrylonitrile–Inhalation of acrylonitrile causes nausea and vomiting, diarrhea, weakness, headache, and jaundice. Skin contact with acrylonitrile has caused epidermal necrolysis.

3. Calcium cyanamide–Ingestion causes flushing of skin and mucous membranes, headache, dizziness, and fall of blood pressure. These symptoms are greatly accentuated by the concomitant ingestion of ethanol. At least one fatality has occurred from ethanol ingestion after calcium cyanamide (calcium carbimide) ingestion.

B. Chronic Poisoning: Repeated inhalation of small amounts of cyanogen chloride causes dizziness, weakness, congestion of lungs, hoarseness, conjunctivitis, loss of appetite, weight loss, and mental deterioration. Similar symptoms have also been reported from inhaling cyanide in low concentrations for 1 year or more. Chronic ingestion of cyanide in the form of cassava is suspected of causing tropical ataxic neuropathy. Thyroid insufficiency also occurs as a result of conversion of cyanide to thiocyanate. A trimer of methylene aminoacetonitrile caused conjunctivitis and respiratory tract inflammation in rubber workers. Workers exposed to acrylonitrile show an increased incidence of cancer. Laetrile has caused agranulocytosis.

C. Laboratory Findings: A severe metabolic acidosis occurs in acute cyanide poisoning.

Prevention

Many individuals cannot detect the odor of cyanide. The exposure limit of cyanide in work rooms must not be exceeded at any time. Emergency treatment kits containing 0.2-mL ampules of amyl nitrite, 10-mL ampules of 3% sodium nitrite, and 25-mL ampules of 25% sodium thiosulfate, with suitable syringes and needles, should be immediately available where cyanide is being used.

Treatment

A. Inhaled Cyanide:

1. Emergency measures–

a. Remove to uncontaminated atmosphere.

b. Give amyl nitrite inhalation, 1 ampule (0.2 mL) every 5 minutes. Stop administration if the systolic blood pressure goes below 80 mm Hg.

c. Give artificial respiration with 100% O_2 in order to maintain high blood O_2 tension. Treatment with hyperbaric O_2 has also been used.

2. Antidote–All cyanide antidotes are toxic, and unnecessary therapy is dangerous, especially in children.

a. Sodium nitrite–As soon as possible, give 3% sodium nitrite solution intravenously at a rate of 2.5–5 mL/min. Stop administration if the systolic blood pressure goes below 80 mm Hg. The administered nitrite forms methemoglobin, which combines with cyanide to form cyanmethemoglobin. The amount of nitrite administered must be based on the hemoglobin level and on the weight of the individual. Table 16–2 gives the amount of sodium nitrite necessary to convert 26% of hemoglobin to methemoglobin. Further administration of nitrite should

Table 16–2. Variation of sodium nitrite and sodium thiosulfate dose with hemoglobin concentration.[*]

Hemoglobin (g/dL)	Initial Dose Sodium Nitrite (mg/kg)	Initial Dose Sodium Nitrite 3% (mL/kg)	Initial Dose Sodium Thiosulfate 25% (mL/kg)
7	5.8	0.19	0.95
8	6.6	0.22	1.10
9	7.5	0.25	1.25
10	8.3	0.27	1.35
11	9.1	0.30	1.50
12	10.0	0.33	1.65
13	10.8	0.36	1.80
14	11.6	0.39	1.95

[*]Reproduced, with permission, from Berlin DM Jr: The treatment of cyanide poisoning in children. *Pediatrics* 1970;46:793.

be based on methemoglobin determinations, and the total methemoglobin should not exceed 40%.

b. Sodium thiosulfate–Follow sodium nitrite with 25% sodium thiosulfate solution intravenously at a rate of 2.5–5 mL/min. Thiosulfate converts cyanide to thiocyanate. The dose of thiosulfate should be based on hemoglobin determination as with nitrite (see Table 16–2).

c. In some countries, dicobalt edetate (Kelocyanor) is available. Give 300–600 mg as a loading dose. An additional 300 mg can be given if symptoms of cyanide poisoning persist. The toxicity of dicobalt edetate is greater in the absence of cyanide. The drug should not be given without clear evidence of cyanide poisoning.

B. Ingested Cyanide:

1. Emergency measures–

a. Give amyl nitrite inhalation, 1 ampule (0.2 mL) every 5 minutes.

b. Gastric lavage (see p 24) should be delayed until nitrite and thiosulfate antidotes have been given.

c. Give artificial respiration with 100% O_2 in order to maintain high blood O_2 tension (see above). Use of hyperbaric O_2 remains controversial.

2. Antidote–Treat as for inhaled cyanide (see above).

C. Ingested Calcium Cyanamide: There is no known antidote. After gastric lavage, treat symptomatically.

Prognosis

In acute cyanide poisoning, survival for 4 hours is usually followed by recovery.

Beamer WC, Shealy RM, Prough DS: Acute cyanide poisoning from laetrile ingestion. *Ann Emerg Med* 1983;**12**:449.

Blanc P et al: Cyanide intoxication among silver-reclaiming workers. *JAMA* 1985;**253**:367.

Holzbecher MD, Moss MA, Ellenberger HA: The cyanide content of laetrile preparations, apricot, peach, and apple seeds. *J Toxicol Clin Toxicol* 1984;**22**:341.

Koerselman W, van der Graaf M: Acrylonitrile: A suspected human carcinogen. *Int Arch Occup Environ Health* 1984;**54**:317.

Litovitz PL et al: Cyanide poisoning treated with hyperbaric oxygen. *Am J Emerg Med* 1983;**1**:94.

Marbury TC et al: Combined antidotal and hemodialysis treatments for nitroprusside-induced cyanide toxicity. *J Toxicol Clin Toxicol* 1982;**19**:475.

Way JL: Cyanide intoxication and its mechanism of antagonism. *Annu Rev Pharmacol Toxicol* 1984;**24**:451.

HYDROGEN SULFIDE, OTHER SULFIDES, MERCAPTANS, CARBON DISULFIDE, & PROPANE SULTONE

Hydrogen sulfide is released spontaneously by the decomposition of sulfur compounds and is found in petroleum refineries, tanneries, mines, and rayon factories. It is produced by bacterial action on sewage effluents containing sulfur compounds when dissolved O_2 has been consumed owing to excessive organic loading of surface water. Such compounds are used by the canning industry as antioxidants during certain seasons and in many instances are discharged to surface waters, where they drastically reduce dissolved O_2. Carbon disulfide is used as a solvent, especially in the rayon industry. Mercaptans are released in petroleum refining and are used as warning odors in liquified propane, butane, and natural gas. Phenylmercaptan and p-chlorophenyl mercaptan are used as pesticides. Calcium polysulfide (Vleminckx's solution), sodium sulfide, ammonium sulfide, and thioacetamide release hydrogen sulfide in contact with water or acids. Propane sultone is used as a chemical intermediate.

Hydrogen sulfide (H_2S) is a gas. Carbon disulfide (CS_2) is a liquid that boils at 46 °C. It ignites at the temperature of boiling water (100 °C). Ethylmercaptan (C_2H_5SH) and methylmercaptan (methanethiol, CH_3SH) are gases.

The exposure limit for hydrogen sulfide is 10 ppm; carbon disulfide, 10 ppm; methylmercaptan, butylmercaptan, ethylmercaptan, and phenylmercaptan, 0.5 ppm; perchloromethylmercaptan, 0.1 ppm; phosphorus pentasulfide, 1 mg/m³; and allylpropyl disulfide, 2 ppm. No exposure limit for propane sultone has been established. Community air should not exceed 0.03 ppm of hydrogen sulfide. The approximate fatal dose of carbon disulfide by ingestion is 1 g; of soluble sulfides, 10 g. The lethal dose of 2-mercaptoethanol in rats is 300 mg/kg. Ingested sulfur is converted to sulfides in the gastrointestinal tract, and ingestion of 10–20 g has caused irritation of the gastrointestinal tract and renal injury.

Hydrogen sulfide causes both anoxic effects and damage to the cells of the central nervous system by direct action. Carbon disulfide damages chiefly the central nervous system, the peripheral nerves, and the hemopoietic system. The mercaptans are severe irritants.

There are no characteristic pathologic findings in sudden fatalities from hydrogen sulfide poisoning; if death is delayed 24–48 hours, pulmonary edema and congestion of the lungs are found. Ingestion of carbon disulfide causes congestion and edema of the gastrointestinal tract. The characteristic unpleasant (rotten egg) odor is noticeable at autopsy. In deaths from carbon disulfide, degenerative changes may be found in the brain and spinal cord. Prolonged exposure to small concentrations of carbon disulfide has caused cerebrovascular changes.

Clinical Findings

The principal manifestation of poisoning with these compounds is irritation.

A. Acute Poisoning:

1. Hydrogen sulfide is detectable by odor at 0.05 ppm, and 0.1 ppm causes irritation and sensory loss. Fifty ppm creates an unpleasant odor, but shortly the smell diminishes. After exposure to concentrations above 50 ppm, symptoms are gradually progressive, with painful conjunctivitis, appearance of a halo around lights, headache, isomnia, nausea, rawness in the throat, cough, dizziness, drowsiness, and pulmonary edema. Concentrations above 500 ppm cause immediate loss of consciousness, depressed respiration, and death in 30–60 minutes.

2. Exposure to carbon disulfide at concentrations from 100 to 1000 ppm causes symptoms progressing from restlessness, irritation of the mucous membranes, blurred vision, nausea and vomiting, and headache to unconsciousness and paralysis of respiration. If consciousness returns, irritability, muscle spasms, visual disturbances, and even psychotic behavior are observed during recovery.

3. Skin contact with carbon disulfide causes reddening and burning and, later, cracking and peeling. If the liquid remains in contact with the skin for several minutes, a second-degree burn may result.

4. Ingestion of carbon disulfide or soluble sulfides causes vomiting, headache, cyanosis, respiratory depression, fall of blood pressure, loss of consciousness, tremors, convulsions, and death.

5. Ethylmercaptan, methylmercaptan, and other mercaptans in high concentrations cause cyanosis, convulsions, hemolytic anemia, fever, coma, and irreversible depression of cerebral function. Perchloromethylmercaptan is a severe pulmonary irritant. Allyl propyl disulfide (onion oil) is a mild pulmonary and mucous membrane irritant.

6. Phosphorus pentasulfide is an eye and skin irritant. It liberates hydrogen sulfide on contact with water.

B. Chronic Poisoning:

1. Hydrogen sulfide–Prolonged exposure causes persistent low blood pressure, nausea, loss of appetite, weight loss, impaired gait and balance, conjunctivitis, and chronic cough.

2. Carbon disulfide–Continued exposure by inhalation or skin absorption first causes bizarre sensations in the extremities and then sensory loss and muscular weakness. Later symptoms are irritability, memory loss, blurred vision, loss of appetite, insomnia, mental depression, partial blindness, dizziness, weakness, and parkinsonian tremor. Examination may reveal vascularization of the retina, dilatation of reti-

nal arterioles, and blanching of the optic disk. The corneal and pupillary reflexes may be diminished or lost. The mortality rate from coronary heart disease is increased in workers exposed to carbon disulfide. The incidence of abortions, sterility, and amenorrhea is increased in exposed women.

3. Propane sultone–Single exposures have been carcinogenic in several animal species.

C. Laboratory Findings:

1. The differential count may reveal a decrease in polymorphonuclear leukocytes and an increase in lymphocytes.

2. Hematuria and proteinuria may be present.

3. Hepatic cell function may be impaired as shown by appropriate tests (see p 75).

Prevention

The exposure limit must be observed at all times. The odor of carbon disulfide or hydrogen sulfide should not be relied upon to give adequate warning. Loss of the sense of smell occurs rapidly. Workers should alternate between jobs requiring exposure to carbon disulfide and jobs in uncontaminated air. Airline face masks must be worn when entering highly contaminated areas. A safety harness and lifeline attended by a responsible person are necessary.

Treatment

A. Acute Poisoning:

1. Emergency measures–

a. Remove from exposure.

b. Give artificial respiration with O_2 if respiration is affected.

c. Remove swallowed poison by gastric lavage or emesis (see pp 21–28), using a saturated sodium bicarbonate solution to reduce gastric acidity and to prevent the formation of hydrogen sulfide, which is more rapidly absorbed.

d. Stimulants may induce ventricular arrhythmias.

2. Antidote–Amyl nitrite or sodium nitrite (see p 254) can be used to aid in the formation of sulfmethemoglobin, thus removing sulfide from combination in tissues. Pyridoxine, 25 mg/kg intravenously, or 10% urea, 1 g/kg intravenously, has been suggested as a sulfide acceptor.

3. General measures–

a. Treat pulmonary edema (see p 65).

b. Keep patient at bed rest for 3–4 days. Reduce sensory input in instances of delirium or excitement.

B. Chronic Poisoning: Remove from further exposure.

Prognosis

In hydrogen sulfide poisoning, if the patient survives for the first 4 hours, recovery is assured. In carbon disulfide poisoning, gradual improvement takes place over several months, but complete recovery may never occur.

Beauchamp RO Jr et al: A critical review of the literature on hydrogen sulfide toxicity. *CRC Crit Rev Toxicol* 1984;**13**:25.

Corsi G et al: Chronic peripheral neuropathy in workers with previous exposure to carbon disulphide. *Br J Ind Med* 1983;**40**:209.

Hagley SR, South BL: Fatal inhalation of liquid manure gas. *Med J Aust* 1983;**2**:459.

Ravizza A et al: The treatment of hydrogen sulfide intoxication: Oxygen versus nitrites. *Vet Hum Toxicol* 1982;**24**:241.

Spyker DA et al: Health effects of acute carbon disulfide exposure. *J Toxicol Clin Toxicol* 1982;**19**:87.

CARBON MONOXIDE

Carbon monoxide is produced by the incomplete combustion of carbon or carbonaceous materials. All flame or combustion devices, including catalytic radiant heaters, are likely to emit carbon monoxide. The worldwide emission of carbon monoxide is approximately 232 million tons each year, of which the USA contributes 88 million tons. The total amount emitted each year would be sufficient to raise the concentration in the lower atmosphere about 0.03 ppm, but a biologic scavenging process prevents the lowest oceanic levels from rising above 0.03–0.10 ppm.

The exhaust from incomplete combustion of natural gas or petroleum fuels may contain as much as 5% carbon monoxide. An unvented natural gas heater may emit as much as 1 cu ft/min, which is enough to make the air in a small room dangerous within minutes. The exhaust from gasoline internal combustion engines contains 3–7% carbon monoxide. A gasoline vehicle with no emission control device emits 2.7 lb of carbon monoxide per gallon of fuel, or 80 g per mile at 15 miles per gallon. Present standards for new cars require limitation of carbon monoxide emission to 0.5%. A diesel vehicle emits 0.074 lb of carbon monoxide per gallon of fuel, or 7 g per mile at 5 miles per gallon. Smoke from cigarettes, pipes, and cigars is also a potent source of carbon monoxide, containing 4%.

The industrial exposure limit for carbon monoxide is 35 ppm. An adverse level of carbon monoxide for community air has been set at 9 ppm for a continuous period of 8 hours. As examples of community air pollution levels, Burbank, California, exceeded 20 ppm for 583 hours and 10 ppm for 6044 hours in 1967, whereas San Francisco exceeded 20 ppm for 20 hours and 10 ppm for 264 hours in the same year.

Carbon monoxide combines with hemoglobin to form carboxyhemoglobin, which is incapable of carrying O_2, and tissue anoxia results. One part of carbon monoxide in 200 parts of O_2 or 1000 parts of air will cause approximately 50% saturation of hemoglobin with carboxyhemoglobin. A human who breathes air with the lowest possible values of carbon monoxide will still have about 1% of red blood cell hemoglobin combined with carbon monoxide. An individual's exhaled air will contain about 3 ppm of carbon monoxide, which comes from the breakdown of hemoglobin liberated when red blood cells die at the end of their life span of about 120 days. A person who inhales smoke from 20 cigarettes during 1 day will have at least 6% of hemoglobin saturated with carbon monoxide. Garage employees working in an atmosphere containing 7–240 ppm carbon monoxide were found to have 3–15% of their hemoglobin combined with carbon monoxide. In laboratory experiments, subjects exposed to 50 ppm for 30 minutes had 3% saturation of hemoglobin with carbon monoxide. The relationship is such that a concentration in air of 6 ppm carbon monoxide will increase the amount of hemoglobin in combination with carbon monoxide by 1%. The time required for this equilibrium to occur is thought to be about 8 hours, although direct measurement has not been made at these low concentrations.

Hemoglobin has an affinity for carbon monoxide 210 times greater than for O_2. In addition, the presence of carbon monoxide increases the stability of the hemoglobin-O_2 combination. Thus, the presence of carbon monoxide reduces the availability of O_2 to the tissues in 2 ways: (1) by direct combination with hemoglobin to reduce the amount of hemoglobin available to carry O_2 and (2) by preventing the release of some of the O_2 at the low O_2 pressure present in body tissues. As an example, a patient with anemia having a hemoglobin level of 50% of normal and with no carbon monoxide will have about twice as much O_2 available to tissues as will the patient with normal hemoglobin who has 50% of hemoglobin combined with carbon monoxide. The patient with anemia may have only slight symptoms, whereas the patient with carbon monoxide poisoning is likely to die. Inhaling the smoke from one cigarette reduces the amount of O_2 available to the tissues by about 8%, the equivalent of going from sea level to an altitude of 4000 ft. This effect could play a role in coronary insufficiency.

In addition to the strong affinity of carbon monoxide for hemoglobin, carbon monoxide also combines with the myoglobin of muscles and with certain enzymes. Interference with the operation of the cytochrome oxidase system is postulated to be the major toxic effect of carbon monoxide; consequently, hyperbaric O_2 administration is recommended for management of serious carbon monoxide poisoning—even after the carboxyhemoglobin level returns toward normal. Mice are able to survive with all of their red blood cell hemoglobin combined with carbon monoxide if the O_2 pressure is sufficiently high.

The visual ability of subjects watching a faint background to distinguish differences in light intensity is impaired when only 4% of the hemoglobin is combined with carbon monoxide. This same level of saturation is also able to interfere with certain psychologic tests (eg, choosing the correct letter, choosing the correct color, crossing t's). Errors in arithmetic and in the ability to underline plural words did not occur until 8–10% saturation of hemoglobin. The ability to discriminate time duration was reduced after exposure to carbon monoxide at 50 ppm for 90 minutes. The pulse rate during exercise at sea level was not affected when 6% of the hemoglobin was combined with carbon monoxide, but it was increased when 13% was combined. On the other hand, 4% saturation of hemoglobin significantly increased the O_2 debt incurred during severe exercise.

Pathologic examination in fatal cases of carbon monoxide poisoning reveals microscopic hemorrhages and necrotic areas throughout the body. Intense congestion and edema of the brain, liver, kidneys, and spleen also occur. The tissues may be bright red. Microscopic examination reveals damage to nerve cells, especially in the cerebral cortex and medulla. Myocardial damage may occur at carboxyhemoglobin levels of 25–50%.

Clinical Findings

The principal manifestation of carbon monoxide poisoning is dyspnea.

A. Acute Poisoning: (From inhalation.) The absorption of carbon monoxide and the resulting symptoms are closely dependent on the concentration of carbon monoxide in the inspired air, the time of exposure, and the state of activity of the person exposed.

1. A concentration of 100 ppm (0.01%) will not produce symptoms during an 8-hour exposure. Cardiovascular changes can be detected in some individuals at carboxyhemoglobin levels above 5%.

2. Exposure to 500 ppm (0.05%) for 1 hour during light work may cause no symptoms or only slight headache and shortness of breath. The blood will contain approximately 20% carboxyhemoglobin. A longer exposure to the same concentration, or greater activity, will raise the blood saturation to 40–50%, with symptoms of headache, nausea, irritability, increased respiration, chest pain, confusion, impaired judgment, and fainting on increased exertion. Cyanosis and pallor occur.

3. Concentrations over 1000 ppm (0.1%) cause unconsciousness, respiratory failure, and death if exposure is continued for more than 1 hour. The blood will contain 50–90% carboxyhemoglobin. Hyperactivity, bizarre behavior, and convulsions can occur during the recovery pe-

riod. Myonecrosis, neuropathy, renal failure, thrombotic thrombocytopenic purpura, and retrobulbar neuritis with neuroretinal edema have occurred after severe poisoning. In 7% of fatal carbon monoxide poisonings, the carboxyhemoglobin level is below 40%.

B. Chronic Poisoning: Chronic poisoning in the sense of accumulation of carbon monoxide in the body does not occur. After the blood carboxyhemoglobin level has returned to normal, susceptibility to carbon monoxide is not increased unless cerebral damage was incurred. However, repeated anoxia from carbon monoxide absorption will cause gradually increasing central nervous system damage, with loss of sensation in the fingers, poor memory, positive Romberg's sign, and mental deterioration. Deaths due to cardiovascular disease are slightly increased in those exposed to low levels of carbon monoxide.

C. Laboratory Findings:

1. The white blood cell count may be normal or may be elevated to 18,000 or higher.

2. The blood level of carboxyhemoglobin should be measured spectrophotometrically.

3. Proteinuria may be present.

4. An ECG is useful to indicate possible myocardial damage.

5. Radiologic evidence of perihilar and intra-alveolar edema indicates a poor prognosis.

Prevention

The air concentration of carbon monoxide must be kept below the exposure limit at all times by proper ventilation. All combustion devices must be vented to the outside air. These devices include flame water heaters, stoves, gas refrigerators, and internal combustion engines.

Treatment

A. Emergency Measures:

1. Remove from exposure.

2. Give 100% O_2 by mask until the blood carboxyhemoglobin is reduced below the dangerous level. The carboxyhemoglobin level should fall 50% in 1–2 hours. If the blood carboxyhemoglobin level exceeds 20%, consider hyperbaric O_2 administration.

3. If respiration is depressed, give artificial respiration with 100% O_2 until respiration is normal.

B. Antidote: Give O_2 as under Emergency Measures.

C. General Measures:

1. Maintain normal body temperature.

2. Maintain blood pressure (see p 66).

3. Give 20% mannitol, 1 g/kg intravenously over 20 minutes, to reduce cerebral edema.

4. Give prednisolone, 1 mg/kg intravenously or intramuscularly every 4 hours, or other corticosteroid, for cerebral edema.

5. If hyperthermia is present, reduce body temperature by application of cooling blankets.

6. Treat bacterial aspiration pneumonia with organism-specific chemotherapy.

7. Bed rest for 2–4 weeks is useful in order to minimize late neurologic complications.

8. Control convulsions or hyperactivity with diazepam, 0.1 mg/kg slowly intravenously. Later, phenytoin may be used.

Prognosis

If the victim recovers, symptoms regress gradually. If a high blood saturation persists for several hours, tremors, mental deterioration, and abnormal behavior may persist or reappear after a symptom-free interval of 1–2 weeks. These symptoms of central nervous system damage may be permanent. Complete recovery is not likely if symptoms of mental deterioration persist for 2 weeks.

Atkins EH, Baker EL: Exacerbation of coronary artery disease by occupational carbon monoxide exposure: A report of two fatalities and a review of literature. *Am J Ind Med* 1985;**7**:73.

Cramer CR: Fetal death due to accidental maternal carbon monoxide poisoning. *J Toxicol Clin Toxicol* 1982;**19**:297.

Mofenson HC, Caraccio TR, Brody GM: Carbon monoxide poisoning. (Clinical conference.) *Am J Emerg Med* 1984;**2**:254.

Olson KR: Carbon monoxide poisoning: Mechanisms, presentation, and controversies in management. *J Emerg Med* 1984;**1**:233.

Watson A et al: Anoxic hepatic and intestinal injury from carbon monoxide poisoning. *Br Med J* 1984;**289**:1113.

17 | Atmospheric Particulates

The federal maxima for suspended particulates in the atmosphere are 75 $\mu g/m^3$ for the annual mean and 260 $\mu g/m^3$ for the 24-hour average. Certain regions have established 60 $\mu g/m^3$ as the annual mean maximum and 150 $\mu g/m^3$ as the maximum 24-hour average.

Particles small enough to remain suspended in the air (aerosols) are formed by grinding, crushing, or burning or by condensation or coalescence. Methods of measurement of the amount of airborne particulate matter consist of the following:

(1) Dust fall is measured in tons per square mile.

(2) Sulfate deposition is measured in mg/100 cm^2.

(3) Coefficient of haze (COH) is determined by drawing 1000 linear feet of air through filter paper; the percentage of light transmission of the resulting spot is read and converted to a number ranging from zero at 100% transmission to 70 at 20% transmission. (The filter will not trap particles smaller than 0.3 μm.)

(4) A high-volume air filter draws air through a 9 × 12 inch sheet of filter paper for 24 hours; the amount of collected material is weighed and reported in $\mu g/m^3$ of air passed through the filter. (The filter will not trap particles smaller than 0.3 μm.)

(5) Visibility or visual range is an indication of light scattering or light absorption in the atmosphere; for a given weight of material, particles in the range of 0.1–1 μm have the greatest effect on visibility.

(6) Size analysis: In addition to the quantity of particulate matter suspended in the air, the size of the particles is of utmost importance for their effect on humans. Only those particles ranging from 0.1 to 10 μm are effectively trapped in the lungs. Larger particles are removed by the upper respiratory tract, and smaller particles are not trapped to a significant extent.

Measurement of atmospheric particulates is still in a primitive stage of development. The only routine measurements widely used are coefficient of haze and high-volume air filters. These tests do not collect toxicologically significant particles less than 0.3 μm in diameter. Of all measurements that can be made routinely, visual range most nearly reflects the quantity in the air of particles in the size range taken up by the human lung. Up to the present time, estimates of visual range have been based on observer sightings of landmarks at various distances and have been done as part of airport weather programs and not as part of air pollution control programs. The sight path for visual range measurements must be horizontal and near the ground in order to correlate with human exposure.

Routine determination of the quantitative distribution of the substances present in the various size fractions of the air-suspended particulates is not being made. The constituents include lead (see p 230), vanadium, chromium, beryllium (see p 224), other metals, silica (see below), carbon particles, organic compounds, motor oil, soil, asbestos, sulfates, sulfuric acid droplets, metal sulfates, glass particles, pollen, microorganisms, and plant and animal products.

Organic particulates can be divided into benzene-soluble substances (mostly organic compounds with high molecular weights) and nonbenzene-soluble substances (plant pollens, microorganisms, and other plant and animal products). The plant and animal products are important in allergic reactions, while the benzene-soluble substances include those with carcinogenic potential such as benzo(α)pyrene and other polycyclic hydrocarbons. These are emitted during incomplete combustion and are also present in the dust from asphalt roads.

Experimental studies have shown that extracts of airborne particulate matter are more likely to induce cancer if injected under the skin of experimental animals than if instilled into the lungs. Part of the reason for such a lack of activity in the lung may be the short time the particulate extracts remain in the lung. If hematite or carbon particles are added to the material instilled into the lung, the carcinogenic potency is increased. This action may result from adsorption and retention of the material in the lung. The carcinogenic effect in animals is characterized by a latent period of 12–24 months, or 50–80% of the animal's lifetime.

When the carcinogenic potency of airborne particulate matter from different regions was compared, that from Alabama was found to be more carcinogenic than that from Los Angeles. The lung cancer death rate was higher in Alabama than in Los Angeles in a study made on mortality rates for 1949–1951. These data do not reflect the great increase in air pollution in Los Angeles since 1950, the effect of which may require 40–50 years to become manifest, since the peak of deaths from lung cancer does not occur until age 55.

SILICA

Dust containing silica is produced during rock cutting, drilling, crushing, grinding, mining, abrasive manufacture, pottery making, processing of diatomaceous earth, and volcanic eruptions. Talcum powder contains magnesium silicate. Many substances containing silica are capable of causing silicosis. Particles less than 5 μm in diameter ap-

Table 17—1. Effects of particulates.*

	Exposure Limit (mg/mg³ Respirable)	Clinical Findings	X-Ray	Prognosis†
Aluminum alkyls	2	Irritation.		
Aluminum oxide (Al₂O₃), emery, bauxite	10	Mild irritation to skin and mucous membranes.	No change.	Nonprogressive.
Aluminum powder	10	Interstitial emphysema, nonnodular fibrosis.	Fibrosis.	Progressive.
Aluminum pyro powder	5	As above.	Fibrosis.	Progressive.
Aluminum welding fumes	5	Irritation.		
Asphalt (petroleum fumes)	5	None.	No change.	No disease.
Barite (barium sulfate)	10	None.	Nodulation of lungs.	Nonprogressive.
Carbon black	3.5	Possible lung cancer.		
Coal dust	2	Gradual progression of respiratory impairment.	Nodulation or "reticulation."	Nonprogressive in early stages.
Coal tar	0.2	Photosensitizers and irritants, lung cancer, acne.		
Coke oven emissions	0.15	Lung and kidney cancer.		
Cotton dust	0.2	Progressive dyspnea, emphysema, weakness (byssinosis).	Emphysema.	Nonprogressive in early stages.
Dusts, nuisance	10	Irritation.	No change.	No change.
Glass fiber	10	Skin irritation, no lung involvement.	No change.	No disease.
Grain dust	4	Sensitizer, asthma.	Pneumonia.	Nonprogressive.
Graphite	2.5	Dyspnea, cough, ventricular hypertrophy.	Nodulation.	Progressive.
Iron oxide	5	Asymptomatic.	Stippling to numerous small round shadows.	Nonprogressive.
Mica, soapstone	3, 20‡	Similar to silicosis (see p 268).	Fibrosis, pleural calcification.	Progressive.
Mineral oil mist	5	Pneumonitis, possible carcinogen.	Pneumonia.	Nonprogressive.

*None of these dusts are toxic when ingested.
†After withdrawal from exposure.
‡Million particles per cubic foot.

Table 17—1 (cont'd). Effects of particulates.*

	Exposure Limit (mg/mg³ Respirable)	Clinical Findings	X-Ray	Prognosis†
Mineral wool fiber	10	None.	No change.	No change.
Paraffin wax fume	2	Pneumonitis, possible carcinogen.	Pneumonia.	Nonprogressive.
Perlite	10	None.	No change.	No change.
Petroleum mist	5	Lipid pneumonia.	Diffuse infiltration.	
Silicon	10	Deposits in eyes, ears, skin, nose, with possible injury.	No change.	No change.
Silicon carbide	10	Pulmonary fibrosis.	Fibrosis.	Nonprogressive.
Sugar cane dust		Cough, dyspnea, hemoptysis, chills and fever, weakness, weight loss.	Miliary mottling.	Nonprogressive after acute stage. Cortisone is helpful in severe involvement.
Talc	2	Similar to silicosis (see p 268). Massive inhalation in children may cause acute bronchitis and bronchiolitis with plugging of small bronchi and cardiopulmonary failure.	Fine fibrosis, calcification of pericardium.	Progressive.
Tin metal, oxide	2	Asymptomatic.	Marked stippling.	Nonprogressive.
Titanium dioxide	10	Pulmonary irritation.	Slight fibrosis?	Nonprogressive.
Wood dust Hard	1	Conjunctivitis, lacrimation, keratitis, irritation of the upper respiratory passages, cancer.	No change.	Nonprogressive.
Soft	5			

*None of these dusts are toxic when ingested.
†After withdrawal from exposure.

pear to be the most important in causing silicosis. The exposure limit for dusts, such as tripoli, containing crystalline quartz is 0.1 mg of respirable particles of quartz per cubic meter of air. Cristobalite and tridymite have an exposure limit of 0.05 mg/m³. For diatomaceous earth and silica gel, the total respirable mass should not exceed 10 mg/m³ of air; for precipitated silica, the respirable mass should not exceed 5 mg/m³.

Silica particles smaller than 5 μm in diameter are taken up from alveoli by phagocytic cells that then travel along the lymph channels toward the lymph nodes. Some of these phagocytes do not reach the lymph nodes but collect in nodules along the lymph channels. These nodules then gradually increase in size through proliferation of fibrous tissue to form the silicotic nodule. Pathologic examination reveals nodular fibrosis of the lungs.

Progression of tuberculosis is greatly increased in silicosis, but susceptibility is apparently not increased.

Clinical Findings

The principal manifestation of silicosis is dyspnea.

A. Acute Pneumoconiosis: Acute pneumoconiosis from overwhelming exposure to silica dust has occurred.

B. Chronic Pneumoconiosis: Breathing silica dust in concentrations greater than the exposure limit for 6 months to 25 years causes progressive dry cough, shortness of breath on exertion, and decreased chest expansion. As the disease progresses, the cough becomes productive of stringy mucus, vital capacity decreases further, and shortness of breath becomes more severe. If the patient gets tuberculosis, the course is rapidly downhill, with increased cough, dyspnea, and weight loss, if the disease is not treated.

C. X-Ray Findings: Radiologic examination of the chest reveals first a diffuse granular appearance. As the disease progresses, the fibrosis becomes linear and later definitely nodular, especially in the inner midlung fields. If tuberculosis is superimposed on the original disease, large nodules, cavities, and pneumonic changes are found. X-rays alone should not be relied upon to make the diagnosis of silicosis, since other pneumoconioses may give a similar radiologic appearance.

D. Laboratory Findings: The vital capacity is gradually reduced as the disease progresses.

Prevention

Frequent quantitative dust counts and analyses must be made in work requiring exposure to dust. Particle counts must be kept within safe limits. Workers exposed to dust should have yearly chest examinations.

Airline face masks and protective suits must be worn in situations where dust cannot be controlled (eg, sandblasting). Wetting processes to control dusts must be used wherever feasible. Dust-producing operations should be segregated.

Accidental spilling of baby powder on infants' faces during diaper changing has resulted in death; care must be taken to avoid such spills.

Treatment

A. Specific Measures: Exposure to silica dust must be reduced to a safe amount. Complete change of occupation is not advisable (see Prognosis).

B. General Measures:

1. Activity should be restricted to an amount that does not produce dyspnea. However, exercise to tolerance is important for rehabilitation.

2. Administration of bronchodilators such as epinephrine, 1:1000; isoproterenol, 1:100; terbutaline, 1:1000; or phenylephrine, 1:100, by aerosol may improve effectiveness of positive-pressure breathing therapy.

Prognosis

A worker who develops silicosis need not in every case be removed from occupational exposure, which might involve intolerable family upheavals and economic hardship. However, exposure to silica must be reduced to a safe amount as described above.

A radiologic appearance identical with that seen in silicosis may be produced by dusts which do not cause progressive disease. Workers should not be frightened with the diagnosis of silicosis unless their histories indicate sufficient exposure to silica.

Silicosis may appear and progress more than 5 years after exposure is discontinued. Removal from exposure does not stop progression of the disease. Individuals with minimal silicosis who avoid tuberculosis, acute pulmonary infections, and excessive exertion will live approximately normal life spans if further silica exposure is avoided. Tuberculosis may progress in patients with silicosis in spite of therapy. Severe attacks of purulent bronchial pneumonia are frequent in persons with silicosis, and emphysema is likely to progress gradually.

ASBESTOS

Although diffuse fibrosis of the lungs was first reported in 1907 in asbestos workers and bronchogenic cancer was reported to be associated with asbestosis in 1935, only since 1960 has disease associated with asbestos been recognized in the general population. At that time, pleural calcification was found in farm families in Finland who lived near an asbestos mine. At present, in communities in Finland where anthophyllite asbestos mines are located, up to 9% of chest x-ray films show pleural calcification as compared to 0.5% in nonasbestos-producing communities. Another disease, mesothelioma of the pleura, has been found in the general population in an area of South Africa where crocidolite asbestos is an important mining product. In a study in London, the exposure history of patients with mesothelioma was investigated. Of the 45 patients who had not worked with asbestos, 9 had lived in a household with asbestos workers and 11 had lived within half a mile of an asbestos plant as much as 20 years previously. In New York City, 24 out of 28 lungs examined carefully were found to contain significant numbers of chrysotile fibers. Again in London, a similar study found that almost 80% of lungs contained chrysotile fibers, and in these lungs it was the most abundant of all fibers detected. The relationship between asbestos found in some metropolitan water supplies and human disease is unknown.

The word **asbestos** is used for any mineral that breaks down into fibers. The most commonly used form, chrysotile, is fibrous serpentine, a magnesium silicate containing 40% silica. Its fibers are tubular in section and range down to 0.015 μm in diameter, which is invisible in the ordinary microscope. Another form, crocidolite, is fibrous riebeckite, a sodium ferro-ferrisilicate containing 51% silica. Its fibers range down to 0.08 μm in diameter. Amosite is fibrous grunerite, a magnesium ferrosilicate containing 49% silica. Fibers of this form range down to 0.1 μm in diameter. Other forms include anthophyllite and tremolite-actinolite. Uses of the various forms of asbestos in cloth, brake linings, cement products, paper, flooring, gaskets, and paint amount to 3 million tons per year in the USA.

Corrective measures to limit asbestos exposure in mines and mills in the USA and Canada have been in force for many years. The exposure limits for particles longer than 5 μm (given in particles per milliliter of air) are as follows: amosite, 0.5; chrysotile, 2; crocidolite, 0.2; other forms, 2. In contrast to efforts made in and around mines and mills, little effort has been made to limit exposure of the general population or of workers in the applications industries (such as those applying insulation or coatings for fire protection or rust prevention). Atmospheric sampling for asbestos and examination of material is difficult, since the fibers are extremely small. Electron microscopy, with magnification of at least 20,000 times (and preferably 40,000 times), is necessary to recognize the fibers of chrysotile. If samples are collected by filtration, the pore size for most filters is 0.3 μm or larger, and the efficiency of collection must be carefully determined. The following levels have been found in urban air: In New York City, Manhattan had asbestos levels of 25–60 ng/m^3 of air; the Bronx had 25–28 ng/m^3; and Staten Island had 11–21 ng/m^3. One nanogram of chrysotile asbestos could represent 1 million fibrils. In Manhattan, asbestos fireproofing has been commonly sprayed in buildings, resulting in widespread dissemination of asbestos over much of the region. Rural areas of Pennsylvania had levels of 10–30 ng/m³ of air.

Pathologic findings include linear fibrosis of the lungs, pleural adhesions, and tumors and calcification of the pleura.

Clinical Findings

The principal manifestation of asbestosis is dyspnea.

A. Pulmonary Fibrosis: The most common disability, fibrosis of the lung, ordinarily has its onset 20–40 years after the beginning of exposure. Symptoms include difficulty in breathing, clubbing of the fingers, and reduction of vital capacity. The disease can develop with as little as 13 years of exposure, and one group exposed to concentrations in the atmosphere above the recommended limit had an incidence of fibrosis of 38%.

The incidence of pulmonary fibrosis after asbestos exposure is increased by smoking. Nonsmokers who had been exposed to asbestos for 20 years did not have pulmonary fibrosis, whereas 29 out of 45 smokers who had been exposed for the same length of time demonstrated pulmonary fibrosis on radiologic examination.

B. Pleural Effusion: Sudden spontaneous pleural effusion sometimes occurs in workers exposed to asbestos years before the diagnosis of asbestosis can be made. Onset of pleural effusion can be as soon as 3–4 years after the beginning of exposure to asbestos.

C. Cancer: Cancers of the mesothelial lining of the pleural cavity are rare except as a result of occupational exposure to asbestos. In addition to cases associated with crocidolite mining in South Africa, many more have occurred in Great Britain in cities where there are factories for processing asbestos or ports at which asbestos was unloaded. Prior to 1962, only 4 cases of mesothelioma had been found in Great Britain; by 1965, the number reached 160, and by 1969 a total of 622 were reported. At present, about 60 new cases are detected yearly.

In a group of men who applied asbestos insulation for 15 years or more, the mortality rate from cancer of the lung and pleura was 9 times that of a comparable age group in the male population as a whole. The study group consisted of 152 asbestos workers who had 15 or more years of exposure. In this group, there were 46 deaths, of which 12 resulted from cancer of the lung and pleura and 7 from cancer of the gastrointestinal tract or peritoneum. The mortality rate from gastrointestinal tract cancer was not considered to be increased over the incidence in the nonexposed population. The mean duration of exposure to asbestos was 26 years for the total group and 32 years for those who died. In another study, the number of deaths in 21,755 white male workers in 3 asbestos products industries was compared with that in 6281 white males in a nonasbestos industry. Cancer of the respiratory system was significantly increased in all of the asbestos industries—asbestos cement products, asbestos friction materials, and asbestos textiles—as compared to the nonasbestos industry. The mortality rate from respiratory diseases in the asbestos building products industry and the asbestos friction products industry was twice that of the nonasbestos industry. The asbestos textile industry had a respiratory disease mortality rate more than 4 times that of the nonasbestos industry. Most of this increase could be accounted for by the incidence of asbestosis.

Asbestos as a contaminant of rice has been suggested as the cause of the high incidence of stomach cancer in Japan. The Japanese prefer rice that has been treated with talc after milling. This talc has been found to contain asbestos. Preliminary reports from Australia indicate that asbestos is also responsible for cancer of the large bowel.

D. X-Ray Findings: Radiologic examination of the chest reveals a diffuse increase in density of the lungs and pleural calcification.

Prevention

Frequent quantitative dust counts and analyses must be made in work requiring exposure to asbestos. Particle counts must be kept within safe limits. Workers should have chest roentgenograms taken yearly. Nonsmokers are much less susceptible to asbestos disease.

Treatment

Exposure to asbestos must be reduced below the exposure limit. Activity should be restricted to an amount that does not produce dyspnea. Daily exercise to tolerance is important for rehabilitation.

Prognosis

After onset of symptoms, asbestosis progresses more rapidly than silicosis (see p 268).

References

General References

Anderson HA, Selikoff IJ: Pleural reactions to environmental agents. *Fed Proc* 1978;**37**:2496.

Biological effects of mineral fibers and particulates. *Environ Health Perspect* 1980;**34**:1.

Bouhuys A: Epidemiology of environmental lung disease. *Yale J Biol Med* 1979;**52**:191.

Bouhuys A: Priorities in prevention of chronic lung diseases. *Lung* 1979;**156**:129.

Gee JBL, Morgan WKC, Brooks SM: *Occupational Lung Disease*. Raven Press, 1984.

Hook GER (editor): Pulmonary toxicology. *Environ Health Perspect* 1984;**55**:1.

Leineweber JP: Fiber toxicology. *J Occup Med* 1981;**23**:431.

Morgan WKC, Seaton A: *Occupational Lung Diseases*. Saunders, 1975.

Witschi H, Coté MT: Primary pulmonary responses to toxic agents. *CRC Crit Rev Toxicol* 1977;**5**:23.

Asbestos

Bégin R et al: Radiographic assessment of pleuropulmonary disease in asbestos workers. *Br J Ind Med* 1984;**11**:373.

Berry G: Mortality of workers certified by pneumoconiosis medical panels as having asbestosis. *Br J Ind Med* 1981;**38**:130.

Browne K: Asbestos-related mesothelioma: Epidemiological evidence for asbestos as a promoter. *Arch Environ Health* 1983;**38**:261.

Castleman BI: The case for criminal sanctions in preventing occupational diseases. Exhibit A: Asbestos. *Dangerous Properties of Industrial Materials Report* (Sept) 1980;**1**:8.

Churg A: Lung cancer cell type and asbestos exposure. *JAMA* 1985;**253**:2984.

Council on Scientific Affairs: A physician's guide to asbestos-related diseases. *JAMA* 1984;**252**:2593.

Craighead JE, Mossman BT: Pathogenesis of asbestos-associated diseases. *N Engl J Med* 1982;**306**:1446.

Davis DL, Mandula B: Airborne asbestos and public health. *Annu Rev Public Health* 1985;**6**:195.

Finkelstein MM: A study of dose-response relationships for asbestos associated disease. *Br J Ind Med* 1985;**42**:319.

Millette JR et al: Asbestos. *Environ Health Perspect* 1984;**53**:1.

Mitchell RS et al: Evaluation for compensation of asbestos-exposed individuals. (2 parts.) *J Occup Med* 1985;**27**:95, 189.

Mossman B et al: Asbestos: Mechanisms of toxicity and carcinogenicity. *Annu Rev Pharmacol Toxicol* 1983;**23**:595.

Coal

Legg SJ et al: Lung mechanics in relation to radiographic category of coal workers' simple pneumoconiosis. *Br J Ind Med* 1983;**40**:28.

Ruckley VA et al: Comparison of radiographic appearances with associated pathology and lung dust content in a group of coal workers. *Br J Ind Med* 1984;**41**:459.

Weeks JL, Fox M: Fatality rates and regulatory policies in bituminous coal mining, United States 1959–1981. *Am J Public Health* 1983;**73**:1278.

Cotton & Other Organic Particulates

Battista G et al: A case-referent study on nasal cancer and exposure to wood dust in the province of Siena, Italy. *Scand J Work Environ Health* 1983;**9**:25.

Beck GJ et al: A prospective study of chronic lung disease in cotton textile workers. *Ann Intern Med* 1982;**97**:645.

Beck GJ et al: The relationship of respiratory symptoms and lung function loss in cotton textile workers. *Am Rev Respir Dis* 1984;**130**:6.

Brinton LA et al: Nasal cancer in textile and clothing industries. *Br J Ind Med* 1985;**42**:469.

Engleberg AL et al: Medical and industrial hygiene characterization of the cotton waste utilization industry. *Am J Ind Med* 1985;**7**:93.

Gerhardsson MR et al: Respiratory cancers in furniture workers. *Br J Ind Med* 1985;**42**:403.

Holness DL et al: Respiratory function and exposure-effect relationships in wood dust–exposed and control workers. *J Occup Med* 1985;**27**:501.

Morgan WKC et al: Byssinosis. *Am Rev Respir Dis* 1982;**126**:354.

Stellman SD, Garfinkel L: Cancer mortality among wood workers. *Am J Ind Med* 1984;**5**:343.

Silica

Cooper WC, Sargent EN: A 26-year radiographic follow-up of workers in a diatomite mine and mill. *J Occup Med* 1984;**26**:456.

Gerhardsson L, Ahlmark A: Silicosis in women. *J Occup Med* 1985;**27**:347.

National Institute of Occupational Safety and Health: Silica flour: Silicosis. *Current Intelligence Bulletin* 1981;**36**:1.

Uber CL, McReynolds RA: Immunotoxicology of silica. *CRC Crit Rev Toxicol* 1982;**10**:303.

Other Particulates

Dazies D, Cotton R: Mica pneumoconiosis. *Br J Ind Med* 1983;**40**:22.

McDowall ME: A mortality study of cement workers. *Br J Ind Med* 1984;**41**:179.

Peters JM et al: Pulmonary effects of exposures in silicon carbide manufacturing. *Br J Ind Med* 1984;**41**:109.

Rom WN et al: Pneumoconiosis and exposures of dental laboratory technicians. *Am J Public Health* 1984;**74**:1252.

Saracci R, Simonato L: Manmade vitreous fibers and workers' health: An overview of the epidemiological evidence. *Scand J Work Environ Health* 1982;**8**:233.

Skulberg KR et al: Mica pneumoconiosis. *Scand J Work Environ Health* 1985;**11**:65.

Thun MJ: Renal toxicity in uranium mill workers. *Scand J Work Environ Health* 1985;**11**:83.

Weill H et al: Respiratory health in workers exposed to man-made vitreous fibers. *Am Rev Respir Dis* 1983;**128**:104.

IV. Household Hazards

BROMATES

Bromates are used as neutralizers in cold waves. On contact with acids such as gastric hydrochloric acid, potassium bromate releases hydrogen bromate, which is an irritating acid.

The fatal dose of bromate is estimated to be 4 g, or 100 mL of a 3% solution. Ingestion of 0.5 g by a 6-year-old boy caused deafness and renal failure. The usual neutralizer contains 15 g of bromate, which is diluted in 500 mL of water to make a 3% solution.

About 10 fatalities from bromate poisoning have been reported.

Bromates are extremely irritating and injurious to tissues, especially those of the central nervous system and kidneys. The pathologic findings include kidney damage and hemolysis.

Clinical Findings

The principal manifestations of acute bromate poisoning are vomiting and collapse. Chronic poisoning has not been reported.

A. Symptoms and Signs: (From ingestion.) Vomiting, diarrhea, abdominal pain, oliguria or anuria, lethargy, deafness, coma, convulsions, low blood pressure, and fast pulse. Cyanosis due to methemoglobinemia and hematuria due to hemolysis may occur as late reactions.

B. Laboratory Findings: Hematuria and proteinuria; elevated nonprotein nitrogen during oliguria or anuria; methemoglobinemia.

Prevention

Nonpoisonous cold wave neutralizers are available and should be used. If poisonous neutralizers are used they must be stored and used safely.

Treatment

A. Emergency Measures: Remove poison by gastric lavage or emesis (see pp 21–28). The gastric lavage or emetic should contain 30–50 g of sodium bicarbonate and 50 g of sodium thiosulfate for each liter of water. At the end of gastric lavage, give 15 mL of Fleet's Phospho-Soda or 10 g of sodium sulfate in 200 mL of the sodium bicarbonate–sodium thiosulfate solution. The prompt use of peritoneal dialysis or of hemodialysis has also been suggested.

Table 18–1. Miscellaneous cosmetics.

Cosmetic Substance	Active Chemical	Remarks	Treatment
Cold wave lotion (For cold wave neutralizer, see potassium bromate, p 277, and perborate, p 360.)	Thioglycolates, thioglycerol.	Gastrointestinal irritation occurs after ingestion. May cause sensitivity dermatitis with edema, burning of skin, itching, and papular rash; hypoglycemia, CNS depression, convulsions, and dyspnea are possible.	Sensitivity dermatitis will disappear on discontinuing the use of cold wave preparations.
Cuticle remover	Potassium hydroxide, 5%.	See p 211.	See p 213.
Depilatories	Barium sulfide (see p 119), thioglycolates (see above), alkalies.	Gastrointestinal irritation occurs after ingestion.	Treat as for alkalies (see p 213).
Eyelash dye	Naphthylamine, phenylenediamines, toluenediamines, and other aromatic amino compounds.	Sensitivity dermatitis or irritation of eyes may occur (see p 144). Not likely to cause serious poisoning after ingestion of usual household preparations.	Discontinue use.
Face powder	Pigments, talc.	Sensitivity dermatitis, pneumoconiosis (see p 267).	Discontinue use.
Hair dyes, permanent	Naphthylamines, phenylenediamines, toluenediamines, and other aromatic amino compounds.	Excessive use may cause liver damage and skin sensitization (see p 144). Serious acute poisoning is rare after ingestion of usual household preparations.	See p 146.
Hair dyes, temporary	Silver, 0.1%; mercury, 0.1%; lead, 0.1%; arsenic, 0.1%; bismuth, 0.1%; pyrogallol, 1%; denatured alcohol, 50%.	The small quantity of toxic ingredients present in hair dyes makes acute poisoning unlikely.	Remove poison (see p 21). Give dimercaprol if symptoms occur (see p 84).
Hair lighteners	Ethanol, 25%; hydrogen peroxide, 6%; potassium persulfate, 10%.	Mucous membrane and gastrointestinal irritation with nausea and vomiting and diarrhea.	Discontinue further exposure.

Table 18–1 (cont'd). Miscellaneous cosmetics.

Cosmetic Substance	Active Chemical	Remarks	Treatment
Hair spray lacquer (wave set)	Vegetable gums, synthetic gum, polyvinylpyrrolidone, carboxymethylcellulose, polyvinyl alcohol, denatured alcohol (50%).	Sensitivity dermatitis may occur. Inhalation causes pulmonary granulomatosis with increase in size of hilar lymph nodes and infiltration in the lung that sometimes resembles sarcoidosis.	Discontinue further exposure.
Hair straighteners	Sodium hydroxide (up to 15%).	See p 211.	See p 213.
Hair tonic	Capsicum, 0.5% Ethanol, 75%	See p 434. See p 170.	See p 434. See p 174.
Lip dye, lipstick	Eosin, other pigments.	Cheilitis, facial dermatitis, or stomatitis.	Discontinue use.
Perfume	Alcohol (to 90%).	See p 168.	See p 169.
Tanning agents	Dihydroxyacetone, dyes.	Sensitivity dermatitis may occur.	Discontinue use.

B. Antidote: Give sodium thiosulfate, 1 mL/kg intravenously as a 10% solution.

C. General Measures:

1. Relieve gastric irritation by giving milk or cream every hour.

2. In the presence of cyanosis and respiratory difficulty, give O_2. If methemoglobin level is above 30%, give methylene blue cautiously, beginning with half the usual amount (see p 78).

3. Treat dehydration by giving 5% dextrose in water. Use caution in the administration of electrolytes, depending on the state of kidney function.

D. Special Problems: Treat anuria (see p 72).

Prognosis

Deafness and renal impairment may be permanent. About 10% of those severely poisoned have died.

DEMULCENTS & PROTECTIVES

Many nontoxic compounds are used as skin protectives, as skin softeners, and as ingredients in cosmetics. The following compounds are not irritating, and toxic doses by ingestion would have to be in excess of 2 g/kg. Skin sensitization is unusual. Aspiration or inhalation of any of these products could cause a chemical pneumonitis. Implantation of any of these substances will cause foreign body reaction.

Algin
Allantoin
Aluminum hydroxide
Calcium carbonate
Calcium phosphate
Caprylates
Carbowax
Chlorophyll
Cleansing cream
Hair dye, vegetable
Hair oil, cream
Hand lotion, cream
Hydroxyethyl cellulose

Kaolin
Lanolin
Makeup, liquid
Methylcellulose
Monoacetin
Neatsfoot oil
Paraffin
Polysorbate
Polyvinyl acetate
Polyvinylpyrrolidone
Red oil
Rosi
Rouge

Sesame oil
Silicone
Sorbic acid
Spermaceti
Starch
Stearic acid
Titanium oxide
Triacetin
Umbelliferone
Zinc oxide

Food Poisoning | 19

BOTULISM

Botulinus toxin is a heat-labile protein that can be destroyed by boiling at 100 °C for 1 minute or heating in water at 80 °C for 10 minutes.

Botulism is caused by the exotoxin produced by the anaerobic growth of *Clostridium botulinum* at pH above 4.6 and temperatures above 3 °C. Such growth frequently occurs in underprocessed, nonacid canned foods. Seven antigenic types of toxin occur—A, B, C, D, E, F, and G; types A, B, and E are the most important. The foods most often responsible are meats, fish, and vegetables; olives and fruits are occasionally responsible. Botulism can occur in infants fed honey, fresh fruit or vegetables, or other foods containing the spores. Exotoxin production then occurs in the gut. Wound botulism also occurs.

The fatal dose of a contaminated food may be 0.1 mL.

Botulinus toxin causes paralysis of muscles by blocking the transfer of nerve impulses at the motor end plate. Other cells appear to be affected also. Pathologic findings are congestion and hemorrhages in all organs and especially in the central nervous system. Degenerative changes occur in the liver and kidneys.

Clinical Findings

The principal manifestations of acute botulism are vomiting, double vision, and muscular paralysis.

In adult poisoning, the symptoms begin 8 hours to 8 days after ingestion, with nausea and vomiting and sometimes diarrhea and abdominal distress, progressing to muscle involvement with marked fatigability, ptosis, dysarthria, blurred or double vision, dilated pupils, difficulty in swallowing, weakness, paralysis of the respiratory muscles, and quadriplegia. Gastrointestinal symptoms may be absent. Deep tendon reflexes are not abolished. Pupillary response to light may be diminished or lost. The toxin can be identified in food, blood, feces, stomach contents, or tissues.

In infants, there is progressive paralysis that may result in respiratory compromise. The paralysis gradually disappears after 3–4 weeks.

Prevention

A temperature of 115 °C is required to destroy the spores of *C botulinum*. This temperature can only be reached by pressure cooking. Process canned foods according to the methods approved by the Department of Agriculture as described in *Home Canning of Fruits and Vegetables*, Catalog No. A1. 77:8; and *Home Canning of Meat*, Catalog No. A1. 77:6. The pamphlets are obtainable from the Superintendent of Documents, US Government Printing Office, Washington, DC 20402.

Boil or pressure cook suspect canned foods for 15 minutes before serving.

If poisoning occurs in any member of a family or a group, treat every person who may have eaten the suspect food. Do not wait for symptoms to develop. Label, seal, and store suspect food in such a way that others will not be poisoned.

Treatment

A. Emergency Measures:

1. Immediately upon suspecting food poisoning, remove the toxin by emesis using sodium bicarbonate or activated charcoal if the patient is asymptomatic; otherwise, use airway-protected gastric lavage (see pp 21–28). Follow by catharsis with Fleet's Phospho-Soda, 30–60 mL diluted 1:4, unless the patient has diarrhea.

2. Draw blood for toxin determination in serum.

3. Notify the local health department.

B. Antidote: Give type ABE botulinus antitoxin unless type A or type B has been identified. Dosage is 1 vial intravenously every 4 hours until the symptoms no longer progress or until the toxin can no longer be demonstrated in the patient's serum. Serum sensitivity must be tested by injecting 0.1 mL of a 1:10 dilution of antitoxin in saline intradermally; wait 15 minutes before giving dose. Centers for Disease Control in Atlanta can advise on the use of antitoxin; telephone (404) 239-3670 during the day, (408) 329-2888 at night.

C. General Measures: Treat respiratory depression by artificial respiration. In respiratory paralysis, maintain respiration by use of a body respirator or other mechanical aid. Artificial respiration may be lifesaving in cases of botulism not amenable to treatment by other means; it should be continued until all vital signs have definitely ceased. Prevent pulmonary aspiration by aseptic tracheal cleansing. If pneumonia develops, treat with organism-specific chemotherapy.

Prognosis

Approximately 50% of those with severe poisoning die. Those who survive recover completely, but residual weakness may persist for more than a year. The mortality rate in infants is less than 5%.

Green J et al: Human botulism (type F). *Am J Med* 1983;**75**:893.

MacDonald KL et al: Botulism and botulism-like illness in chronic drug abusers. *Ann Intern Med* 1985;**102**:616.

MacDonald KL et al: Type A botulism from sauteed onions: Clinical and epidemiologic observations. *JAMA* 1985;**253**:1275.

Morris JG Jr et al: Infant botulism in the United States: An epidemiological study of cases occurring outside of California. *Am J Public Health* 1983;**73**:1385.

Ruthman JC et al: Type A botulism. *Am J Emerg Med* 1985;**3**:203.

Schmidt-Nowara WW et al: Early and late pulmonary complications of botulism. *Arch Intern Med* 1983;**143**:451.

Sonnabend OAR et al: Continuous microbiological and pathological study of 70 sudden and unexpected infant deaths: Toxigenic intestinal *Clostridium botulinum* infection in 9 cases of sudden infant death syndrome. *Lancet* 1985;**1**:237.

Tacket CO et al: Equine antitoxin use and other factors that predict outcome in type A foodborne botulism. *Am J Med* 1984;**76**:794.

BACTERIAL FOOD POISONING

Bacterial food poisoning is caused by toxins elaborated during the growth of staphylococci or other organisms (Table 19–1) in foods kept at warm temperatures. Food poisoning typically occurs when food is allowed to stand at room temperature after it is cooked, either because spores that survive heating regrow or because the standing food is allowed to be contaminated. Reheating the food will not destroy staphylococcal toxins and may or may not destroy *Clostridium perfringens* toxins. Toxins from *Vibrio parahaemolyticus* and *Bacillus cereus* are destroyed by heating at 80 °C. The foods most often responsible for this type of poisoning are ham, tongue, sausage, dried meat, fish products, milk and milk products (including cream and cream-filled bakery goods), and eggs.

Bacterial food poisoning is ordinarily self-limited, since the bacteria do not continue to grow in the presence of normal bacterial flora. Symptoms presumably arise from the local effects of toxins. The mortality rate is approximately 1%.

Table 19–1. Bacterial food poisoning.

Source	Incubation Period (Hours)	Duration (Days)	Occurrence
Staphylococcus	1–6	1–2	Carrier contamination.
Clostridium perfringens	8–22	1–2	Spore growth.
Bacillus cereus	1–16	1	Spore growth.
Vibrio parahaemolyticus	4–96	1–7	Sea water contamination.

Clinical Findings

The principal manifestations of acute bacterial food poisoning are vomiting and diarrhea. Chronic poisoning has not been reported.

A. Symptoms and Signs: Nausea and vomiting, diarrhea, abdominal cramps or pain, and weakness occur; the incubation period varies depending on the organisms (Table 19–1). The symptoms ordinarily progress for 12–24 hours and then regress. Abdominal pain and tenesmus may be severe. Prostration, mild fever, dehydration, and shock sometimes occur.

B. Laboratory Findings: The blood count may reveal hemoconcentration. Urinalysis may reveal a trace of protein. Diagnosis is based on recovery of organisms from food, stomach contents, or feces.

Prevention

If foods containing meats, milk or milk products, fish, or eggs are not eaten immediately after being cooked, they should be chilled quickly and stored under refrigeration. Raw seafoods should not be eaten after storage. Seafoods should be protected from seawater contamination after cooking. Food handlers with skin or eye infections should not work until after recovery.

Treatment

A. Emergency Measures: Control severe vomiting by administration of chlorpromazine (Thorazine), 25–100 mg rectally or intramuscularly, or other antiemetic. Repeat every 4 hours as necessary.

B. General Measures: Place the patient at bed rest and give nothing by mouth until vomiting has subsided for 4 hours. Then give oral fluids as tolerated for 12–24 hours before beginning regular diet. If vomiting and diarrhea are severe, maintain fluid balance by giving 5% dextrose in saline intravenously. Diarrhea is self-limited and should not be suppressed.

Prognosis

If the patient lives for 48 hours, recovery is likely.

Goldfrank L, Weisman R: Bacterial food poisoning. *Postgrad Med* (Sept) 1982;**72**:171.

CHEMICAL FOOD POISONING

Storage of foods such as fruit juice or sauerkraut in containers lined with cadmium, copper, zinc, or antimony (enameled metal pans) will lead to acute gastric irritation manifested by nausea and vomiting and diarrhea. The disease usually lasts 24–48 hours. If necessary, atropine,

0.5 mg, and bismuth subcarbonate, 5 g, may be given orally to relieve abdominal distress. If symptoms are persistent and indicate metal poisoning, specific treatment may be necessary. (See cadmium, p 226; antimony, p 220; copper, p 430; zinc, p 430.) Food poisoning may also occur when meat preservatives that contain sodium nitrite are used excessively or erroneously in place of salt (see p 384).

20 | Miscellaneous Chemicals

BLEACHING SOLUTIONS
(Clorox, Purex, Sani-Clor)

Bleaching solutions are 3–6% solutions of sodium hypochlorite in water. The solution used for chlorinating swimming pools is 20% sodium hypochlorite. These solutions are about as corrosive as similar concentrations of sodium hydroxide. Upon contact with acid gastric juice or acid solutions, they release hypochlorous acid, which is extremely irritating to skin and mucous membranes but apparently is rapidly inactivated by blood serum and has low systemic toxicity. Buffering the acid by the administration of antacids offers a rapid means of reducing the irritating effect. Do not use acid antidotes in the treatment of sodium hypochlorite poisoning. Sodium thiosulfate immediately reduces hypochlorite to nontoxic products but may produce hydrogen sulfide in contact with acid.

The fatal dose for children is estimated to be about 30 mL if emesis does not occur.

Clinical Findings

The principal manifestation of acute poisoning with bleaching solutions is severe irritation with vomiting. Chronic poisoning does not occur.

Inhalation of hypochlorous acid fumes causes severe pulmonary irritation with coughing and choking followed by pulmonary edema. Ingestion causes irritation and corrosion of mucous membranes with pain and vomiting. Systemic effects include fall of blood pressure, delirium, and coma. Edema of the pharynx and larynx may be severe. Aspiration causes severe tracheobronchial irritation and exudation. Esophageal stenosis may occur later. Perforation of the esophagus or stomach has occurred but is rare. Prolonged skin contact with bleaching solution causes irritation.

Treatment

A. Emergency Measures:

1. Remove bleaching solution from the skin by flooding with water.

2. Dilute and decompose swallowed bleaching solution by giving milk, melted ice cream, or beaten eggs. Antacids such as milk of magnesia or aluminum hydroxide gel are also useful. Do not use emesis, lavage, or acid antidotes.

B. General Measures: Treat as for esophageal lesions due to sodium hydroxide poisoning (see p 213).

Prognosis

Recovery is likely if treatment is started early. Experience has shown that far less significant problems arise than would have been expected.

SOAPS & DETERGENTS

Soaps and detergents can be grouped into 3 general classes that differ in toxic effects: anionic detergents, nonionic detergents, and cationic detergents.

Anionic Detergents

The anionic household detergents (hand dishwashing liquids, hair shampoo) are sulfonated hydrocarbons or phosphorylated hydrocarbons. Powdered, flake, or bar soaps are made of sodium, potassium, or ammonium salts of fatty acids. Laundry compounds (All, Tide, Cheer, etc) have added water softeners such as sodium phosphate, sodium carbonate, or sodium silicate (see p 211).

The anionic detergents irritate the skin by removing natural oils, causing redness, soreness, and papular dermatitis. In sensitive persons they also cause thickening of the skin with weeping, cracking, scaling, and blistering. Ingestion causes oropharyngeal irritation, abdominal discomfort, diarrhea, intestinal distention, and occasionally vomiting. Fatalities from ingestion have not been reported. Animal experiments on anionic detergents without additives indicate that the LD50 ranges from 1 to 5 g/kg. The maximum safe amount for children may be estimated at 0.1–1 g/kg. The following are typical compounds: alkyl sodium sulfate, sodium lauryl sulfate, sodium alkyl phosphate, sodium aryl alkyl sulfonate, dioctyl sodium sulfosuccinate (docusate), and sodium oleate. The presence of enzymes does not increase the toxicity, but the enzymes are potent sensitizers.

In pregnant women, concentrated soap enema at term has caused colitis and possible fetal injury.

Skin eruptions are treated by removal from further exposure. For ingestion of detergents or soap, give fluids and allow vomiting to occur. Flush skin or eyes with water. For laundry compounds containing sodium phosphate or sodium carbonate, see p 213.

Table 20–1. Miscellaneous chemicals.

Common Name	Poisonous Ingredient	Remarks	Treatment
Aquarium products	Sodium chloride. Copper sulfate. Sodium hydroxide. Potassium permanganate.	See p 454. See p 430. See p 211. See p 365.	See p 454. See p 431. See p 213. See p 365.
Baking powder	Tartaric acid (50%).	Renal injury is possible from more than 1 g/kg orally. Tetany from reduction of ionic calcium.	Give 10 mL of 10% calcium gluconate IV.
Baking soda	Sodium bicarbonate.	Causes alkalosis in doses over 5 g/kg. Alkalosis can also occur from skin application.	Treat alkalosis by giving fluids (see p 49).
Bleach, powdered	N-Chlorosuccinimide; 1,3-dichloro-5,5-dimethylhydantoin (exposure limit 0.2 mg/m³); dichloroisocyanurate; sodium perborate (see p 360); trichloroisocyanate. These products also contain 10–20% sodium carbonate (see p 211).	Bronchospasms; mild inflammation and edema of eyes and upper respiratory tract; irritation or corrosion of stomach. Large ingested doses (0.5–1 g/kg) may cause weakness, lethargy, tremors, salivation, lacrimation, dyspnea, and coma.	Remove by gastric lavage or emesis.
Carpet backing	Latex (rubber) emulsion.	Intestinal obstruction is possible.	Gastric lavage and catharsis.
Chlorinated lime	Calcium hypochlorite (10–70% available chlorine).	Irritating in lower strengths; 70% preparation may cause corrosion and severe local injury.	Emesis. Treat as for bleaching solution (see p 286).
Cleaners, abrasive	Sodium phosphates.	See p 211.	See p 213.
Cleaners, liquid	Sodium phosphates. Kerosene. Pine oil. Glycerol ethers.	See p 211. See p 189. See p 432. See p 175.	See p 213. See p 191. See p 433. See p 177.
Cleaning solvents (inflammable)	Petroleum hydrocarbons.	Also called Stoddard solvent or French dry cleaner. See Kerosene (p 189).	See p 191.
Cleaning solvents (noninflammable, "safe")	Carbon tetrachloride. Trichloroethylene.	"Safe" only because it is noninflammable.	See p 149. See p 153.
Cloth-marking ink	Aniline	Produces methemoglobinemia by skin absorption or ingestion.	See p 146.

Table 20—1 (cont'd). Miscellaneous chemicals.

Common Name	Poisonous Ingredient	Remarks	Treatment
Crayons, industrial	Lead chromate.	See p 228.	See p 229.
Dishwashing compounds (machine)	Sodium polyphosphates, sodium carbonate, sodium silicates.	Irritating and corrosive to mucous membranes (see p 211). Cause hypocalcemia with shock, cyanosis, slow pulse, tetany.	Give 5 mL of 10% calcium gluconate IV and repeat as necessary.
Drain cleaners (eg, Drano)	Sodium hydroxide (90%). Sulfuric acid (100%).	See p 211. See p 198.	See p 213. See p 201.
Dyes, cloth	Synthetic dyes, salt.	May produce gastric irritation or skin sensitization.	Remove.
Dyes, fish bait	Chrysoidin.	Urinary bladder irritant and carcinogen.	Avoid.
Dye remover	Sodium hydrosulfite (80%). Sodium carbonate (20%).	See p 209. See p 211.	See p 201. See p 213.
Fertilizer	Ammonium nitrate, phosphate, and metal salts.	Produce mild gastric irritation and possibly methemoglobinemia (see p 77).	Dilute with milk or water.
Fireworks	Arsenic. Mercury. Antimony. Lead. Thiocyanate. Phosphorus.	See p 221. See p 238. See p 220. See p 230. See p 382. See p 243.	See p 223. See p 241. See p 221. See p 234. See p 383. See p 248.
Fluorescent lamps	Beryllium salts. Mercury.	See p 224. See p 238.	See p 225. See p 241.
Fuel tablets	Metaldehyde. Methenamine.	See p 185. See p 408.	See p 186. See p 408.
Furniture polish	Turpentine. Petroleum hydrocarbons.	See p 432. See p 189.	See p 433. See p 191.
Indelible pencils	Triphenylmethane dyes.	Injurious to tissues. Puncture wound or eye contamination causes pain, edema, and necrosis. Treat eye contamination by washing with water for at least 15 minutes. Repeated instillation of 1% fluorescein solution *(must be sterile)* will remove the dye by forming a soluble salt (see p 29). Treat puncture wounds by surgical debridement.	
Ink eradicator	Sodium hypochlorite (5%)	See p 286.	See p 286.
Ink, writing	Synthetic dyes, ferrous sulfate, tannic acid.	May produce gastric irritation.	Give demulcents.

Table 20—1 (cont'd). Miscellaneous chemicals.

Common Name	Poisonous Ingredient	Remarks	Treatment
Matches: Safety	Potassium chlorate.	See p 371.	See p 372.
Striking surface, safety	Red phosphorus.	See p 243.	See p 248.
Strike-anywhere	Phosphorus sesquisulfide (p 243). Potassium chlorate (p 371).	May cause nausea and vomiting.	Remove by gastric lavage or emesis.
Moth repellant	p-Dichlorobenzene. Naphthalene.	See p 164. See p 194.	See p 149. See p 195.
Paints	Potentially toxic metallic compounds as pigments.		See pp 227 and 234.
Oil type	Ill effects from single ingestion caused by the vehicle (see Petroleum Distillates, Xylene). After multiple ingestions of dry paint, lead poisoning is possible.		See pp 191 and 193. See p 234.
Emulsion type (latex base)	These contain water as a vehicle and a variety of pigments and suspending agents, none of which are seriously toxic. The single acute toxic dose is more than 5 mL/kg. Large doses might cause gastrointestinal irritation without systemic toxicity.		Remove by gastric lavage.
Paint, lacquer, and varnish removers	Benzene. Petroleum hydrocarbons. Methylene chloride. Methanol.	See p 192. See p 189. See p 155. See p 168.	See p 193. See p 191. See p 156. See p 169.
Photographic developers	Metol, hydroquinone, p-phenylenediamine, and other amino compounds.	Any of these compounds may sensitize the skin. The resulting dermatitis is characterized by weeping, crusting, and itching.	Avoid further contact with the particular developer or compound responsible for the dermatitis.
Photographic fixative	Sodium thiosulfate.	Possible release of hydrogen sulfide on contact with acid (see p 256).	
Plastic casting resin	Polyester monomer (65%). Styrene monomer (34%).	Irritating to skin and mucous membranes.	Remove by washing.
Plastic resin hardener	Methyl ethyl ketone peroxide (60%). Dimethyl phthalate (40%).	Corrosive to skin, mucous membranes, and eyes. See p 122.	Remove by washing or cautious gastric lavage. Avoid emesis.
Stamp pad inks	Aniline dyes.	May produce gastric irritation, skin sensitization, methemoglobinemia.	Remove. See p 78.
Steam iron cleaner	Tetrasodium edetate (20%); sodium carbonate (20%).	Doses over 1 mL/kg cause tetany by reduction of ionic calcium.	Give 10 mL of 10% calcium gluconate IV.
Water colors	Gum cambogia (gamboge).	See p 437.	See p 439.

Additives in soaps or detergents, including deodorants, may be skin sensitizers. Enzyme additives cause asthma.

Nonionic Detergents

These compounds are only slightly irritating to the skin and are apparently harmless by ingestion. Single doses of 20 g by mouth produce no symptoms. The following are typical examples: alkyl aryl polyether sulfates, alcohols, or sulfonates; alkyl phenol polyglycol ethers; polyethylene glycol alkyl aryl ethers; and sorbitan monostearate.

No treatment is necessary.

Cationic Detergents

See p 369.

V. Medicinal Poisons

Analgesics, Antipyretics, & Anti-inflammatory Agents | 21

SALICYLATES

Aspirin (acetylsalicylic acid) is present in many analgesic tablets. Salicylic acid is used in corn applications and in dermatologic ointments or as sodium salicylate for internal use. Methyl salicylate (oil of wintergreen) is the active ingredient in many skin liniments and ointments used for analgesic purposes. Salicylamide, salsalate (Disalcid), and sodium thiosalicylate are less toxic than aspirin and are used as weak analgesics given orally.

The fatal dose of any salicylate is estimated to be 0.2–0.5 g/kg. In children, the number of deaths caused by salicylates has declined precipitously over the past 20 years; this is largely attributed to the use of child-proof containers. Toxic effects appear at varying plasma levels depending on the duration of poisoning (Fig 21–1) but are uncommon below 30 mg/dL. Ingestion of 1 teaspoon of methyl salicylate (4 g of salicylate) has been fatal to a $2\frac{1}{2}$-year-old child. The exposure limit for salicylates in work atmospheres is 5 mg/m^3.

An association is now thought to exist between salicylate administration during certain viral infections (eg, varicella, influenza) and the occurrence of Reye's syndrome; however, the exact nature of the relationship is not clear.

Salicylates in toxic doses stimulate the central nervous system directly to cause hyperpnea and also produce a metabolic derangement with accumulation of organic acids. During hyperpnea, loss of CO_2 compensates for the metabolic increase in organic acids to maintain the blood pH at nearly 7.4, although in some instances arterial pH may rise. The urine remains continuously below pH 7. Renal losses of sodium and potassium accompanying organic acid excretion, accumulation of organic acid metabolites from the salicylate-induced metabolic derangement, and ketosis from starvation and dehydration bring on metabolic acidosis especially in children under 4 years of age. Acidemia increases the fraction of un-ionized salicylic acid, facilitating its entry into the brain. Blood P_{CO_2}, bicarbonate, and pH fall progressively, indicating inadequate buffering capacity in the blood. In severe poisoning in small children or adults with renal failure, hyperkalemia may become a problem.

At therapeutic doses, salicylates interfere with platelet aggregation, causing a prolongation of bleeding time. At toxic doses, salicylates lower plasma prothrombin by interfering with vitamin K utilization in the liver. In the presence of gastric acid, aspirin produces direct mucosal injury and consequent bleeding. The presence of alcohol increases mucosal injury. Salicylates are absorbed readily from the gastrointestinal tract, more rapidly in the presence of alkalinizing agents such as sodium bicarbonate. Elimination of salicylates by the body is almost entirely by means of renal excretion; thus, renal function must be adequate. In the presence of normal renal function, approximately 50% of a toxic dose will be excreted within the first 24 hours. Excretion is about 3–10 times as rapid if the urine is alkaline. If renal function is adequate and urine is alkaline, serum salicylate will fall to half the initial level in about 6 hours.

The pathologic findings in deaths from salicylate poisoning are erosion and congestion of the gastrointestinal tract and edema, hemorrhages, and degenerative changes in the kidneys, brain, lungs, and liver.

Clinical Findings

The principal manifestations of salicylate poisoning are hyperpnea and disturbed acid-base balance.

A. Acute Poisoning: (From ingestion or skin absorption.)

1. Mild–Burning pain in the mouth, throat, or abdomen; slight to moderate hyperpnea; lethargy; vomiting; tinnitus; hearing loss; and dizziness.

2. Moderate–Severe hyperpnea, marked lethargy, excitability, delirium, fever, sweating, dehydration, incoordination, restlessness, and ecchymoses.

3. Severe–Severe hyperpnea, coma, convulsions, cyanosis, oliguria, uremia, pulmonary edema, and respiratory failure. Some of the symptoms may result from hypoglycemia.

Severe reactions characterized by rhinorrhea, bronchiolar constriction, and circulatory collapse occur rarely, especially in asthmatics, after doses of 0.3–1 g.

B. Chronic Poisoning: (From ingestion or skin absorption.) Tinnitus, abnormal bleeding (gastric or retinal), gastric ulcer, weight loss, mental deterioration, skin eruptions. Liver damage can occur in normal patients but is more likely in patients with systemic lupus erythematosus, juvenile rheumatoid arthritis, rheumatic fever, alcoholism, and possibly rheumatoid arthritis.

C. Laboratory Findings:

1. Determination of the blood salicylate level (Fig 21–1) is essen-

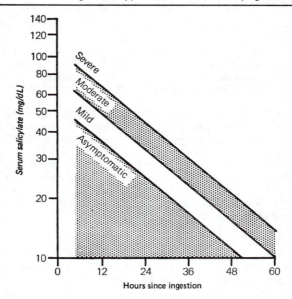

Figure 21–1. Nomogram relating serum salicylate concentration and expected severity of intoxication at varying intervals following ingestion of a single dose of salicylate. (Redrawn and reproduced, with permission, from Done AK: Salicylate intoxication. *Pediatrics* 1960;26:800.)

tial for the treatment of salicylate poisoning. (*Note:* Fig 21–1 does not apply to chronic poisoning.) The relationship between serum salicylate levels (in mg/dL) in the first 6 hours after poisoning is as follows: less than 45, not intoxicated; 45–65, mild intoxication; 65–90, moderate intoxication; 90–120, severe intoxication; above 120, usually lethal. The serum salicylate level may continue to rise for 6–10 hours after ingestion as a result of intestinal absorption. The ferric nitrate method of determining serum salicylate levels does not indicate the presence of salicylamide.

2. Blood bicarbonate below 8 meq/L indicates significant acidosis and disturbances in carbohydrate metabolism.

3. Other blood chemistry values that must be known for adequate treatment of severe salicylate poisoning include arterial pH; serum chloride, potassium, and sodium; and blood glucose.

4. Hematuria and proteinuria may be present.

5. To test for salicylates in urine, add a few drops of tincture of ferric chloride to 5 mL of boiled, acidified urine. A violet color indicates a phenolic compound (salicylate). Since this test is sensitive, it

only indicates that the patient has taken salicylates; it does not indicate the quantity.

6. Phenistix can be used to give semiquantitative indications of serum salicylate levels above 20 mg/dL. A Phenistix dipped into separated plasma or serum gives a tan color with levels below 40 mg/dL; a deeper brown color at 40–90 mg/dL; and a purple color above 90 mg/dL.

7. Prothrombin levels may drop below 20% of normal.

8. Long-term aspirin administration may result in abnormal liver function tests, including elevated alkaline phosphatase, SGOT, and SGPT levels.

9. Chronic salicylate administration increases urine cellular content, increases creatinine excretion, and reduces glomerular filtration rate.

10. Blood loss in stools may vary from 1 to 3 g/d during chronic aspirin administration.

Prevention

Salicylates should not be given to children with varicella, influenza, or certain other viral infections. Make certain that parents understand the proper dosage of salicylates for children. Do not apply salicylic acid ointment repeatedly over a large part of the body surface. If salicylates are prescribed, parents should be advised against giving additional salicylates.

Treatment

A. Emergency Measures:

1. Remove salicylates by emesis with syrup of ipecac unless respiration is depressed. Do not use apomorphine. Delay absorption of the remaining poison by giving activated charcoal. If respiration is depressed, use airway-protected gastric lavage. Enteric-coated tablets can be removed by lavage with 1% sodium bicarbonate. Gastric lavage and catharsis will remove significant amounts of salicylates up to 12 hours after ingestion.

2. If blood pressure is low, give blood, 10–15 mL/kg by transfusion over a period of 1 hour.

3. Treat respiratory depression by administering artificial respiration with O_2.

4. If convulsions occur and hypoglycemia is not a contributing factor, the administration of succinylcholine as well as artificial respiration with O_2 is probably the safest means of control. Central nervous system depressant agents such as barbiturates or diazepam must be administered cautiously.

B. General Measures: Intravenous alkaline fluids are used to alkalinize the urine rather than to reverse the acidosis per se.

1. Draw blood for initial measurement of bicarbonate, chloride, potassium, sodium, glucose, and arterial pH levels.

2. In mild poisoning with adequate urine output and no vomiting, give milk and fruit juice orally every hour up to a total of 100 mL/kg in the first 24 hours.

3. In severe poisoning, begin hydration in the first hour with intravenous fluid, 400 mL/m^2. A 5% dextrose solution containing sodium bicarbonate, 75 meq/L, is satisfactory. After the first hour, the same solution can be continued at one-third the initial rate until urine flow begins, dehydration is corrected, or evidence of renal insufficiency appears (rising blood urea nitrogen). After urine flow is established, add potassium, 30 meq/L of administered fluid, depending on the measured potassium deficit. Discontinue administration of potassium when serum levels reach 5 meq/L. If renal function is adequate, fluid administration should be approximately 3 L/m^2/24 h. Excessive fluid administration in the presence of fluid retention can lead to cerebral edema with blurring of the optic disk, periorbital edema, and central nervous system depression. In the presence of fluid retention, give 20% mannitol, 5 mL/kg slowly intravenously; or furosemide, 0.25–1 mg/kg orally or intravenously.

4. Maintenance of alkaline urine greatly speeds the excretion of salicylates but is difficult in chronically poisoned infants. Further adjustment of sodium and potassium in fluids should be based on serum sodium and potassium determinations.

5. Coma persisting after the salicylate level has returned to normal indicates the possibility of cerebral edema. This must be treated by the administration of osmotic diuretics such as mannitol. Corticosteroid administration may also be helpful.

6. In the presence of pneumonia, give organism-specific chemotherapy.

C. Special Problems:

1. In the presence of abnormal bleeding or hypoprothrombinemia, give phytonadione, 10 mg intramuscularly. Fresh blood or platelet transfusion may be necessary.

2. Do not give barbiturates, paraldehyde, morphine, or other central nervous system depressants.

3. If renal function is impaired, dialysis must be used to remove salicylates. If peritoneal dialysis is used, add 5% human albumin to the dialysate. Potassium chloride, 5 meq/L, should be added to the dialysate unless the serum potassium level is elevated.

4. Reduce hyperpyrexia by tepid sponging. Do not use alcohol for sponging. Elevated body temperature must not be allowed to persist.

Prognosis

If the blood bicarbonate level can be maintained above 15 meq/L, recovery is likely. Chronic poisoning responds very slowly to treatment.

Aaron TH, Muttitt ELC: Reactions to acetylsalicylic acid. *Can Med Assoc J* 1982;**126**:609.

Curtis RA et al: Efficacy of ipecac and activated charcoal/cathartic: Prevention of salicylate absorption. *Arch Intern Med* 1984;**144**:48.

Fisher CJ et al: Salicylate-induced pulmonary edema: Clinical characteristics in children. *Am J Emerg Med* 1985;**3**:33.

Gaudreault P et al: The relative severity of acute versus chronic salicylate poisoning in children. *Pediatrics* 1982;**70**:566.

Gordon IJ et al: Algorithm for modified alkaline diuresis in salicylate poisoning. *Br Med J* 1984;**289**:1039.

Halpin TJ: Reye's syndrome and medication used. *JAMA* 1982;**248**:687.

PHENACETIN

Phenacetin (acetophenetidin) was formerly a component of many proprietary medications. In the USA, it has been almost entirely replaced by acetaminophen. Phenacetin is metabolized in the body to the active compound acetaminophen, and the parent molecule of phenacetin precipitates methemoglobinemia. In western Europe, where the drug is still available, chronic ingestion has been associated with chronic renal failure. In the USA, this sequela was extremely rare even when phenacetin was widely available.

The fatal dose of phenacetin is about 1 g/kg.

ACETAMINOPHEN

Acetaminophen (paracetamol) is used alone or in combination with other drugs in a number of proprietary analgesic compounds. Phenacetin has been almost entirely replaced by acetaminophen.

The popularity of acetaminophen has increased dramatically over the past decade; over 40% of the analgesics now sold contain acetaminophen. Acetaminophen poisoning is becoming common in the USA, and in Great Britain more than 5000 patients with acetaminophen poisoning are admitted annually to hospitals, and 50–100 die. Most fatalities from acetaminophen have occurred in adults who have intentionally taken 10 g or more (140 mg/kg).

Toxic doses of acetaminophen can injure the liver, kidneys, heart, and central nervous system. Liver damage from acetaminophen develops within hours as a result of oxidation of acetaminophen to toxic metabolites (epoxides); these damage the liver after the detoxifying agent glutathione has been depleted. N-Acetylcysteine, cysteamine, and methionine can act as glutathione precursors and are thought to block the formation of toxic oxidation products of acetaminophen. Acetaminophen is rapidly absorbed. Thirty minutes after ingestion of 1 g of acetaminophen, 10 g of activated charcoal reduces total absorption by only 30%.

Clinical Findings

The principal manifestation of poisoning with acetaminophen is hepatic failure. It does not cause acid-base disturbances such as those that occur with the salicylates.

A. Acute Poisoning: (From ingestion.) Ingestion of 150 mg/kg or more causes nausea and vomiting, drowsiness, confusion, liver tenderness, low blood pressure, cardiac arrhythmias, jaundice, and acute hepatic and renal failure. Deaths have resulted from liver necrosis up to 2 weeks after ingestion.

B. Chronic Poisoning: Hepatic damage has been reported after daily ingestion of acetaminophen for a year or more, but this is rare.

C. Laboratory Findings:

1. Plasma acetaminophen levels peak $2\frac{1}{2}$–4 or more hours after ingestion of the drug. In acute acetaminophen poisoning, unless the amount ingested is known to be less than 100–150 mg/kg body weight, the plasma acetaminophen level should be determined 3–4 or more hours after ingestion in order to determine treatment (Fig 21–2). The initial level and levels determined at intervals thereafter should be plotted on semilogarithmic paper to determine the relative potential for toxicity and the disappearance half-time (half-life) of the drug (see p 98). A half-life greater than 4 hours indicates liver damage. Fatalities are unlikely unless the 4-hour plasma acetaminophen level is above 300 μg/mL. Liver damage is likely in all patients with 4-hour plasma acetaminophen levels above 300 μg/mL, in 40% of those with 250–300 μg/mL, in 25% of those with 150–250 μg/mL, and in 5% of those with 120–150 μg/mL. Levels below 120 μg/mL are nontoxic. About 25% of patients with 4-hour plasma acetaminophen levels above 300 μg/mL will have acute renal failure.

2. Liver damage is indicated by serum aspartate aminotransferase (SGOT) or alanine aminotransferase (SGPT) levels above 40 IU/L, a prothrombin time ratio above 1.3 compared to normal, or a plasma bilirubin level above 1 mg/dL. Liver damage is severe if aspartate or alanine aminotransferase levels exceed 1000 IU/L.

3. Urine may contain protein, casts, hemoglobin, or red blood cells.

Treatment

A. Emergency Measures: Remove ingested drug by emesis with syrup of ipecac unless respiration is depressed. Do not use apomor-

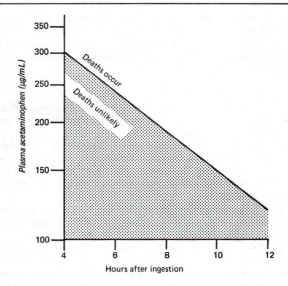

Figure 21-2. Nomogram relating plasma acetaminophen concentration with time. (Adapted from Prescott LF et al: Cysteamine, methionine, and penicillamine in the treatment of paracetamol poisoning. *Lancet* 1976;2:109.)

phine. Activated charcoal interferes with absorption of N-acetylcysteine, but opinion is divided as to the clinical significance of this. Give a saline cathartic. If respiration is depressed, use airway-protected gastric lavage (see pp 21–28). Efforts to remove acetaminophen are useless after 4 hours.

B. Antidote: (Best given within 10 hours after ingestion.)

1. If the 4-hour plasma acetaminophen level (Fig 21–2) exceeds 150 μg/mL, administration of N-acetylcysteine (available as Mucomyst) is suggested. N-Acetylcysteine is given orally, 140 mg of 20% solution per kilogram as a loading dose, followed by 70 mg/kg every 4 hours for 3 days. Some physicians use a shorter course of treatment. It may be necessary to administer the drug via a nasogastric tube. Adverse effects include nausea and vomiting.

2. Cysteamine hydrochloride and methionine have also been suggested, but these may be less effective and are more toxic. They are not available for use in the USA.

C. General Measures:

1. Keep patient warm and quiet.

2. If the prothrombin time ratio exceeds 3.0, give phytonadione,

1–10 mg intramuscularly. Fresh plasma or clotting factor concentrates may be necessary.

3.   Forced diuresis may be harmful; peritoneal dialysis, hemodialysis, and hemoperfusion are ineffective.

4.   Give 5% dextrose intravenously for the first 48 hours.

Prognosis

In acute poisoning, patients who survive will probably recover. In chronic poisoning, recovery is the rule.

Bateman DN et al: Adverse reactions to N-acetylcysteine. *Lancet* 1984;**2**:228.

Lieh-Lai MW et al: Metabolism and pharmacokinetics of acetaminophen in a severely poisoned young child. *J Pediatr* 1984;**105**:125.

Mant TGK et al: Adverse reactions to acetylcysteine and effects of overdose. *Br Med J* 1984;**289**:217.

Prescott LF, Critchley JA: The treatment of acetaminophen poisoning. *Annu Rev Pharmacol Toxicol* 1983;**23**:87.

Renzi FP et al: Concomitant use of activated charcoal and N-acetylcysteine. *Ann Emerg Med* 1985;**14**:568.

Rumack BH: Acetaminophen overdose in young children. *Am J Dis Child* 1984;**138**:428.

PYRAZOLONES: AMINOPYRINE, ANTIPYRINE, PHENYLBUTAZONE

Aminopyrine (Pyramidon), antipyrine (Phenazone), phenylbutazone (Butazolidin), dichloralphenazone (Midrin), and dipyrone (Novaldin) are used as analgesics for the treatment of rheumatic diseases and other painful conditions. Sulfinpyrazone (Anturane) is used in the treatment of gout.

The acute fatal dose for these drugs is 5–30 g, but fatalities from acute poisoning have been rare. Leukopenic reactions occur in about 1% of users, and fatalities from agranulocytosis have followed doses as small as 1 g. At least 300 deaths from agranulocytosis due to aminopyrine poisoning have been reported.

In large doses, the pyrazolones stimulate the central nervous system. Only antipyrine is likely to cause methemoglobinemia. These drugs produce agranulocytosis presumably on the basis of a sensitivity reaction. Patients who have had leukopenia following the use of one of the pyrazolones may have recurrences following doses as low as 1–10 mg. These drugs also cause retention of water and sodium chloride, presumably by affecting the kidney.

Pathologic findings in fatalities from acute poisoning include degenerative changes in the kidney, liver, and brain. After antipyrine poisoning, the blood may be chocolate-colored owing to methemoglobin formation. In agranulocytosis, myeloid elements are absent from the bone marrow. Perforation of a preexisting peptic ulcer is sometimes seen.

Clinical Findings

The principal manifestations of poisoning with the pyrazolones are mental disturbances and leukopenia.

A. Acute Poisoning: (From ingestion or rectal instillation.) Dizziness, mental disturbances, cyanosis, nausea and vomiting, epigastric pain, tinnitus, difficulty in hearing, and coma and convulsions, with thready pulse.

B. Chronic Poisoning: (From ingestion.)

1. Moderate toxicity–Phenylbutazone in therapeutic doses causes the following toxic reactions in 20–50% of patients: epigastric pain, vomiting, anorexia, edema, oliguria, urticaria, and cyanosis. The other agents of this class are likely to produce similar findings.

2. Severe toxicity or hypersensitivity–Severe manifestations of toxicity or hypersensitivity from therapeutic doses of any of these compounds occur in about 1% of patients and include the following:

a. Leukopenia, aplastic anemia, or agranulocytosis, with sore throat, fever, and pharyngeal membrane.

b. Liver damage, with jaundice and enlargement of liver and spleen.

c. Exfoliative dermatitis.

d. Gastric or duodenal erosion, with perforation or bleeding.

e. Adrenal necrosis.

f. Thrombocytopenia purpura.

g. Acute leukemia, at least 25 cases of which have occurred in patients who have taken phenylbutazone.

3. Anuria with uremia occurs most often when there is preexisting renal disease and when doses greater than 600 mg/d are given. Acute renal failure has followed single doses of antipyrine.

4. Aminopyrine causes agranulocytosis in about 1% of patients.

5. Antipyrine causes exfoliative dermatitis in about 0.1% of patients. The incidence of drug rash is almost 3% after administration of dipyrone.

C. Laboratory Findings:

1. White blood cell count is low; granulocytes are markedly diminished; red blood cell count is low.

2. Blood urea nitrogen levels may be elevated.

3. Hepatic cell function may be impaired as shown by appropriate tests (see p 75).

4. Stools may reveal frank or occult blood.

5. Methemoglobinemia.

Prevention

(1) Avoid the use of pyrazolones for simple analgesic or antipyretic effects.

(2) Use minimum effective doses of pyrazolones. Daily doses of phenylbutazone over 400 mg or of aminopyrine or antipyrine over 1 g are likely to induce toxicity.

(3) Perform white blood cell count at least once a week for the first 2 months and then once a month during prolonged therapy.

Treatment

A. Acute Poisoning:

1. Emergency measures–Delay absorption of ingested drug by giving tap water, milk, or activated charcoal and then remove by gastric lavage or emesis followed by catharsis (see pp 21–28).

2. General measures–

a. If cyanosis is severe, give methylene blue (see p 78).

b. Control convulsions (see Table 4–3).

c. Treat oliguria (see p 72).

B. Chronic Poisoning:

1. Immediate measures–Discontinue medication at the first symptom.

2. General measures–Give low-salt, high-protein, high-carbohydrate, low-fat diet.

3. Special problems–

a. Treat agranulocytosis (see p 79).

b. Treat liver damage (see p 77).

c. Treat gastroduodenal perforation surgically.

d. Treat gastroduodenal bleeding by transfusions and bed rest.

e. Treat anuria (see p 72).

f. In exfoliative dermatitis, prevent infections by means of organism-specific chemotherapy.

Prognosis

Approximately 10% of severe reactions end fatally. If the patient survives for 1 month, recovery is to be expected.

CINCHOPHEN & NEOCINCHOPHEN

Cinchophen and neocinchophen, popular in the past as analgesics, antipyretics, and uricosuric agents in the treatment of gout, are still used in patent medicines, proprietary mixtures, and prescriptions.

The acute fatal dose of either drug is 5–30 g, although fatalities from liver damage have followed repeated doses of as low as 1 g/d for 1–2 weeks. Fatalities from acute poisoning have been rare, but at least 250 deaths have followed the repeated medicinal use of cinchophen.

Table 21–1. Miscellaneous drugs used in painful conditions.

Drug	Clinical Findings and Treatment
Gold compounds Aurothioglucose (Solganal) Gold sodium thiosulfate Gold sodium thiomalate (Myochrysine)	Skin rash, stomatitis, pruritus, herpes, papular eruptions, nausea and vomiting, diarrhea, metallic taste, proteinuria, hematuria, uremia, nephrosis, hepatitis, fever, exfoliative dermatitis, photosensitivity, granulocytopenia, thrombocytopenic purpura, hypersensitivity pneumonitis, and aplastic anemia. **Remarks:** Patients should avoid exposure to sunlight, x-rays, and ultraviolet radiation while under treatment with gold compounds. **Treatment:** Give dimercaprol (see p 84) or penicillamine (see p 87).
Nonsteroidal anti-inflammatory agents Diflunisal (Dolobid) Fenoprofen (Nalfon) Ibuprofen (Motrin) Indomethacin (Indocin) Meclofenamate (Meclomen) Mefenamic acid (Ponstel) Naproxen (Naprosyn) Piroxicam (Feldene) Sulindac (Clinoril) Tolmetin (Tolectin)	Gastrointestinal irritation with erosion and hemorrhage or perforation, kidney damage, liver damage, heart damage, hemolytic anemia, agranulocytosis, thrombocytopenia, aplastic anemia, and meningitis can possibly occur with any of these drugs. Other symptoms include headache, dizziness, tinnitus, confusion, blurred vision, mental disturbances, skin rash, stomatitis, edema, reduced retinal sensitivity, corneal deposits, and hyperkalemia. Naproxen has caused cough, eosinophilia, and pulmonary infiltration. Sudden death has occurred after indomethacin in children. **Remarks:** Indomethacin and mefenamic acid are contraindicated and the others possibly hazardous in children. **Treatment:** Discontinue use. Remove oral overdoses by emesis if patient is alert, by gastric lavage if patient is depressed. Activated charcoal is useful. Treat symptomatically (see p 298).

Neocinchophen is considered less dangerous, but it is also less effective. About 1% of those who take cinchophen have acute liver damage.

The acute effects of large doses of these drugs are similar to those from salicylates (see p 295) and appear to be due to the acidic nature of the molecule. The high incidence of liver damage apparently is due to increased susceptibility in certain individuals, which cannot be explained entirely by the development of sensitivity, since some patients have developed liver involvement after the first dose of cinchophen. Although gastric ulceration has not been reported in humans, it is readily produced when cinchophen is administered to dogs.

The pathologic findings in delayed deaths from cinchophen or neocinchophen are acute yellow atrophy of the liver and fatty degeneration in the kidneys and heart.

Clinical Findings

The principal manifestations of poisoning with these compounds are hyperpnea, acidosis, and jaundice.

A. Acute Poisoning: (From ingestion.) Gastrointestinal irritation, epigastric discomfort, anorexia, diarrhea, vomiting, hyperpnea, tinnitus, hyperthermia, delirium, convulsions, and coma. The possibility of gastric ulceration of perforation should be considered.

B. Chronic Poisoning: (From ingestion.) Jaundice, anorexia, abdominal discomfort, and painful enlargement of the liver. Within 1–4 weeks, the size of the liver decreases, abdominal ascites forms, and the patient may die in hepatic coma.

C. Laboratory Findings:

1. Hematuria and proteinuria may be present in either acute or chronic poisoning.

2. In acute poisoning, a blood bicarbonate level below 10 meq/L indicates significant acidosis.

3. Evaluate liver function by appropriate tests (see p 75).

Prevention

These drugs should never be included in proprietary mixtures for use without prescription. The high incidence of fatal liver damage associated with these drugs makes their use in the treatment of gout dangerous.

Treatment

Treat as for salicylate poisoning (see p 298). If gastric perforation occurs, surgical closure will be necessary. For chronic poisoning, discontinue the use of any drug or proprietary medication that may contain cinchophen or neocinchophen. Treat liver damage (see p 77).

Prognosis

Approximately 25% of patients with liver damage from cinchophen die with acute yellow atrophy.

INTERACTIONS
(See p 17.)

If corticosteroids are withdrawn during continuing salicylate therapy, salicylate toxicity can occur.

Phenylbutazone decreases excretion of hydroxyhexamide, the active metabolite of acetohexamide. Phenylbutazone and congeners and indomethacin potentiate the effects of warfarin, tolbutamide, chlorpropamide, and phenytoin by displacement from binding sites. Salicylate, phenylbutazone and congeners, and indomethacin enhance the effects of cortisone by displacement.

Salicylates enhance the effects of coumarin anticoagulants and hypoglycemic drugs. Salicylates potentiate the effects of methotrexate by protein displacement.

Probenecid raises the blood level of indomethacin by blocking indomethacin excretion. If indomethacin and furosemide are given together or if beta-blocking agents and indomethacin are given together, the response to the drugs is altered.

Salicylamide may greatly potentiate the hepatic toxicity of acetaminophen.

PHARMACOKINETICS & TOXIC CONCENTRATIONS
(See p 89.)

	pKa	t½	Vd	% Binding	Toxic Concentration (µg/mL)
Acetaminophen	9.5	2–7	0.7–1	25	150 (at 4 hours)
Aminopyrine	5.0	2–7		15	
Aspirin	3.5	2–24	0.1, 0.3*	50–75	500
Fenoprofen	4.5	1.5–3	0.1	99	
Ibuprofen	4.4	2	0.14	99	
Indomethacin	4.5	4–12	0.34–1.57	92–99	
Naproxen	5	10–17	0.09	98–99	
Oxyphenbutazone	4.7	27–64		99	
Phenacetin		0.7–1.25	1–2.1	30	
Phenylbutazone	4.5	29–175	0.02, 0.25*	98	120
Sulfinpyrazone	2.8	2–3		98–99	
Sulindac		7		93	
Tolmetin	3.5	5.3	0.04	90	

*For children.

References

Barry WS, Meinzinger MM, Howse CR: Ibuprofen overdose and exposure in utero: Results from a postmarketing voluntary reporting system. *Am J Med* 1984;**77(1A)**:35.

Blackshear JL et al: Identification of risks for renal insufficiency from nonsteroidal anti-inflammatory drugs. *Arch Intern Med* 1983;**143**:1130.

Clive DM et al: Renal syndromes associated with nonsteroidal anti-inflammatory drugs. *N Engl J Med* 1984;**310**:563.

Heyd J, Simmeran A: Gold-induced lung disease. *Postgrad Med J* 1983;**59**:368.

Lanza FL: Endoscopic studies of gastric and duodenal injury after use of ibuprofen, aspirin, and other nonsteroidal anti-inflammatory agents. *Am J Med* 1984;**77(1A)**:19.

Anesthetics | 22

COCAINE

Cocaine is used as a local anesthetic on mucous membranes.

The fatal dose after application to mucous membranes may be as low as 30 mg. While ingested cocaine is much less toxic than cocaine taken or administered by other routes, including application to mucous membranes, it is still a serious problem. Fatalities have also occurred when ingested rubber balloons or plastic bags containing large quantities of cocaine have broken.

In toxic doses, cocaine first stimulates and then depresses the central nervous system in descending order from the cortex to the medulla. The pathologic findings in fatal cases of cocaine poisoning are congestion of the gastrointestinal tract, brain, and other organs.

Clinical Findings

The principal manifestations of cocaine poisoning are convulsions and circulatory failure.

A. Acute Poisoning: (From ingestion, injection, or absorption through mucous membranes or skin abrasions.) The initial symptoms are restlessness, excitability, hallucinations, tachycardia, dilated pupils, chills or fever, sensory aberrations, abdominal pain, vomiting, numbness, and muscular spasms. These are followed by irregular respirations, convulsions, coma, and circulatory failure. Death may occur almost immediately after the use of cocaine or may be delayed 1–3 hours. Fatal pulmonary edema has occurred after intravenous administration of the free cocaine base.

B. Chronic Poisoning: (From ingestion, injection, or absorption through mucous membranes or skin abrasions.) Hallucinations, mental deterioration, weight loss, and change of character. The use of cocaine as snuff can cause perforation of the nasal septum.

C. Laboratory Findings: These are noncontributory.

Prevention

Avoid using more than 50 mg (1 mL of 5% solution) of cocaine on mucous membranes. Less should be used for patients under age 20 years. Cocaine should never be injected. It should always be kept labeled.

Treatment

A. Acute Poisoning:

1. Emergency measures–

a. Maintain airway and respiration. Delay absorption of ingested drug by giving activated charcoal and then remove from the stomach by gastric lavage or emesis (see pp 21–28). Limit absorption from an injection site by tourniquet or ice pack. Efforts to remove the drug after 30 minutes are probably useless.

b. Control convulsions by giving diazepam, 0.1 mg/kg orally or slowly intravenously, or 2.5% thiopental sodium slowly intravenously. Be prepared to give artificial respiration. Tachycardia and other cardiac arrhythmias can be controlled by giving propranolol, 1 mg slowly intravenously; repeat up to a total dose of 8 mg. Lidocaine, 1 mg/min intravenously, may also be useful in treating cardiac arrhythmias.

2. General measures–

a. Succinylcholine may be necessary if convulsions interfere with respiration.

b. Maintain blood pressure with fluids. Vasopressors are hazardous.

c. For hypertensive reactions, give phentolamine, 5 mg slowly intravenously.

d. Treat for the possible presence of morphinelike substances (see p 327).

e. Treat hyperthermia (see p 50).

B. Chronic Poisoning: Discontinue use of the drug. There are usually no withdrawal symptoms following cocaine withdrawal such as those that occur after morphine withdrawal.

Prognosis

If the patient survives the first 3 hours after acute poisoning, recovery is likely.

Caruana BS et al: Cocaine-packet ingestion: Diagnosis, management, and natural history. *Ann Intern Med* 1984;**100**:73.

Itkonen J et al: Pulmonary dysfunction in "freebase" cocaine users. *Arch Intern Med* 1984;**144**:2195.

McCarron MM, Wood JD: The cocaine "body packer" syndrome: Diagnosis and treatment. *JAMA* 1983;**250**:1417.

Mittleman RE: Death caused by recreational cocaine use. *JAMA* 1984;**252**:1889.

PROCAINE & OTHER LOCAL ANESTHETICS
(Tables 22–1 and 22–2)

A large number of local anesthetics are used by injection or on skin or mucous membranes. Procaine, lidocaine, and other local anesthetic agents are used for antiarrhythmic effects. They are rapidly absorbed from mucous membranes.

For maximum safe doses, see Tables 22–1 and 22–2. Local anesthetics ordinarily have no systemic effects when ingested, since they are rapidly hydrolyzed. Excessive doses may cause methemoglobinemia, since even the hydrolytic products are still capable of forming methemoglobin.

After injection or surface application, large doses induce severe circulatory collapse by direct depression of blood vessel tone or by an effect on the central nervous system. Blood pressure lowering effects are more pronounced after intravenous injection in patients with heart or liver disease. In large doses, local anesthetics first stimulate and then depress the central nervous system. In pregnant patients, these agents cross the placenta and are not readily metabolized by the liver of the fetus.

The pathologic findings in fatal cases of poisoning are not characteristic.

Table 22—1. Local anesthetics for injection.
(For clinical findings and treatment, see p 312 and above.)

Drug	Maximum Adult Dose by Injection or Topical Application	
	mg	mL
Bupivacaine (Marcaine)	250	25 of 1%
Butethamine (Monocaine)	750	75 of 1%
Chloroprocaine (Nesacaine)	750	75 of 1%
Dibucaine (Nupercaine)*	25	5 of 0.5%
Etidocaine (Duranest)	750	75 of 1%
Hexylcaine (Cyclaine)	500	50 of 1%
Isobucaine (Kincaine)	750	75 of 1%
Lidocaine (Xylocaine)	500	50 of 1%
Mepivacaine (Carbocaine)	400	40 of 1%
Meprylcaine (Oracaine)	750	75 of 1%
Metabutethamine (Unacaine)	750	75 of 1%
Piperocaine (Metycaine)	750	37.5 of 2%
Prilocaine (Citanest)	600	60 of 1%
Procaine (Novocaine)	1000	100 of 1%
Propoxycaine (Blockain)	100	10 of 1%
Tetracaine (Pontocaine)	50	10 of 0.5%

*Necrosis following injection; severe itching and weeping dermatitis frequent when used on skin or mucous membranes.

Table 22–2. Local anesthetics for topical use.
(For treatment, see p 313.)

	Maximum Adult Dose For Surface Use			Additional Clinical Findings (See below.)
	mg	mL		
Amolanone (Amethone)	100	30	of 0.33%	
Benoxinate (Dorsacaine)	100	25	of 0.4%	
Benzyl alcohol	5000	100	of 5%	Irritation, tissue injury.
Butacaine sulfate	100	5	of 2%	
Butyl aminobenzoate	5000	25	of 20%	Sensitivity dermatitis.
Cyclomethycaine (Surfacaine)	500	25	of 2%	
Dimethisoquin (Quotane)	100	10	of 1%	Sensitivity dermatitis.
Diperodon (Diothane)	100	10	of 1%	
Dyclonine (Dyclone)	100	20	of 0.5%	
Ethyl aminobenzoate (benzocaine)	5000	25	of 20%	Cyanosis from methemoglobinemia.
Naepaine	100	2.5	of 4%	
Orthoform	5000	25	of 20%	Irritation, inflammation, tissue injury.
Phenacaine (Holocaine)	50	5	of 1%	
Pramoxine (Tronothane)	200	20	of 1%	
Proparacaine (Ophthaine)	5	1	of 0.5%	

Clinical Findings

The principal manifestations of poisoning with these agents are fall of blood pressure and convulsions.

A. Acute Poisoning: (From injection, ingestion, or application to mucous membranes.) Dizziness, cyanosis due to methemoglobinemia, fall of blood pressure, muscular tremors, convulsions, coma, irregular and weak breathing, cardiac standstill, and bronchial spasm. Ingestion of 300–600 mg of lidocaine has caused convulsions and respiratory failure in a 17-month-old-child, and rapid intravenous injection of 2 g has caused cardiac arrest in an adult. Mepivacaine has been injected into an unborn baby's head during administration of caudal anesthesia; this caused asphyxia, cyanosis, bradycardia, and convulsions and resulted in death.

B. Hypersensitivity: Hypersensitivity reactions sometimes occur after repeated applications of local anesthetics to skin or mucous membranes. The findings are itching, erythema, excoriation, edema, and vesiculation.

C. Laboratory Findings: The ECG may show atrioventricular block.

Prevention

Do not use doses larger than the suggested maximum doses (Tables 22–1 and 22–2) either topically or by injection. Hypersensitivity can be tested by applying the local anesthetic to the nasal mucosa on a cotton pledget for at least 5 minutes prior to injection. Signs of discomfort such as irritation, burning, or swelling indicate hypersensitivity. However, tests of hypersensitivity may be unreliable. If procaine or lidocaine is administered parenterally for the treatment of cardiac irregularities, give only by slow intravenous infusion with electrocardiographic monitoring and stop at the first untoward sign.

Treatment

A. Acute Poisoning:

1. Emergency measures–Remove ingested drug by induced emesis followed by activated charcoal. Limit absorption from injection site by a tourniquet and ice pack (see p 28). Maintain airway and give artificial respiration with O_2 until convulsions or depression is controlled and blood pressure and pulse return to normal. Efforts to remove the drug are probably useless after 30 minutes.

2. Special problems–

a. Control convulsions with diazepam, 0.1 mg/kg intravenously, or give succinylcholine chloride (see Table 4–3). Perform artificial respiration with O_2 until convulsions are controlled (see p 52), and continue giving O_2 until blood pressure and pulse return to normal. Adequate arterial O_2 saturation must be maintained. If convulsions are not continuous, the administration of O_2 may be sufficient to maintain the patient until the blood level of local anesthetic falls.

b. Treat methemoglobinemia with methylene blue, 1%, 0.1 mL/kg intravenously over 10 minutes.

3. General measures–

a. Treat hypoxia (see p 57).

b. Do not give stimulants.

c. Treat blood pressure fall by placing the patient in a head-down position; give intravenous saline or blood transfusion (see p 66).

d. Exchange transfusions may be necessary in newborns with local anesthetic toxicity.

B. Hypersensitivity Reactions:

1. Remove from further exposure.

2. Treat dermatitis (see p 83).

Prognosis

Survival for 1 hour indicates that the patient will recover.

Bryant CA et al: Pitfalls and perils of intravenous lidocaine. *West J Med* 1983;**139**:528.

Lovejoy FJ Jr: Fatal benzyl alcohol poisoning in neonatal intensive care units. *Am J Dis Child* 1982;**136**:974.

Mofenson HC et al: Lidocaine toxicity from topical mucosal application. *Clin Pediatr* 1983;**22**:290.

Rothstein P et al: Prolonged seizures associated with the use of viscous lidocaine. *J Pediatr* 1982;**101**:461.

VOLATILE & GASEOUS ANESTHETICS

Ether (diethyl ether, ethyl ether), chloroform, divinyl ether (Vinethene), ethyl chloride, halothane (Fluothane), methoxyflurane (Penthrane), and trifluoroethylvinyl ether (fluroxene, Fluoromar) are volatile liquid anesthetic agents. Ethylene, cyclopropane, and nitrous oxide are gases.

Volatile and gaseous anesthetics are used to produce general anesthesia.

Fatal doses of liquid anesthetic agents by ingestion or inhalation are approximately as follows: ether, 30 mL; chloroform, 10 mL; divinyl ether, 30 mL; halothane, 10 mL; methoxyflurane, 10 mL; fluroxene, 10 mL; enflurane, 10 mL. The exposure limit for chloroform is 10 ppm (NIOSH 2 ppm); for diethyl ether, 400 ppm; for enflurane, 75 ppm; for halothane, 50 ppm.

Approximately 500 fatalities that are at least partly due to the administration of anesthetic agents occur each year. The overall fatality rate following administration of anesthetic agents is approximately 0.5–1 per 10,000. The incidence of hepatic necrosis following halothane administration is 1 per 10,000 after a single administration, which is not significantly different from that found with other anesthetic agents. The incidence of hepatic necrosis after halothane administration rises to 7 per 10,000 after multiple exposures. Hepatic necrosis after halothane administration is assumed to be an autoimmune response.

The gaseous and volatile anesthetics depress all functions of the central nervous system in descending order from the cortex to the medulla. Excessive amounts stop respiration. If O_2 is diminished and the percentage of inspired CO_2 is increased, irregularities of ventricular contraction, ventricular fibrillation, and damage to internal organs are likely to occur. Patients who die several days following chloroform, ethyl chloride, halothane, or divinyl ether administration may show fatty degeneration and other degenerative changes in the liver, heart, and kidneys. The pathologic findings in deaths from cyclopropane, ether, or ethylene are not characteristic. Chloroform is a carcinogen in animals.

Clinical Findings

The principal manifestations of poisoning with these agents are unconsciousness and respiratory failure.

A. Acute Poisoning: (From inhalation or ingestion.) Excitement followed by unconsciousness and paralysis of respiration. Cardiac irregularities occur with cyclopropane, chloroform, and halothane if CO_2 in the inspired air is increased. Cardiac arrest also occurs. Convulsions in anesthesia are caused by increased CO_2 in alveolar air. Reduction of blood pressure during anesthesia is greatest with halothane, chloroform, methoxyflurane, and cyclopropane. Cyanosis and respiratory depression are greatest with halothane and cyclopropane. Uncontrollable hyperthermia occurs rarely during or after anesthesia; this is a genetically determined response. Severe to fatal liver necrosis has been associated with single or repeated administration of halothane and fluroxene. High-output renal failure with polyuria, increased blood urea nitrogen, and hypernatremia has followed administration of methoxyflurane. Fatalities have occurred; these result from fluoride released by metabolic degradation of methoxyflurane. Nitrous oxide without adequate O_2 can cause fatal cardiac arrhythmias and anoxic brain damage with headache, cerebral edema, and permanent mental deficit.

B. Chronic Poisoning: (From inhalation.) Repeated anesthesia with chloroform, methoxyflurane, halothane, or divinyl ether increases the likelihood of liver or kidney damage. Repeated industrial exposure to chloroform at levels above 10 ppm has caused liver damage. Chloroform is a carcinogen in animals.

C. Laboratory Findings: In patients with jaundice following the use of liver-damaging anesthetic agents, appropriate tests show impairment of liver function (see p 75).

Prevention

Avoid prolonged or repeated use of organ-damaging anesthetics. Maintain adequate oxygenation and CO_2 removal during the administration of volatile anesthetics. Alveolar O_2 concentration should always be 18% or higher. Monitor rectal temperature every hour during the recovery period.

Treatment

A. Emergency Measures: Establish airway and maintain respiration. Remove volatile anesthetic by forced ventilation.

B. General Measures:

1. Maintain blood pressure by intravenous saline or blood transfusion (see p 66).

2. Maintain body warmth.

3. Maintain adequate airway by removing secretions from trachea by catheter suction.

4. Prevent hypoxia (see p 57).

5. If hyperthermia occurs, lower body temperature by application of wet towels. For malignant hyperthermia, give dantrolene sodium,1 mg/kg every 15 minutes intravenously to a total of 10 mg/kg, and procainamide, 15 mg/kg intravenously over 10 minutes. Give normal saline intravenously at a rate of 1 L every 10 minutes for 30 minutes. Lavage stomach, urinary bladder, rectum, and peritoneum with iced saline. Treat acidosis with intravenous sodium bicarbonate. Monitor serum total base, serum potassium, and arterial pH and treat appropriately. Maintain urine output at 1–2 L daily with furosemide and mannitol. After the first day, give dantrolene, 1 mg/kg orally daily for 3 days.

C. Special Problems: Treat liver damage by high-carbohydrate, low-protein, low-fat diet.

Prognosis

Recovery from immediate respiratory depression is usually permanent. Liver damage caused by chloroform may progress to cirrhosis and death.

Drug reactions during anaesthesia. (Editorial.) *Lancet* 1985;**1**:1195.

Neuberger J et al: Halothane anaesthesia and liver damage. *Br Med J* 1984;**289**:1136.

Schwartz RH, Calihan M: Nitrous oxide: A potentially lethal euphoriant inhalant. *Am Fam Physician* (Nov) 1984;**30**:171.

INTERACTIONS
(See p 17.)

Cyclopropane, enflurane, and halothane sensitize the myocardium to catecholamines.

Diethyl ether increases the risk of heart failure and hypotension from propranolol.

Procaine enhances the effect of muscle relaxants.

Enzyme induction (see p 17) enhances metabolism of anesthetic agents containing fluorine and increases their toxicity.

Quinidine, procainamide, lidocaine, propranolol, and phenytoin reduce cardiac contraction and thus increase the possibility of heart failure during anesthesia.

PHARMACOKINETICS & TOXIC CONCENTRATIONS
(See p 89.)

	pK$_a$	t½	V$_d$	% Binding	Toxic Concentration (µg/mL)
Bupivacaine	8.1	2.7	1	95	
Cocaine		2.5			0.1
Etidocaine	7.7	2.7	1.9	94	
Lidocaine	7.9	1.3–2.3	1.3–1.7*	65	7
Mepivacaine	7.5	1.9	1.2	75	
Prilocaine	7.9			50	

*For children.

23 | Depressants

SEDATIVES, HYPNOTICS, & ANTICONVULSANTS

A large number of drugs cause sedation or hypnosis by depression of the central nervous system. Overdosage with these or with some anticonvulsant drugs leads to coma and respiratory failure. Fatal doses for most nonbarbiturate depressants and antiepileptics except chloral hydrate are in the range of 0.1–0.5 g/kg. For chloral hydrate, the fatal dose may be as small as 30 mg/kg. For barbiturates, see Table 23–2.

The hypnotics and sedatives cause progressive depression of the central nervous system in descending order from cortex to medulla. After toxic doses, the respiratory center is depressed and respiratory exchange is diminished, resulting in tissue anoxia. Pathologic findings in fatalities from central nervous system depressants include pulmonary edema, pneumonia, and cerebral edema.

Clinical Findings

The principal manifestations of poisoning with most of these agents are coma and slowing of the respiratory rate.

A. Acute Poisoning: (From ingestion or injection.) Early symptoms are sleepiness, mental confusion, and unsteadiness; these are followed rapidly by coma with slow, shallow respiration; flaccid muscles; hypotension; cyanosis; hypothermia or hyperthermia; and absent reflexes. Duration of coma is dependent on dose as well as on the specific medication taken (Table 23–2). In prolonged coma, moist rales are heard in the lower lung fields and can be an indication of pulmonary edema. Atelectasis or aspiration pneumonia with signs of lung consolidation and fever can also occur. Carbon dioxide retention under these conditions causes acidosis and, via effects on the carotid body, can lead to hypotension. Death occurs most often from pneumonia, pulmonary edema, or refractory hypotension. Cerebral edema contributes to the persistence of coma. Bullous lesions occurring over pressure points indicate usually that coma has lasted 12 hours or more. Intravenous injection of any barbiturate may cause severe respiratory depression, laryngospasm, excitement, and severe fall of blood pressure. Combination with ethanol causes effects that appear to be more than additive.

B. Chronic Poisoning: (From ingestion.) Symptoms of chronic intoxication are skin rash, mental confusion, ataxia, dizziness, drowsiness, hangover, emotional lability or depression, irritability, poor judgment, neglect of personal appearance, and other behavior disturbances. Prolonged use of any of these drugs will cause the above mental changes; many have habit-forming potentialities. In addition, reactions peculiar to each type of drug may occur (Tables 23–1, 23–2, 23–3). Sudden withdrawal from prolonged use of large amounts of barbiturates, methyprylon, glutethimide, and other sedatives causes anxiety, insomnia, dizziness, weakness, nausea and vomiting, muscular twitchings, tremors, and convulsions. The risk of teratogenicity is reported to be increased 2- to 3-fold with administration of antiepileptic drugs. Serious ocular effects, including microphthalmos, prominent iris vessels, and coloboma, are reported to occur in 11% of infants in utero when the mother has been taking hydantoins.

C. Laboratory Findings:

1. The serum potassium level may be low in prolonged coma.

2. Blood P_{CO_2} may be elevated.

3. Drug blood levels associated with severe coma are related to the duration of action of the barbiturate. For barbiturates with which the coma lasts 1–3 days, the blood drug level associated with severe poisoning is 1–3 mg/dL. For those with which coma may last up to 5 days, the blood level is above 3 mg/dL. Blood levels of glutethimide over 3 mg/dL are also associated with serious poisoning. For phenobarbital and barbital, the blood level associated with severe poisoning is 5–8 mg/dL or higher. The severity of symptoms does not necessarily correlate well with the blood drug level.

Prevention

Depressant drugs should not be self-administered by emotionally unstable individuals and should be stored safely. Prescription containers should have a warning label and a child-proof cap. They should not be left where repeat doses can be taken inadvertently while the patient is falling asleep. Prescriptions usually should not be refillable.

Many physicians advocate that every patient who takes an overdose of barbiturates should be seen by a psychiatrist.

Treatment

The following therapeutic recommendations apply to severe depression from any of the compounds listed in Tables 23–1, 23–2, and 23–3.

A. Emergency Measures:

1. Maintain adequate airway–Intubate if comatose. Remove mucous secretions from the trachea by suction with a soft rubber catheter. If respiratory difficulty is present, use an oropharyngeal airway. In the

Table 23–1. Nonbarbiturate depressants.

Drug	Clinical Findings (In Addition to Those on p 318)
Carisoprodol (Soma)	Paralysis, visual disturbances, excitement, skin rash, asthma, fever, hypotension.
Chloral hydrate, tri- clofos (Triclos)	Acute: Gastric irritation, rapid circulatory collapse, cardiac arrhythmias. Chronic: Kidney, liver, and heart damage; psychosis; leukopenia.
Ethchlorvynol (Placidyl)	Fatigue, headache, confusion, nausea, vomiting, hemolysis, pulmonary edema, acidosis, liver damage, pancytopenia.
Ethinamate (Valmid)	Thrombocytopenia, liver impairment.
Glutethimide (Doriden)	Nausea, pancytopenia, thrombocytopenia, leukopenia, peripheral neuritis, osteomalacia, paresthesia, toxic psychosis, laryngospasm, nystagmus, double vision, pupillary dilatation, dry mouth, ileus, cerebellar ataxia, cerebral edema, convulsions.
Meprobamate (Equanil, Miltown)	Chills, fever, peripheral edema, vascular collapse, cardiac arrest, aplastic anemia, nonthrombocytopenic purpura with petechiae and ecchymoses. Convulsions on withdrawal.
Methaqualone (Quaalude)	Nausea, gastric irritation, vomiting, paresthesia, aplastic anemia, pulmonary edema, convulsions.
Methyprylon (Noludar)	Nausea, vomiting, headache, dizziness, possibly leukopenia.

Table 23–2. Depressants: Barbiturates.
(For treatment of overdoses, see below.)

Drug	Estimated Fatal Dose (g)	Duration of Coma (Days) (See p 318.)
Allobarbital (Dialog)	2	3
Amobarbital (Amytal)	1.5	5
Aprobarbital (Alurate)	2	5
Barbital*	2	5
Butabarbital	2	3
Heptabarbital (Medomin)	2	3
Hexobarbital (Evipal)	2	2
Mephobarbital (Mebaral)†	2	5
Metharbital (Gemonil)	2	5
Methohexital (Brevital)	1	3
Pentobarbital (Nembutal)	1	3
Phenobarbital (Luminal)	1.5	7
Probarbital (Ipral)	2	3
Secobarbital (Seconal)	2	3
Talbutal (Lotusate)	2	5
Thiamylal (Surital)	1	1
Thiopental (Pentothal)‡	1	1

*Not metabolized. Excreted by kidney.
†Liver damage and agranulocytosis reported.
‡Stored in fat.

Table 23—3. Depressants: Antiepileptics.*†

Drug	Clinical Findings (In Addition to Those on p 318)
Carbamazepine (Tegretol)	Aplastic anemia, agranulocytosis, abnormalities in liver function tests, jaundice, fatal hepatitis, urinary retention, skin rash, gastrointestinal upset, heart failure, hypertension, lens opacities. (Also like amitriptyline.)
Ethotoin (Peganone)	Nausea, vomiting, rash, diarrhea, lymphadenopathy.
Methsuximide (Celontin) and ethosuximide (Zarontin)	Periorbital edema, proteinuria, hepatic dysfunction, fatal bone marrow aplasia, delayed onset of coma.
Mephenytoin (Mesantoin)	Hemolytic anemia, aplastic anemia, visual disturbances, lymph gland enlargement, fever.
Phenacemide (Phenurone)	Liver damage, aplastic anemia, leukopenia, behavioral effects, renal impairment, skin rash, suicidal tendencies.
Phensuximide (Milontin)	Nausea, vomiting, muscular weakness, hematuria, casts, nephrosis.
Phenytoin (diphenylhydantoin, Dilantin)	Swelling of gums, fever, liver and kidney damage, agranulocytosis, adenopathy, aplastic anemia, pulmonary changes, lupus erythematosus, lymph gland enlargement, epidermal necrolysis, cardiac irregularities, peripheral nerve damage, tremor, drug psychosis, rigidity.
Primidone (Mysoline)	Painful gums, excessive fatigue.
Trimethadione (Tridione) and paramethadione (Paradione)	Neutropenia, hematuria, agranulocytosis, nephrosis, photophobia, lupus, myasthenia, blurred vision.

*For treatment of overdoses, see p 319.

†Precautions: Perform white count and urinalysis at least monthly or immediately on occurrence of upper respiratory infection, sore throat, or other change in status.

presence of laryngeal stridor, laryngeal edema, or other restriction in airway, place an endotracheal airway with low-pressure, high-volume cuff (7–7.5 mm in diameter in adult females and 8–8.5 mm in diameter in adult males). The cuff pressure should be just sufficient to ensure a proper seal. The cuff of the endotracheal tube should be placed just below the vocal cords, with the tip above the bifurcation (the position should be checked by x-ray). The tube is then tied firmly with strong tape at the level of the patient's mouth to prevent movement due to the patient's activity. Respiratory or cardiac arrest sometimes occurs during intubation and must be anticipated.

2. Maintain adequate O_2 intake and CO_2 removal. Arterial P_{O_2} should be 70–100 mm Hg, and P_{CO_2} should be below 40 mm Hg. If respiration is depressed, give O_2 as necessary to maintain adequate arterial oxygenation, and ventilate the patient. Avoid O_2 concentrations above 50% if possible. Either of the following methods is usually adequate for this purpose: (1) nasal catheter at a flow rate of 4–6 L/min or (2) oronasal mask with a flow rate of 2–4 L/min. Minute volume should exceed 4 L/min. If cyanosis or CO_2 retention is present, give artificial res-

piration. If artificial ventilation is used, an hourly check of tidal volume is necessary.

3. In conscious patients, delay absorption of the drug by giving activated charcoal. Follow by gastric lavage and catharsis (see pp 21–28). Avoid induction of emesis. If respiration is depressed, place a cuffed endotracheal tube before doing gastric lavage. For catharsis, 30–60 mL of 50% sodium sulfate or Fleet's Phospho-Soda diluted in 200 mL of water can be given. The chances of removing a significant amount of drug are better if treatment is started within 2 hours after ingestion. Since the remaining drug in the gastrointestinal tract can contribute to relapse after initial improvement, repeated gastric lavage and catharsis combined with charcoal administration are useful, especially in ethchlorvynol and glutethimide poisoning. Glutethimide and meprobamate are fat-soluble and markedly slow gastric emptying; thus, gastric lavage is useful whenever the patient is seen. In comatose patients, any of these procedures increases the hazard of aspiration pneumonia or cardiac arrest.

4. Maintain blood pressure (see below).

B. Antidote: No specific antidote is known for the sedative and hypnotic drugs. Analeptic drugs such as pentylenetetrazol (Metrazol), picrotoxin, caffeine, bemegride (Megimide), ethamivan (Emivan), and amphetamine are absolutely contraindicated. In the presence of severe respiratory depression these drugs are not effective; they do not shorten the duration of depression but only stimulate the medullary centers for short periods of time, and the initial stimulation will be followed by greater depression. Complications of stimulant therapy are cardiac failure, cardiac arrhythmias, hyperthermia, convulsions, delayed psychosis, and kidney damage with anuria.

C. General Measures: Several procedures are to be carried out under 24-hour supervision by a physician who has had training in resuscitation techniques. Check and record the following every hour: rate and quality of the pulse, blood pressure, reaction of the pupils, respiration rate, temperature, color of the skin (cyanosis), reflexes (corneal, pupillary, tendon), and response to painful stimuli (pinching or pinprick).

1. Elevate the patient's head (15 degrees) to reduce cerebral venous pressure and the possibility of cerebral edema. Maintain pharyngeal suction if necessary. Give intermittent positive-pressure respiration to help prevent pneumonia.

2. Every 2 hours, turn the patient and massage skin. Use an oscillating bed, if available.

3. Endotracheal suction should be done hourly, or oftener if necessary. Prior to suction, ventilate with O_2 for 3 minutes. Introduce catheter without suction, apply suction, and remove catheter slowly while rotating gently. Do not jiggle the catheter. The procedure should

be completed in not more than 15 seconds. Do not use endotracheal suction in the presence of pulmonary edema.

4. If renal function is adequate, give fluids up to 40 mL/kg daily at a rate not exceeding 3 mL/kg/h (eg, 0.2% sodium chloride in 5% dextrose with 20 meq of potassium chloride added per liter) to maintain a daily urine output of 15–30 mL/kg. Measure serum potassium, chloride, and sodium levels daily and adjust intravenous fluid as necessary. Forced alkaline diuresis to 10–15 L/d is only marginally useful in phenobarbital poisoning, and associated pulmonary edema is a significant hazard.

5. Urine output exceeding 0.5 mL/kg/h in the absence of diuretics indicates adequate tissue perfusion; blood pressure should be maintained at this level, usually 85–90 mm Hg. Maintain blood pressure by administering 5% plasma or low-molecular-weight dextran while monitoring central venous pressure (normal, 5–8 cm of water). Low pressure indicates a need for fluid replacement, and rising pressure indicates too rapid fluid administration. Excessive administration of fluids may lead to pulmonary edema. In hypotension that does not respond to fluid administration, give dopamine hydrochloride, 200 mg in 500 mL of 0.9% saline, at a rate of 0.5 mL/80 kg/min (2.5 μg/kg/min). The rate of infusion must be monitored carefully to maintain blood pressure at the lowest level that will give adequate renal perfusion. A peristaltic infusion pump or pediatric microdrip may be necessary to adjust the infusion rate accurately. Vasopressor-induced arrhythmias are most common after barbiturates, hydantoins, or chloral hydrate.

6. The role of hemodialysis, peritoneal dialysis, and extracorporeal resin or charcoal hemoperfusion in the treatment of depressant poisoning is not yet clearly established. The recovery rate is better than 99% in patients treated with intensive supportive care. The hazards from dialysis are significant. For short-acting drugs, dialysis can only increase the removal rate by 10–20%. For longer-acting drugs, dialysis is more likely to be helpful; blood drug levels can be used as an indication. The following blood levels are indications for the use of dialysis therapy: for aprobarbital, amobarbital, talbutal, and allobarbital, 10 mg/dL; for barbital and phenobarbital, 15 mg/dL. Dialysis has not reduced the mortality rate in poisoning due to ethchlorvynol, glutethimide, or methaqualone. Conditions that increase the hazard of dialysis therapy include hypotension that has not responded to therapy, pulmonary edema, and reduced renal function.

D. Special Problems:

1. Treat hypothermia by application of blankets. Avoid rapid warming or burning of the patient by hot pads or hot-water bottles. Administer intravenous fluids at 37 °C and gases at 40 °C. Administration of 40% moistened O_2 at 40 °C improves cardiac function and reduces the risk of hypothermic ventricular fibrillation.

2. Treat hyperthermia by applying wet towels, ice packs, or cooling blanket until the patient's rectal temperature is down to 38 °C.

3. Treat pulmonary edema (see p 65).

4. Monitor urine output and prevent bladder distention by placing an indwelling catheter. Maintain strictly accurate fluid input/output chart to facilitate monitoring electrolyte and fluid balance.

5. Treat aspiration pneumonia with organism-specific chemotherapy.

6. Neonatal or addict withdrawal convulsions from any depressant can be treated by paraldehyde, 0.2 mL/kg rectally in oil or intramuscularly. In hyperactive states, avoid use of depressants (eg, diazepam), since they may induce sudden apnea.

Prognosis

Determine prognosis by the severity of the clinical findings.

A. Mild: Patient can be aroused. No treatment is necessary.

B. Moderate: Patient cannot be aroused. Respiration is full and regular. No cyanosis or pulmonary edema is present. Blood pressure is normal. Recovery occurs in 24–48 hours with good nursing care and adequate fluid balance.

C. Severe: Coma with slow, shallow, irregular respiration; cyanosis; absence of all reflexes; low blood pressure; hypothermia of 0.5–2 °C; dilated pupils; and absence of response to painful stimuli. The mortality rate should be less than 5%. Recovery of consciousness may require 3–5 days.

NARCOTIC ANALGESICS
(Table 23–4)

Narcotic analgesics control severe pain by their depressant effect on the brain.

Fatalities have occurred from overdosage during therapeutic use, accidental ingestion, or intentional misuse. Overdoses of heroin in addicts caused more than 1200 deaths in narcotic addicts in New York City in 1970, and the number of deaths in the USA may exceed 10,000 per year. Accidental ingestion of methadone has led to the death of many children. Naloxone appears to be a pure antagonist, and doses of naloxone above 5 g have not caused death.

The narcotic analgesics produce variable effects on the central nervous system depending on the drug, the susceptibility of the patient, and the dosage. For example, morphine and most of the other opium derivatives except codeine depress the cortex and medullary centers and stimulate the spinal cord. Codeine, on the other hand, is somewhat less de-

Table 23—4. Narcotic depressants and antagonists.*

Drug	Fatal Dose† (g)	Clinical Findings (In Addition to Those on p 326)
Alphaprodine (Nisentil)	0.1	
Anileridine (Leritine, Apodol)	0.5	
Apomorphine	0.1	Violent emesis, cardiac depression.
Butorphanol (Stadol)	0.1	
Codeine	0.8	Convulsions.
Dextromethorphan (dormethan, Romilar)	0.5	Dizziness.
Dihydrocodeine	0.5	
Diphenoxylate (Lomotil)	0.2	Constipation.
Ethylmorphine (Dionin)	0.5	Irritation.
Fentanyl (Sublimaze)	0.002	Muscle rigidity.
Heroin	0.2	
Hydrocodone (Dicodid, Hycodan)	0.2	Tremors.
Hydromorphone (Dilaudid)	0.2	
Levallorphan (Lorfan)‡	0.2	Restlessness.
Levopropoxyphene (Novrad)	1	
Levorphanol (Levo-Dromoran)	0.1	
Loperamide (Imodium)	0.5	Nausea, vomiting.
Meperidine (pethidine, Demerol, Dolantin)	1	Fainting, edema.
Methadone (Dolophine, Adanon)	0.1	
Metopon	0.2	Agitation.
Morphine	0.2	
Nalbuphine (Nubain)	0.3	
Nalorphine (Nalline)‡	0.2	Restlessness, hallucinations.
Naloxone (Narcan)‡		
Naltrexone (Trexan)‡		Liver damage.
Omnopon (Pantopon)	0.3	
Opium *(Papaver somniferum)*	0.3	
Oxycodone (Percodan)	0.5	
Oxymorphone (Numorphan)	0.05	Restlessness.
Paregoric (camphorated tincture of opium)	60	
Pentazocine (Talwin)	0.3	Nausea.
Phenazocine (Prinadol)	0.2	
Piminodine (Alvodine)	0.5	
Propoxyphene (Darvon)	0.5	Nausea, vomiting, skin rash, ptosis, convulsions.
Sufentanil (Sufenta)	0.002	

*For treatment, see p 327.

†Estimated for an adult. May be much higher (up to 10 times) in narcotic addicts and much lower (1/20) in infants.

‡Narcotic antagonist. Naloxone is a pure antagonist. Doses up to 5 g have not caused death.

pressing to the cortex and medullary centers but more stimulating to the spinal cord. Methadone, alphaprodine, and levallorphan are similar to morphine in their depressant effects on the cortex and medullary centers in toxic doses.

The pathologic findings in death from narcotic analgesics are not characteristic.

Clinical Findings

The principal manifestations of poisoning with these drugs are slowing of respiration and coma.

A. Acute Poisoning: (From ingestion or injection.) Toxic doses of the narcotic analgesics cause unconsciousness; pinpoint pupils (dilated with anoxia); slow, shallow respiration; cyanosis; weak pulse; hypotension; spasm of gastrointestinal and biliary tracts; and in some cases pulmonary edema, spasticity, and twitching of the muscles. Death from respiratory failure may occur within 2–4 hours after oral or subcutaneous administration or immediately after intravenous overdose. Convulsions may accompany codeine, meperidine, apomorphine, propoxyphene, or oxymorphone poisoning. The metabolite of meperidine, normeperidine, has significantly greater excitatory effect than meperidine. Metabolites of other drugs may also be more convulsant than the parent drugs. Convulsions are more likely with high doses, renal impairment, alkaline urine, the presence of enzyme-inducing drugs, or the presence of phenothiazines.

B. Chronic Poisoning: (From ingestion or injection.) The findings in chronic poisoning or addiction are not marked. Pinpoint pupils and rapid changes in mood may occasionally be observed, and the addict is usually not well integrated socially.

C. Withdrawal Symptoms: All the narcotic analgesics have strong addicting potentialities. The addict's craving is partly psychologic and partly due to fear of the severe consequences of withdrawal. Sudden withdrawal from morphine or other narcotic analgesics causes yawning; lacrimation; pilomotor reactions; severe gastrointestinal disturbance with cramps, vomiting, diarrhea, or constipation; sweating; fever; chills; increase in respiratory rate; insomnia; tremor; and mydriasis. Death is rare. The narcotic antagonist naltrexone can precipitate withdrawal symptoms that may be life-threatening.

D. Laboratory Findings: The abrupt production of withdrawal symptoms after the administration of levallorphan or nalorphine will indicate dependence. Analysis of urine or blood can also be used to determine drug use.

Prevention

Narcotic analgesics should be used with caution in children under 12 years of age.

Repeated doses of narcotic analgesics must be avoided in the treatment of injuries and other chronic painful conditions unless the benefit to be derived, such as in terminal illness, outweighs the danger of inducing addiction.

The use of narcotic analgesics must be avoided except on clear-cut indications in psychoneurotic, psychopathic, and emotionally unstable patients, since the danger of addiction may be greater in such patients.

The combination of monoamine oxidase inhibitor drugs (see p 415) with any narcotic analgesic may cause coma with hyperthermia, respiratory failure, convulsions, cerebral edema, and unstable blood pressure. The combined use of LSD (see p 426) and narcotic analgesics is also dangerous to life.

Treatment

A. Acute Poisoning:

1. Emergency measures–

a. Maintain respiration with artificial respiration and then give antidote as prescribed below.

b. In fully conscious patients, remove swallowed poison by thorough gastric lavage or emesis (see pp 21–28). The chances of removing a significant amount of the drug are better if treatment is started within the first 2 hours. If the patient is unconscious or respiration is depressed, emesis is contraindicated and the dangers of unprotected gastric lavage are not justified. If a massive dose has been ingested, catharsis is possibly useful after the patient is awake.

c. Delay absorption of subcutaneously injected narcotic analgesics by use of a tourniquet (see p 28).

d. Treat coma (see p 52) and shock (see p 66).

2. Antidote–For overdoses of any of the narcotic analgesics except levopropoxyphene (Novrad), give naloxone hydrochloride (Narcan), 0.01 mg/kg intravenously. Naloxone does not depress respiration and has a longer duration of action than either nalorphine or levallorphan. It is effective against pentazocine, for which nalorphine and levallorphan are contraindicated. Repeat injection of the antagonist only as necessary to maintain response to stimuli. If an effective increase in pulmonary ventilation is not achieved with the first dose, the dose may be repeated every 2–3 minutes until respiration returns to normal and the patient responds to stimuli. The dose of naloxone may need to be 0.1–0.2 mg/kg in massive overdoses of narcotic analgesics. Observe the patient closely for the first 24–48 hours in the case of methadone overdose. Naloxone is safe to use as a test in coma of unknown origin in which a narcotic is suspected. In addicts or newborns of addicted mothers, injection of naloxone can precipitate acute, severe withdrawal. Naloxone does not antagonize convulsant effects of some narcotics and may enhance meperidine seizures.

3. General measures–Maintain body warmth and adequate fluid intake. Treat shock.

4. Other measures–Dialysis is obviated by the availability of antagonists. Stimulants are contraindicated.

B. Chronic Poisoning or Addiction:

1. The treatment of chronic poisoning or addiction is best undertaken in hospitals and under the direction of physicians who specialize in these problems. These include private sanatoria and US Public Health Service hospitals at Lexington, Kentucky, and Fort Worth, Texas.

2. If withdrawal is to be attempted, the following principles must be followed:

a. Treatment must be under the supervision of a physician.

b. The patient must be hospitalized if further administration of the drug is planned.

c. The patient must not be given supplies of narcotic analgesics and must be searched to prevent smuggling; this includes all the opium derivatives as well as the synthetic analgesics.

d. Methadone can be substituted in a dosage sufficient to control symptoms. Give an initial dose of 1 mg/kg orally once daily and reduce dosage by 50% every 2–3 days. When the dosage reaches approximately 5% of the initial dose, the drug may be withdrawn completely.

e. In mild addiction, if the patient is adequately prepared psychologically, total withdrawal of the addicting agent can also be done.

f. Psychologic or other factors leading to addiction in a particular individual must be carefully evaluated and corrected if possible.

g. Supportive care includes the administration of atropine, 0.5–1 mg orally every 6 hours, for severe diarrhea and abdominal cramps.

3. Clonidine, 17 μg/kg/d in divided doses for 10 days, has been used to block the symptoms of rapid withdrawal from narcotic addiction.

4. Since regulation of narcotics is so strict, the physician who prescribes narcotics should be familiar with the Controlled Substances Act of 1970. The Bureau of Narcotics, US Department of Justice, has a pamphlet that describes the Act for physicians.

Prognosis

In acute poisoning, if naloxone can be given, recovery will usually occur within 1–4 hours.

In addiction, continued abstinence is to be expected in only 5–10% of patients.

ANTIHISTAMINES
(Table 23–5)

Many antihistamines are sold both over the counter and by prescription for the treatment of allergies and colds and as sedatives. Some are also used as motion sickness remedies.

At least 20 fatalities have been reported from accidental ingestion in children.

Antihistaminic drugs in toxic doses produce a complex of central nervous system excitatory and depressant effects, partly from atropine-

Table 23–5. Antihistamines and similar drugs.

Name	Fatal Doses
Antazoline	25–250 mg/kg*
Azatadine (Optimine)	25–250 mg/kg*
Bromodiphenhydramine (Ambodryl)	25–250 mg/kg*
Brompheniramine (Dimetane)	25–250 mg/kg*
Buclizine (Bucladin)	25–250 mg/kg*
Carbinoxamine (Clistin)	25–250 mg/kg*
Chlorcyclizine†	25–250 mg/kg*
Chlorpheniramine (Chlor-Trimeton)	25–250 mg/kg*
Chlorphenoxamine (Phenoxene)	25–250 mg/kg*
Clemastine (Tavist)	10–100 mg/kg*
Cyclizine (Marezine)†	25–250 mg/kg*
Cyproheptadine (Periactin)	25–250 mg/kg*
Dexbrompheniramine (Disomer)	25–250 mg/kg*
Dexchlorpheniramine (Polaramine)	25–250 mg/kg*
Dimenhydrinate (Dramamine)	25–250 mg/kg*
Diphenhydramine (Benadryl)	400 mg, 40 mg/kg‡
Diphenylpyraline (Diafen)	5–10 mg/kg*
Doxylamine (Decapryn)	25–250 mg/kg*
Hydroxyzine (Atarax)	25–250 mg/kg*
Meclizine (Bonine)†	25–250 mg/kg*
Methapyrilene	100 mg, 10 mg/kg‡
Orphenadrine (Disipal)	25–250 mg/kg*
Phenindamine	25–250 mg/kg*
Pheniramine (Trimeton)	30 mg/kg‡
Phenyltoloxamine	25–250 mg/kg*
Pyrilamine	1 g, 40 mg/kg‡
Pyrrobutamine (Co-Pyronil)	25–250 mg/kg*
Rotoxamine (Twiston)	25–250 mg/kg*
Thenyldiamine (Thenfadil)	25–250 mg/kg*
Thonzylamine (Neohetramine)	25–250 mg/kg*
Trimethobenzamide (Tigan)	25–250 mg/kg*
Tripelennamine (Pyribenzamine)	25–250 mg/kg*
Triprolidine (Actidil)	25–250 mg/kg*

*Estimated acute fatal dose.

†Shown to cause birth defects in animals, hence contraindicated in pregnancy.

‡Reported acute fatal dose.

like anticholinergic effects. The pathologic findings are not characteristic. Cerebral damage and kidney damage have been observed at autopsy.

Clinical Findings

The principal manifestations of poisoning with these drugs are convulsions and coma.

A. Acute Poisoning: (From ingestion.) Therapeutic doses of antihistaminic drugs cause a high incidence of toxic symptoms and signs, including drowsiness, dryness of the mouth, headache, nausea, tachycardia, urinary retention, and nervousness. Larger doses cause 2 different types of effects—either drowsiness, disorientation, staggering gait, hallucinations, stupor, and coma; or hyperreflexia, tremors, excitement, nystagmus, hyperthermia, and convulsions. Symptoms may vary from patient to patient with the same drug, or a mixture of the above symptoms may be seen in the same patient.

B. Chronic Poisoning: Tripelennamine, methapyrilene, and pyrilamine have caused agranulocytosis or aplastic anemia.

Prevention

Antihistamines should be sold with a poison label and stored safely. Patients should be warned to discontinue medication at the first symptoms.

Treatment

A. Acute Poisoning:

1. Emergency measures–

a. If coma and respiratory depression are present, use resuscitative measures. *Do not use stimulants.*

b. Delay absorption of ingested drug by giving activated charcoal and then remove by airway-protected gastric lavage followed by catharsis (see pp 21–28). Emetics may not work successfully.

c. Maintain blood pressure (see p 66).

2. General measures–Control convulsions by giving diazepam, 0.1 mg/kg slowly intravenously. Physostigmine, 0.5–2 mg intravenously, reverses the anticholinergic central nervous system effects of antihistamines. Give physostigmine diluted in saline over 5 minutes with electrocardiographic control. Atropine, 1 mg, should be available in a syringe to reverse physostigmine toxicity. Physostigmine should not be used in the presence of asthma, cardiac or vascular disease, or intestinal or urinary obstruction. Exchange transfusions are reported to be helpful, but forced diuresis is not.

3. Special problems–Treat agranulocytosis (see p 79). Treat hyperthermia by cooling applications. Dexamethasone, 1 mg/kg intravenously, can also be tried.

B. Chronic Poisoning: Discontinue the drug at the onset of symptoms. For further treatment, see Acute Poisoning, above.

Prognosis

Fewer than 10% of those seriously poisoned have died. Patients who live more than 24 hours will probably survive.

PHENOTHIAZINE DRUGS
(Table 23–6)

Chlorpromazine and related drugs are synthetic chemicals derived in most instances from phenothiazine. They are used as antiemetics, as tranquilizers, and as potentiators of analgesic and hypnotic drugs.

The acute fatal dose for these compounds appears to be in the range of 15–150 mg/kg, although severe symptoms have occurred with doses

Table 23–6. Phenothiazines and related drugs.

Name	Blood Dyscrasias	CNS Effects, Convulsions	Liver Damage
	Reported Toxic Effects		
Acetophenazine (Tindal)	+	+	+
Butaperazine (Repoise)		+	
Carphenazine (Proketazine)	+	+	+
Chlorpromazine (Thorazine)	*	*	*
Chlorprothixene (Taractan)		+	
Ethopropazine (Parsidol)		+	
Fluphenazine (Permitil)	+	+	+
Mesoridazine (Serentil)		+	
Methdilazine (Tacaryl)	+	+	+
Methotrimeprazine (Levoprome)†	+	+	+
Perphenazine (Trilafon)		*	+
Pipamazine (Mornidine)		+	
Piperacetazine (Quide)	+	+	+
Prochlorperazine (Compazine)	+	*	*
Promazine (Sparine)	*	*	*
Promethazine (Phenergan)		+	
Propiomazine (Largon)		+	
Thiethylperazine (Torecan)		+	
Thiopropazate (Dartal)		+	
Thioridazine (Mellaril)	+	+	+
Thiothixene (Navane)	+	+	+
Trifluoperazine (Stelazine)		*	
Triflupromazine (Vesprin)	+	*	+
Trimeprazine (Temaril)	+	+	

*Deaths from toxic reaction reported.
†Prolonged orthostatic hypotension and marked sedation occur.

less than 1 mg/kg. Reported fatal doses are as follows: chlorpromazine, 350 mg in a 4-year-old and 2 g in an adult female; promazine, 1 g in a 2-year-old. Because these compounds enhance the effects of other drugs, administration during acute toxicity from antihistamines, alcohol, barbiturates, or morphine must be done cautiously. At least 25 deaths due to agranulocytosis and several deaths due to liver damage have been reported as due to poisoning with chlorpromazine or related drugs. The incidence of toxic reactions may be as high as 1–5% of patients receiving these drugs for more than 1 month.

The principal pathologic finding in patients who have died with liver damage is cirrhosis of the liver. In patients dying with agranulocytosis, the pathologic findings have been acellular bone marrow and, sometimes, regurgitation of bile into the bile canaliculi with pigment deposition in the parenchymal cells of the liver. Damage to liver cells was not present.

Clinical Findings

The principal manifestations of poisoning with phenothiazines are drowsiness, jaundice, and leukopenia.

A. Acute Poisoning: Usual doses induce drowsiness and mild hypotension in as many as 50% of patients. Larger doses cause drowsiness, severe postural hypotension, hypothermia, tachycardia, dryness of the mouth, nausea, ataxia, anorexia, nasal congestion, fever, constipation, tremor, blurring of vision, stiffness of muscles, urinary retention, and coma. Intravenous injection of solutions containing more than 25 mg/mL of these drugs causes thrombophlebitis and cellulitis in a small number of patients. Hypotension and ventricular arrhythmias are the most common causes of death.

B. Chronic Poisoning: (From ingestion.) Prolonged administration of chlorpromazine or related drugs may produce the following reactions:

1. Leukopenia or agranulocytosis has appeared 4–8 weeks after therapy with doses over 50 mg/d. Findings include ulcerations of the gums, tongue, or pharynx; fever; weakness; disorientation; and anorexia.

2. Jaundice, characteristically obstructive and without evidence of liver cell damage (at least in the early stages), may appear shortly after treatment or may be delayed 2–6 weeks.

3. Generalized maculopapular eruptions with edema, scaling, and pruritus may appear after administration of chlorpromazine but are more likely to appear as sensitivity reactions in medical personnel who handle the preparation or after exposure to sunlight in persons taking the drug.

4. A syndrome similar to paralysis agitans occurs as a result of extrapyramidal and other central nervous system effects. Symptoms in-

clude spasmodic contractions of face and neck muscles with trismus and swallowing difficulties, extensor rigidity of back muscles, oculogyric crisis, carpopedal spasm, intolerable motor restlessness (akathisia) or rhythmic choreoathetoid movements, salivation, convulsions, and endocrine disturbances, including abnormal lactation, interference with menstruation, and increase in thyroid activity. The dosage necessary to produce these effects is highly variable.

5. Prolonged administration of phenothiazines in high doses has caused skin pigmentation and corneal and lens opacities. The exposed areas of the face, neck, and hands show a purplish pigmentation that has the histologic appearance of melanin. Corneal and lens pigmentation or other changes are accompanied by reduction in visual acuity. Chorioretinopathy has been reported after thioridazine.

6. Electrocardiographic abnormalities and sudden death thought to result from ventricular fibrillation have occurred in patients on long-term therapy.

C. Laboratory Findings:

1. Liver function tests in the presence of jaundice reveal elevated serum bilirubin, elevated serum alkaline phosphatase, and the presence of bile in the urine.

2. Serum cholesterol and blood sugar are sometimes elevated.

3. In agranulocytosis, the blood examination reveals white blood cell count decreased below 2000, polymorphonuclear neutrophils diminished or absent from the blood smear, and acellular and aplastic bone marrow.

4. Phenothiazine compounds in urine can be detected by the addition of a few drops of tincture of ferric chloride to urine acidified with dilute nitric acid. A violet color results if phenothiazine compounds are present.

5. An ECG may show a prolonged QT interval and a widened QRS complex.

Prevention

Patients must be warned to discontinue the drug and report for examination immediately upon the appearance of sore throat, fever, jaundice, or other signs of reaction. Severe hypotensive reactions also occur during surgical anesthesia in patients receiving phenothiazines.

Treatment

A. Acute Poisoning:

1. **Emergency measures–**

a. Establish airway and maintain respiration.

b. Discontinue chlorpromazine or related drugs at the first untoward sign until the severity of the reaction can be evaluated. Remove overdoses by gastric lavage or emesis (see pp 21–28). Emetics are not likely to be effective.

c. Treat severe hypotension by giving fluids (see p 66). The use of sympathomimetic amines (norepinephrine, etc) is contraindicated.

d. Monitor ECG.

2. Antidote–

a. Diphenhydramine (Benadryl), 1–5 mg/kg intravenously, will reverse extrapyramidal signs.

b. For ventricular arrhythmias, give phenytoin, 1 mg/kg slowly intravenously, with electrocardiographic control. The injection rate should not exceed 50 mg/min. Phenytoin can be repeated every 5 minutes up to a total dose of 10 mg/kg. Lidocaine is contraindicated. A pacemaker may be necessary.

3. General measures–Control convulsions or hyperactivity with pentobarbital (see Table 4–3). Avoid other depressant drugs.

B. Chronic Poisoning:

1. Immediate measures–Discontinue chlorpromazine at the first sign of jaundice, fever, sore throat, pigmentation, or ocular change.

2. General measures–

a. In the presence of fever, sore throat, pulmonary congestion, or other signs of infection, give organism-specific chemotherapy.

b. For liver damage, no measures have been helpful other than discontinuing the drug.

Prognosis

In agranulocytosis from phenothiazines, recovery is likely if the patient survives for 2 weeks.

In liver damage from phenothiazines, complete recovery usually occurs within 4–8 weeks after discontinuing the drug.

BROMIDES

Sodium bromide (NaBr), potassium bromide (KBr), and ammonium bromide (NH_4Br) are water-soluble salts.

Some nonprescription medications (eg, Bromo-Seltzer, Dr. Miles' Nervine) formerly contained bromides, but none currently available in the USA contain bromides. However, patients may still have access to the older preparations. Some prescription drugs contain bromides. Other preparations that release bromide, such as bromisovalum (Bromural) and carbromal, can lead to chronic bromide toxicity. Well water containing as little as 20 mg of bromide per liter has caused toxicity.

Toxic signs from bromides occur in 1–10% of users, but fatalities from bromides alone are rare.

Bromides displace chlorides from the plasma and cells; this produces depression of the central nervous system.

Pathologic findings are pneumonia and pulmonary edema.

Clinical Findings

The principal manifestation of bromide poisoning is mental confusion.

A. Acute Poisoning: Large doses of bromide cause nausea and vomiting, abdominal pain, coma, and paralysis.

B. Chronic Poisoning: Symptoms from overdosage are confusion, irritability, tremor, memory loss, anorexia, emaciation, headache, slurred speech, delusions, psychotic behavior, ataxia, stupor, and coma. From 1 to 5% of bromide users will have an acneiform papular eruption of the face and hands.

C. Laboratory Findings: Blood bromide levels should be determined in undiagnosed patients who are stuporous or show psychotic or irrational behavior of recent onset. Toxicity can occur at blood bromide levels above 20 mg/dL.

Prevention

Blood bromide levels should be determined monthly during bromide therapy to avoid levels above 50 mg/dL.

Treatment

A. Acute Poisoning:

1. Emergency measures–The delirious patient should be wrapped in a sheet or otherwise restrained.

2. Antidote–Give sodium chloride, 1 g orally every hour in water or as salt tablets; for more severe involvement in which oral medication is impossible, give normal saline, 1 L every 8 hours intravenously to a maximum of 2 L daily. Sodium chloride therapy must be continued until the blood bromide level drops below 50 mg/dL. Simultaneous administration of diuretics is also useful.

3. General measures–Give fluids and food by mouth to maintain nutrition.

B. Chronic Poisoning: Discontinue use.

Prognosis

Patients with bromide poisoning recover completely in 1–6 months.

Table 23-7. Selective depressants.*

Drug	Clinical Findings (In Addition to Those on p 337)
Alprazolam (Xanax)	Hypotension, skin rash.
Baclofen (Lioresal)	Cholinergic effects, nausea, constipation, anorexia, urinary retention, impotence, confusion.
Benzonatate (Tessalon)	Gastrointestinal upset, convulsions.
Benzquinamide (Emet-con)	Pyrexia, autonomic effects, hypertension or hypotension, ventricular arrhythmias, muscle twitching.
Chlordiazepoxide (Librium)	Stimulation, rage reaction, severe generalized dermatitis, syncope without warning, mental confusion, jaundice from liver damage, agranulocytosis, convulsions.
Chlormezanone (Trancopal)	Vertigo, flushing, nausea, drowsiness, depression, weakness.
Chlorphenesin (Maolate)	Leukopenia, agranulocytosis, hypersensitivity reactions. One patient had nausea and drowsiness for 6 hours after 12 g.
Chlorzoxazone (Paraflex)	Constipation or diarrhea, gastrointestinal disturbances with bleeding, liver damage, sensitivity reactions.
Clonazepam (Clonopin)	Hair loss, hirsutism, gastrointestinal disturbances, hepatomegaly, sore gums, dysuria, lymphadenopathy, leukopenia, thrombocytopenia.
Chlophedianol (Ulo)	Nausea, vomiting, excitement.
Clorazepate (Tranxene)	Abnormal liver and kidney function tests, hypotension, skin rash.
Cyclandelate (Cyclospasmol)	Flushing, tingling, sweating.
Dantrolene (Dantrium)	Liver damage, gastrointestinal upset or bleeding, speech and vision disorders, tachycardia.
Diazepam (Valium)	Tinnitus, excitability, rage reaction, hallucinations. Synergism with other depressants. Lactic acidosis from prolonged use, phlebitis.
Dioxyline (Paveril)	Nausea, sweating, flushing, abdominal cramps.
Diphenidol (Vontrol)	Auditory and visual hallucinations, disorientation, confusion, drowsiness, dry mouth, dizziness, skin rash, and, rarely, headache, nausea, indigestion, blurred vision, and hypotension.
Droperidol (Inapsine)	Hypotension, hallucinations, extrapyramidal symptoms, tachycardia, respiratory depression when used with narcotics.
Ethaverine	Nausea, gastrointestinal upset, malaise, hypotension, headache.
Flurazepam (Dalmane)	Hypotension, excitement, skin rash, leukopenia, elevated liver enzymes, jaundice.
Halazepam (Paxipam)	Nausea, vomiting, constipation.
Haloperidol (Haldol)	Extrapyramidal reactions, persistent tardive dyskinesia, depression, headache, confusion, vertigo, grand mal seizures, exacerbation of psychosis, hypotension, leukopenia, endocrine malfunction, skin rash.

*For treatment, see p 338.

Table 23–7 (cont'd). Selective depressants.*

Drug	Clinical Findings (In Addition to Those on p 337)
Ketamine (Ketaject)	Rise in blood pressure and pulse rate, apnea in the presence of increased intracerebral pressure, laryngospasm and respiratory arrest, profuse salivation with respiratory obstruction, EEG changes similar to those of epilepsy. Contraindicated in patients with convulsions. Delirium, hallucinations, excitement, and irrational behavior occasionally occur during recovery. Tonic and clonic movements sometimes resemble seizures.
Lorazepam (Ativan)	Nausea, change of appetite, headache, sleep disturbance.
Loxapine (Daxolin)	Extrapyramidal effects, tardive dyskinesia, hypotension, hypertension, anticholinergic effects, gastrointestinal disturbances, convulsions, CNS depression, hypothermia, rhabdomyolysis, acute renal failure.
Methocarbamol (Robaxin)	Skin rash, conjunctivitis, blurred vision, fever.
Molindone (Moban)	Hypotension, extrapyramidal effects, tardive dyskinesia.
Noscapine (Conar)	Skin rash, nausea, drowsiness.
Oxazepam (Serax)	Syncope, liver or bone marrow damage, sensitivity reactions.
Papaverine	Constipation, increased reflex excitability, liver damage.
Prazepam (Vestran)	Nausea, liver function alterations, psychosis.
Temazepam (Restoril)	Anorexia, diarrhea.
Triazolam (Halcion)	Nausea, vomiting, fatigue, tachycardia.
Valproic acid (Depakene), sodium valproate, divalproex (Depakote)	Gastrointestinal disturbances, hair loss, psychosis, altered bleeding time, altered liver enzymes, fatal hepatic failure.

*For treatment, see p 338.

SELECTIVE DEPRESSANTS
(Table 23–7)

A large number of drugs are used as depressants to relieve anxiety, relax muscle spasm, or inhibit cough. The single dose of any of these compounds that would be fatal in an adult is 0.05–0.5 g/kg. Smaller doses might be dangerous in children or in elderly persons.

Clinical Findings

A. Acute Poisoning: Drowsiness, weakness, nystagmus, diplopia, incoordination, and lassitude, progressing to coma with cyanosis and respiratory depression. Aspiration pneumonia is a frequent complication of coma with respiratory depression. Newborn infants of mothers given any of these drugs may have prolonged effects as a result of slow detoxification.

B. Chronic Poisoning: Drowsiness, depression, weakness, anxiety, ataxia, headaches, blurred vision, gastric upset, and pruritic skin rashes characterized by urticaria or erythematous macular eruptions.

Drug dependence has been reported to result from abuse of many of the selective depressants. Convulsions can occur from abrupt withdrawal.

C. Laboratory Findings: Any of the formed elements of the blood may be decreased in number.

Prevention

The patient should be warned to discontinue medication with these agents at the onset of any unusual symptoms. Severe hypotension may occur when any of these drugs are used. These agents should not be used in pregnancy.

Treatment

A. Acute Poisoning:

1. Emergency measures–

a. Remove drug by ipecac emesis followed by administration of activated charcoal. Airway-protected gastric lavage is necessary in patients with depressed respiration (see pp 21–28).

b. If coma and respiratory depression are present, treat as for depressants (see p 319). Alkaline diuresis has been suggested, but the hazard of pulmonary edema probably outweighs the benefits.

c. Maintain blood pressure.

2. General measures–Avoid concurrent administration of other depressant drugs.

B. Chronic Poisoning: Discontinue the drug at onset of any abnormal hematologic findings. Reduce dosage if drowsiness occurs. Treat withdrawal hyperactivity with low doses of phenobarbital. Propranolol has been useful in withdrawal from benzodiazepines.

Prognosis

Recovery is likely except in patients with aplastic anemia.

NEUROMUSCULAR BLOCKING AGENTS
(Table 23–8)

Agents that block neuromuscular transmission are used to promote relaxation during surgical anesthesia and occasionally to control convulsions. Dosages sufficient to relax peripheral muscles will also dangerously depress respiration. Thus, an effective dose of any of these compounds is potentially a fatal dose if respiration is not maintained by artificial means. The incidence of fatalities during the use of general anesthetic agents is greatly increased by the concomitant use of skeletal neuromuscular blocking agents.

These compounds appear to block neuromuscular transmission by either of 2 methods. The curare derivatives and gallamine triethiodide

Table 23–8. Skeletal neuromuscular blocking agents.

Drug	Initial Dose* (mg/kg)	Maximum Duration (min)	Antidote
Prevents depolarization			
Atracurium (Tracrium)	0.5	45	Edrophonium or neostigmine.
Metocurine iodide (Metubine)	0.1	120	Edrophonium or neostigmine.
Gallamine triethiodide (Flaxedil)	1	60	Edrophonium or neostigmine.
Pancuronium (Pavulon)	0.04	120	Edrophonium or neostigmine.
Tubocurarine chloride (Tubarine, etc)	0.1	120	Edrophonium or neostigmine.
Vecuronium (Norcuron)	0.1	30	Edrophonium or neostigmine.
Augments depolarization			
Succinylcholine chloride (Anectine, etc)	0.1	30	None.

*Dose that causes respiratory paralysis.

paralyze muscles by increasing the resistance of the muscle to depolarization by the acetylcholine released by nerve stimulation. By giving neostigmine or edrophonium, the resistance to depolarization can be partially overcome and the paralysis relieved. Atropine is ordinarily given along with neostigmine to block the effects of neostigmine on other systems. On the other hand, decamethonium bromide and succinylcholine chloride act by depolarizing the muscles, and no drugs are available that will overcome the paralysis thus induced. All of the skeletal neuromuscular blocking agents also depress autonomic ganglia to some extent, leading to fall in blood pressure.

The pathologic findings in deaths from skeletal neuromuscular blockade are not characteristic.

Clinical Findings

Chronic poisoning does not occur. The principal manifestations of acute poisoning (from injection) are respiratory failure and circulatory collapse. Symptoms are heaviness of the eyelids, diplopia, and difficulty in swallowing and talking, followed rapidly by paralysis of the extremities, neck, intercostal muscles, and, lastly, the diaphragm. Venous pooling and vascular dilatation, with severe fall in blood pressure, also occur. Cardiac arrest during succinylcholine administration has occurred after head injury. Symptoms ordinarily progress for 1–10 minutes after the injection is discontinued. The time required for complete recovery is variable, but it may be several hours. Malignant hyperthermia has been reported after the use of succinylcholine. Pancuronium may cause tachycardia.

Prevention

Skeletal neuromuscular blocking agents should be used only when facilities for giving artificial respiration and for controlling circulatory collapse are available. Local anesthetics, general anesthetics, and other drugs may prolong the effect of skeletal neuromuscular blocking agents. Atypical plasma cholinesterase is present in 1 out of 2000 patients, and in these succinylcholine is hydrolyzed slowly and the effect is prolonged.

Treatment

A. Emergency Measures: Intubate. Give artificial respiration and maintain blood pressure (see p 66).

B. Antidote: For curare derivatives or gallamine triethiodide, give either of the following: (1) Edrophonium (Tensilon) chloride, 10 mg (1 mL of 1% solution) intravenously; this may be repeated to a maximum of 30 mg. (2) Neostigmine (Prostigmin) methylsulfate, 1–2 mL of 1:2000 solution intravenously, with atropine, 1 mg. *Caution:* These antidotes may aggravate the circulatory collapse that occurs during muscular paralysis due to skeletal neuromuscular blocking agents.

Prognosis

If spontaneous respiration occurs, recovery is usually permanent.

INTERACTIONS
(See p 17.)

In the presence of tranquilizers or depressants, the action of ketamine may be prolonged. Hypertension and ventricular tachycardia from ketamine may occur if thyroid drugs are being used.

All central nervous system depressants, including ethanol, enhance the central nervous system depressant effects of other central nervous system depressants, anesthetics, tranquilizers, antihistamines, antidepressants, narcotic analgesics, and monoamine oxidase inhibitor antidepressants. Tolerance to one indicates tolerance to the others.

The effect of succinylcholine is enhanced by propanidid, procaine, echothiophate, hexafluorenium, polymyxins, and aminoglycosides.

Allyl barbiturates reduce the cytochrome P-450 enzyme necessary for metabolism of some drugs and chemicals. Excessive response to these drugs may occur.

Hypnotics, antihistamines, and narcotic analgesics slow intestinal absorption.

Phenytoin toxicity can occur in slow acetylators given disulfiram or isoniazid. Phenytoin levels rise and toxicity is possible when diazoxide is withdrawn. Diazepam, coumarins, phenylbutazone, thioridazine, and methylphenidate may increase blood levels of phenytoin, with possible toxicity.

Neuromuscular blockade from tubocurarine type agents is increased by propranolol, procainamide, quinidine, clindamycin, polymyxins, and aminoglycosides and by potassium loss induced by diuretics, carbenoxolone, amphotericin B, corticosteroids, or laxative abuse.

Long-term phenothiazine administration increases and short-term phenothiazine administration decreases anesthetic requirements. Phenothiazines are alpha sympathomimetic blocking agents and cause hypotension. Phenothiazines also alter catecholamine levels in the brain and interact dangerously with monoamine oxidase inhibitors. Vasopressors can be more or less effective in the presence of phenothiazines.

PHARMACOKINETICS & TOXIC CONCENTRATIONS
(See p 89.)

	pK_a	$t\frac{1}{2}$	V_d	% Binding	Toxic Concentration ($\mu g/mL$)
Amobarbital	7.7	12—27	2.5—4	61	30
Baclofen	3.9, 9.6	3—4		30	
Barbital					100
Bromide		168			500
Butabarbital	7.9	37.5	0.8	26	28—73*
Carbamazepine		18—55	1	72	10
Chloral hydrate	10.04	8—35	0.6	70—80	
Chlordiazepoxide	4.6	8—28	0.3—0.5	94—97	8
Chlormethiazole	3.2	3.1—5	5.4	63	
Chlorpheniramine	9.2	12—15		72	
Chlorpromazine	9.3	16—31	40—50	91—99	300*
Clonazepam	1.5, 10.5	20—60	3.1		0.069
Codeine	8.2	2—3	5—10	7	1.1
Dantrolene	7.5	8.7			
Diazepam	3.3	20—96	0.7, 2.6†	98	
Diphenhydramine	8.3	5—8		72	0.1
Diphenoxylate	7.07	2.5	4.6		
Droperidol	7.6	2		85—90	
Ethchlorvynol		35	5—10		85
Ethosuximide	9.3	60	0.7,† 0.9	0	150
Fluphenazine	3.9, 8.05	14			
Flurazepam	1.9	47—100?			0.12*
Glutethimide	9.2	10—100	10—20	54	6

*Fatal.
†For children.

	pK$_a$	t½	V$_d$	% Binding	Toxic Concentration (µg/mL)
Haloperidol	8.7	14–21	17–30	92	42
Hexabarbital	8.2	3–7	1.1		
Ketamine	7.5	3–4			
Loperamide	8.6	9–14			
Lorazepam	1.3, 11.5	10–24	0.9	90	
Loxapine	6.6	3–4			
Meclastine	8.1	35	1.14	96	
Meperidine	8.7	2.4–4	4.3	64	30
Meprobamate		6–17			150
Methadone	8.6	18–97	5–10	85	1.6*
Methapyrilene					12
Methaqualone	2.4	20–60	6	80	10
Methsuximide		10			
Methyprylon					30
Morphine	8.05	10–44?	2.8	35	0.1
Naloxone		1–2			
Nitrazepam	3.2, 10.8	21–28	2.1	85	
Normeperidine		15–20			
Norpropoxyphene		30–36			
Orphenadrine	8.4	10		20	
Oxazepam	1.7, 11.6	10–14	1.6	90	
Paraldehyde		4–10			
Pentazocine	9.0	2–3	3	60–70	
Pentobarbital	7.6	23–30	0.9–1	40–65	10
Perphenazine	7.8	21			
Phenobarbital	7.4	48–144	1	40–60	100
Phenytoin	8.3	10–42	1	89	50
Pimozide	8.6	29		97	
Prazepam		78		85	
Primidone		3.3–12.5	1	0	18
Prochlorperazine	8.1	23			
Promethazine	9.1			7.5	
Propoxyphene	6.3	3–12	1	78	2*
Quinalbarbital	7.9	40		65–75	
Secobarbital		29			30
Thiopental	7.6	3–8		75–90	14
Thioridazine	9.5	16–24			18*
Valproate		8–15	0.15–0.4	90	200+

*Fatal.

References

Barbiturate & Nonbarbiturate Depressants

Berg MJ et al: Acceleration of the body clearance of phenobarbital by oral activated charcoal. *N Engl J Med* 1982;**307**:642.

Kelner MJ, Bailey DN: Ethchlorvynol ingestion: Interpretation of blood concentrations and clinical findings. *J Toxicol Clin Toxicol* 1983;**21**:399.

McCarron MM et al: Short-acting barbiturate overdosage. *JAMA* 1982;**248**:55.

Olson KR et al: Intestinal infarction complicating phenobarbital overdose. *Arch Intern Med* 1984;**144**:407.

Pond SM et al: Randomized study of the treatment of phenobarbital overdose with repeated doses of activated charcoal. *JAMA* 1984;**251**:3104.

Anticonvulsants

Bradbury AJ et al: Dystonia associated with carbamazepine toxicity. *Postgrad Med J* 1982;**58**:525.

deGroot G et al: Charcoal hemoperfusion in the treatment of two cases of carbamazepine poisoning. *J Toxicol Clin Toxicol* 1984;**22**:349.

Earnest MP et al: Complications of intravenous phenytoin for acute treatment of seizures. *JAMA* 1983;**249**:762.

Leslie TJ et al: Cardiac complications of carbamazepine intoxication: Treatment by haemoperfusion. *Br Med J* 1983;**286**:1018.

Nilsson C, Sterner G, Idvall J: Charcoal hemoperfusion for treatment of serious carbamazepine poisoning. *Acta Med Scand* 1984;**216**:137.

Narcotic Analgesics

Brittain JL: China white: The bogus drug. [Methyl fentanyl.] *J Toxicol Clin Toxicol* 1982;**19**:1123.

Carin I et al: Neonatal methadone withdrawal. *Am J Dis Child* 1983;**137**:1166.

Cuddy PG: Management of acute opioid intoxication. *Crit Care Quarterly* 1982;**4(4)**:65.

Cuss FM et al: Cardiac arrest after reversal of effects of opiates with naloxone. *Br Med J* 1984;**288**:363.

Handal KA et al: Naloxone. *Ann Emerg Med* 1983;**12**:438.

Lewis JM et al: Continuous naloxone infusion in pediatric narcotic overdose. *Am J Dis Child* 1984;**138**:944.

Rice TB: Paregoric intoxication with pulmonary edema in infancy. *Clin Pediatr* 1984;**23**:101.

Ruttenber AJ, Luke JL: Heroin-related deaths. *Science* 1984;**226**:14.

Stahl SM, Kasser IS: Pentazocine overdose. *Ann Emerg Med* 1983;**12**:28.

Street-drug contaminant causing parkinsonism. *MMWR* 1984;**33**:351.

Bromides

Iberti TJ et al: Prolonged bromide intoxication resulting from a gastric bezoar. *Arch Intern Med* 1984;**144**:402.

Antihistamines & Phenothiazines

Hausmann E et al: Lethal intoxication with diphenhydramine. *Arch Toxicol* 1983;**53**:33.

Kemper AJ et al: Thioridazine-induced torsade des pointes. *JAMA* 1983;
249:2931.

Ko PT et al: Torsade des pointes, a common arrhythmia induced by medication. *Can Med Assoc J* 1982;**127:**368.

Selective Depressants

Conell LJ, Berlin RM: Withdrawal after substitution of a short-acting for a long-acting benzodiazepine. *JAMA* 1983;**250:**2838.

Cruz FG et al: Neuroleptic malignant syndrome after haloperidol therapy. *South Med J* 1983;**76:**684.

Leung FW, Guze PA: Diazepam withdrawal. *West J Med* 1982;**138:**98.

Olson KR et al: Coma caused by trivial triazolam overdose. *Am J Emerg Med* 1985;**3:**210.

Rosenthal SA et al: Apparent diazepam toxicity in a child due to accidental ingestion of misrepresented Quaalude. *Vet Hum Toxicol* 1984;**26:**320.

Drugs Affecting the Autonomic Nervous System | 24

ATROPINE, HYOSCYAMINE, BELLADONNA, SCOPOLAMINE, & SYNTHETIC SUBSTITUTES

Atropine, scopolamine, related alkaloids, and synthetic substitutes are sold both in prescriptions and in a number of proprietary mixtures for the treatment of gastrointestinal diseases, colds, hay fever, parkinsonism, and asthma. Plants containing atropine and related alkaloids are also occasionally eaten by children. Such plants as *Atropa belladonna* (deadly nightshade, English nightshade), *Hyoscyamus niger* (henbane), and *Datura stramonium* (jimsonweed) contain 0.25–0.5% atropine or related alkaloids. Tincture of belladonna contains 30 mg of atropine alkaloids per 100 mL. Synthetic atropine substitutes are as follows:

Adiphenine (Trasentine)
Anisotropine (Valpin)
Benztropine (Cogentin)
Biperiden (Akineton)
Clidinium (Quarzan)
Cyclopentolate (Cyclogyl)
Dicyclomine (Bentyl)
Eucatropine
Flavoxate (Urispas)
Glycopyrrolate (Robinul)
Hexocyclium (Tral)
Homatropine
Isopropamide (Darbid)
Mepenzolate (Cantil)

Methantheline (Banthine)
Methixene (Trest)
Methscopolamine (Pamine)
Oxybutynin (Ditropan)
Oxyphencyclimine (Daricon)
Oxyphenonium (Antrenyl)
Pentapiperium (Perium)
Poldine (Nacton)
Procyclidine (Kemadrin)
Propantheline (Pro-Banthine)
Thiphenamil (Trocinate)
Trihexyphenidyl (Artane)
Tropicamide (Mydriacyl)

The fatal dose of atropine or scopolamine in children may be as low as 10 mg. Death has occurred from dicyclomine (60 mg/kg) with doxylamine. The fatal dose for other synthetic substitutes would be 10–100 mg/kg. The fatality rate in cases of atropine or scopolamine poisoning is less than 1%.

Atropine and scopolamine paralyze the parasympathetic nervous system by blocking the action on effector cells of the acetylcholine released at nerve endings. Atropine and the various synthetic substitutes also stimulate the central nervous system. Since atropine is almost entirely eliminated by the kidneys, abnormalities of kidney function may lead to toxic reactions in patients receiving atropine. Kidney function must be normal to eliminate the drug.

The pathologic findings are not characteristic. The internal organs may be congested.

Clinical Findings

The principal manifestations of poisoning with these drugs are delirium, fast pulse, and fever.

A. Acute Poisoning: (From ingestion, injection, or application to mucous membranes.) Therapeutic doses of atropine, scopolamine, or other anticholinergic drugs may cause dilated pupils, blurring of vision, rise in intraocular tension, and increased heart rate. Toxic doses (5–10 mg or higher) may cause hot, dry, red skin; dry mouth; disorientation; hallucinations; aggressive behavior; delirium; rapid pulse and respiration; urinary retention; muscular stiffness; fever; convulsions; and coma. Synthetic substitutes in doses of 0.1–1 g may cause similar symptoms. Some synthetic substitutes are similar to antihistamines and are more likely to cause convulsions. In doses above 10 mg, scopolamine also causes respiratory depression and coma.

B. Chronic Poisoning: (From ingestion, injection, or application to mucous membranes.) The above symptoms may occur after repeated therapeutic doses.

Prevention

The dosage of atropine or related compounds must be lowered during periods of hot weather for patients who are taking maximum tolerated amounts, since such patients are most susceptible to heat exhaustion.

Do not give atropine or related drugs to patients with glaucoma. Reduction of dosage is necessary if urinary retention occurs.

Treatment

A. Acute Poisoning:

1. Emergency measures–Maintain airway and respiration. Remove poison from mucous membranes by washing. Delay absorption of ingested material by giving activated charcoal and then remove by gastric lavage (see pp 21–28). Follow with saline catharsis. Efforts to remove these agents are useful for several hours after ingestion, since they depress gastrointestinal motility.

2. Antidote–To reverse life-threatening central and peripheral effects of atropine and substitutes, give physostigmine salicylate intravenously, 1–5 mL of dilution containing 1 mg in 5 mL of saline. The smaller dose is for children, and injection should take not less than 2 minutes. Electrocardiographic control is advisable. Dosage can be repeated every 5 minutes up to a total dose of 2 mg in children and 6 mg in adults every 30 minutes (Table 24–2). Physostigmine is contraindicated in hypotensive reactions. Atropine, 1 mg, should be available for immediate injection if physostigmine causes bradycardia, convulsions, or severe bronchoconstriction.

3. General measures–

a. Monitor ECG.

b. Reduce rectal body temperature to 38 °C by applying wet towels. Dexamethasone, 1 mg/kg slowly intravenously, has been suggested for pyrexia.

c. Control convulsions by giving diazepam.

d. Give fluids orally or intravenously to maintain urine output.

e. If patient does not void, catheterization may be necessary to avoid bladder rupture.

B. Chronic Poisoning: Discontinue medication and treat as for acute poisoning.

Prognosis

A patient who survives for 24 hours will probably recover. Whether physostigmine increases the survival rate in patients poisoned with anticholinergic agents has not been determined.

Brizer DA, Manning DW: Delirium induced by poisoning with anticholinergic agents. *Am J Psychiatry* 1982;**139**:1543.

Goldfrank L et al: Anticholinergic poisoning. *J Toxicol Clin Toxicol* 1982;**19**:17.

Klein-Schwartz W et al: Jimsonweed intoxication in adolescents and young adults. *Am J Dis Child* 1984;**138**:737.

SYMPATHOMIMETIC AGENTS: EPINEPHRINE, EPHEDRINE, AMPHETAMINE, NAPHAZOLINE, & RELATED DRUGS

Epinephrine, ephedrine, and related agents are widely sold on prescription and in proprietary mixtures for the treatment of nasal congestion, asthma, and hay fever.

From 1 to 10% of users of epinephrine or related drugs have reactions from overdosage. See Table 24–1 for estimated fatal doses. Fatalities are rare.

Epinephrine and related drugs stimulate muscle and gland cells innervated by the sympathetic nervous system. They also produce variable stimulatory effects on the central nervous system.

The pathologic findings are not characteristic.

Table 24–1. Sympathomimetic agents: Epinephrine and related drugs.
(See treatment on p 350.)

Drug	MLD* (mg)	Method of Administration
Albuterol (salbutamol, Proventil)	200	Oral.
Amphetamine (Benzedrine)	10	Oral.
Benzphetamine (Didrex)	200	Oral.
Chlorphentermine (Presate)	200	Oral.
Cyclopentamine (Clopane)	200	Mucous membranes.
Dextroamphetamine	20	Oral.
Diethylpropion (Tenuate)	200	Oral.
Dobutamine (Dobutrex)	200	IV.
Dopamine (Intropin)	200	IV.
Ephedrine	200	Oral.
Epinephrine	10	IM or subcut.
Fenfluramine (Pondimin)	200	Oral.
Hydroxyamphetamine (Paredrine)	200	Intranasal.
Isoetharine (Bronkosol)	20	Oral.
Isometheptene (Octin)	200	Oral.
Isoproterenol (Isuprel, Aludrine)	100	Mucous membranes.
Isoxsuprine (Vasodilan)	100	Oral.
Levodopa	1000?	Oral.
Mazindol (Sanorex)	50	Oral.
Mephentermine (Wyamine)	200	Intranasal, oral.
Metaproterenol (Alupent)	20	Oral.
Metaraminol (Aramine)	60	Intranasal, IM.
Methamphetamine (Desoxyn, etc)	100	Oral.
Methoxamine (Vasoxyl)	60	IM, subcut.
Methoxyphenamine (Orthoxine)	200	Oral.
Methylhexaneamine (Forthane)	200	Mucous membranes.
Methylphenidate (Ritalin)	200	Oral.
Naphazoline (Privine)	10	Intranasal.
Norepinephrine (levarterenol, Levophed)	10	IM or subcut.
Nylidrin (Arlidin)	200	Oral.
Oxymetazoline (Afrin)	10	Intranasal.
Pemoline (Cylert)	200	Oral
Phendimetrazine (Plegine)	200	Oral.
Phenmetrazine (Preludin)	200	Oral.
Phentermine (Fastine)	200	Oral.
Phenylephrine (Neo-Synephrine)	100	Intranasal.
Phenylpropanolamine (Propadrine)	200	Intranasal.
Propylhexedrine (Benzedrex)	200	Intranasal, oral.
Protokylol (Ventaire)	100	Oral.
Pseudoephedrine (Afrinol)	200	Oral.
Ritodrine (Yutopar)	200	Oral.
Terbutaline (Bricanyl)	50	Oral.
Tetrahydrozoline (Tyzine)	5	Intranasal.
Tuaminoheptane (Tuamine)	200	Intranasal, oral.
Xylometazoline (Otrivin)	10	Intranasal.

*Estimated for children up to age 2 years. Adult MLD at least 10 times as high.

Clinical Findings

The principal manifestation of poisoning with these drugs is convulsions.

A. Acute Poisoning: (From injection, ingestion, inhalation, or application to mucous membranes.) Nausea and vomiting, nervousness, irritability, tachycardia, cardiac arrhythmias, dilated pupils, blurred vision, chills, pallor or cyanosis, fever, suicidal behavior, mania, opisthotonos, spasms, convulsions, pulmonary edema, gasping respiration, coma, and respiratory failure. A child died with convulsions, hyperthermia, tachycardia, and cardiac arrest after taking diethylpropion, 30 mg/kg. The blood pressure is markedly raised initially but may be below normal later and may be accompanied by persistent anuria. Inhalation or injection of decomposed (pink) epinephrine will cause a psychosislike state with hallucinations and morbid fears. Perivascular or subcutaneous injection of norepinephrine or other epinephrine substitutes causes cutaneous necrosis or slough. Naphazoline, oxymetazoline, tetrahydrozoline, and xylometazoline can cause hypotension and central nervous system depression. Terbutaline given as a uterine relaxant in threatened abortion has caused maternal pulmonary edema when given with corticosteroids and death of the fetus when given in 10 times the usual dose. Dopamine (Intropin) can increase cardiac irritability, with paroxysmal supraventricular tachycardia and other arrhythmias, and can cause hypotension. Gangrene of the extremities has occurred after dopamine administration. Intra-arterial injection of dopamine can cause severe pain, ischemia, and gangrene in the arterial distribution area.

B. Chronic Poisoning: Prolonged nasal use of epinephrine or substitutes leads to chronic nasal congestion. Prolonged oral use of amphetamine or ephedrine or similar drugs in large doses by emotionally unstable individuals may lead to personality changes with a psychic craving to continue the use of the drug. Use of these compounds can also cause reactions of tension and anxiety progressing to psychosis. Abuse of methylphenidate has caused fever with eosinophilia. Long-term use of dextroamphetamine or methylphenidate for control of hyperactivity in children has caused growth retardation. Pemoline is suspected of causing liver damage. Isoxsuprine can cause skin rash. Dobutamine has caused anginal pain and dyspnea.

Levodopa can cause anorexia, nausea, tachycardia, ventricular extrasystoles, depression or agitation, hypotension or hypertension, choreiform or dystonic movements, hallucinations, and toxic psychosis. The maximum dose should not exceed 8 g/d. A combination of carbidopa with levodopa (Sinemet) can cause psychosis, depression, convulsions, nausea, cardiac irregularity, hypotension, gastrointestinal ulceration, and hypertension. Continued use of vasopressors such as norepinephrine to maintain blood pressure in the presence of hypovolemia can lead to acidosis.

C. Laboratory Findings: These are noncontributory.

Prevention

Parents should be warned of the dangers of incautious administration of potent nose drops to infants. Nasal inhalers and amphetamine preparations should be stored safely. Administration of epinephrine or substitutes during or after surgery may lead to ventricular arrhythmias and cardiac arrest.

Treatment

A. Acute Poisoning:

1. Emergency measures–

a. If respirations are shallow or if cyanosis is present, give artificial respiration. Maintain adequate arterial O_2 concentration. Minute volume of respiration should be 1–1.5 L/10 kg. Vasopressors are contraindicated.

b. Remove drug by ipecac emesis followed by activated charcoal. Airway-protected gastric lavage is necessary in hyperactive patients or those with depressed respiration (see pp 21–28).

c. Maintain blood pressure in cardiovascular collapse (see p 66).

2. Antidote–For cutaneous or perivascular injection of norepinephrine, infiltrate the area with 5 mg of phentolamine (Regitine). For hypertensive reactions to epinephrine or substitutes, give phentolamine, 5 mg diluted in saline slowly intravenously, or 100 mg orally. Chlorpromazine is contraindicated except in amphetamine poisoning. In pure amphetamine poisoning, give chlorpromazine, 0.5–1 mg/kg every 30 minutes as needed. Droperidol, 2.5 mg/min intravenously to a total of 10–15 mg, has been suggested for amphetamine and methamphetamine poisoning.

3. General measures–Control convulsions (see p 51). Diazepam is probably safe. Control pyrexia with cooling blanket and dexamethasone, 1 mg/kg slowly intravenously. Acid diuresis may be useful for amphetamine and methamphetamine poisoning.

B. Chronic Poisoning: Discontinue use.

Prognosis

If the patient survives the first 6 hours, recovery is likely. In psychotic reactions resulting from prolonged use, recovery may require weeks or months.

Call TD et al: Acute cardiomyopathy secondary to intravenous amphetamine abuse. *Ann Intern Med* 1982;**97**:559.

Cornelius JR et al: Paranoia, homicidal behavior, and seizures associated with phenylpropanolamine. *Am J Psychiatry* 1984;**141**:120.

Friedman R et al: Seizures in a patient receiving terbutaline. *Am J Dis Child* 1982;**136**:1091.

Howrie DL, Wolfson JH: Phenylpropanolamine-induced hypertensive seizures. *J Pediatr* 1983;**102**:43.

Hyams JS et al: Pseudopheochromocytoma and cardiac arrest associated with phenylpropanolamine. *JAMA* 1985;**253**:1609.

Klein-Schwartz W et al: Central nervous system depression from ingestion of nonprescription eyedrops. *Am J Emerg Med* 1984;**2**:217.

Kurachek SC et al: Inadvertent intravenous administration of racemic epinephrine. *JAMA* 1985;**253**:1441.

Pentel P: Toxicity of over-the-counter stimulants. *JAMA* 1984;**252**:1898.

Sankey RJ et al: Visual hallucinations in children receiving decongestants. *Br Med J* 1984;**288**:1369.

Shnaps Y et al: Methyldopa poisoning. *J Toxicol Clin Toxicol* 1982;**19**:501.

Solomon SL et al: Medication errors with inhalant epinephrine mimicking an epidemic of neonatal sepsis. *N Engl J Med* 1984;**310**:166.

Stecyk O et al: Multiple organ failure resulting from intravenous abuse of methylphenidate hydrochloride. *Ann Emerg Med* 1985;**14**:597.

PARASYMPATHOMIMETIC AGENTS: PHYSOSTIGMINE, PILOCARPINE, NEOSTIGMINE, METHACHOLINE, & RELATED DRUGS

Physostigmine, pilocarpine, neostigmine, and methacholine are used for the treatment of myasthenia gravis, for atonic conditions of the gastrointestinal tract and urinary bladder, and for certain cardiac irregularities.

More than 20 fatalities from these compounds have been reported in the literature. Physostigmine, benzpyrinium, and neostigmine inhibit the esterase responsible for hydrolyzing the parasympathetic effector acetylcholine. Pilocarpine, bethanechol, and methacholine act at the same point as does acetylcholine. As a result of these actions, these drugs stimulate muscles and glands innervated by the parasympathetic nervous system.

The pathologic findings are congestion of the brain, lungs, and gastrointestinal tract. Pulmonary edema may occur.

Clinical Findings

The principal manifestation of poisoning with these drugs is respiratory difficulty.

A. Acute Poisoning: (From ingestion, injection, or application to mucous membranes.) Tremor, marked peristalsis with involuntary defecation and urination, pinpoint pupils, vomiting, cold extremities, hypotension, bronchial constriction with difficult breathing and wheez-

Table 24–2. Parasympathomimetic agents: Physostigmine and related drugs.

Drug	Fatal Dose* (mg)	Method of Administration
Acetylcholine	20	Injection.
Ambenonium (Mytelase)	60	Oral.
Benzpyrinium (Stigmonene)	10	IM.
Bethanechol (Urecholine)	20	Injection.
Carbachol (Miostat)	10	Injection or topical.
Demecarium (Humorsol)	20	Topical.
Echothiophate iodide (Phospholine)	10	Topical.
Edrophonium (Tensilon)	100	Injection.
Metoclopramide (Reglan)	200	Oral.
Methacholine (Mecholyl)	30	Injection.
Muscarine	10	Oral.
Neostigmine (Prostigmin)	60	Oral.
	10	Injection.
Physostigmine (Antilirium)	6	Injection or oral.
Pilocarpine	60	Topical.
Pyridostigmine (Mestinon)	300	Oral.

*Estimated for adult.

ing, twitching of muscles, fainting, slow pulse, convulsions, and death from asphyxia or cardiac slowing. Life-threatening ventricular arrhythmias have occurred after use of physostigmine. Esophageal rupture has occurred from the use of carbachol, a drug similar to bethanechol. Metoclopramide can cause drowsiness, dizziness, and exrapyramidal signs.

B. Chronic Poisoning: Repeated small doses may reproduce the syndrome described under Acute Poisoning.

Prevention

When physostigmine and related drugs are used, atropine should be readily available for immediate use. Do not use physostigmine in the presence of asthma, gangrene, diabetes, cardiac or vascular disease, or mechanical obstruction of the intestines or urogenital tract; in vagotonic states; or in patients receiving choline esters or depolarizing neuromuscular blocking agents such as decamethonium or succinylcholine.

Treatment of Acute or Chronic Poisoning:

A. Emergency Measures: Maintain artificial respiration until antidote can be given.

B. Antidote: Give atropine, 2 mg slowly intravenously. Repeat this dose intramuscularly every 2–4 hours as necessary to relieve respiratory difficulty. For echothiophate only, pralidoxime (see p 117) is also useful.

Prognosis

If atropine can be given, recovery is immediate.

MISCELLANEOUS BLOCKING AGENTS
(Table 24–3)

Sympatholytic agents are used to reduce blood pressure and for other therapeutic purposes. Most of these agents produce postural hypotension, with faintness and tachycardia, dry mouth, cardiac irregularities, and failure of erections. Toxic reactions are controlled by reducing the dosage or discontinuing the drug. Avoid the use of sympathomimetic drugs such as epinephrine, since in some instances the effects of such drugs are greatly intensified in the presence of sympatholytic agents. Abrupt withdrawal of clonidine may cause hyperexcitability, psychosis, cardiac arrhythmias, and rapid rise of blood pressure. Deaths have occurred.

Treatment

In acute toxic reactions to any of the blocking agents, discontinue use. Maintain respiration. Remove overdoses with lavage and activated charcoal. Use sympathomimetic agents cautiously, since their effects may be intensified. Mechanical ventilation and cardiac pacing may be necessary. Atropine may also be helpful. For clonidine overdose, the administration of atropine, diazoxide for hypertension or dopamine infusion for hypotension, and maximum diuresis with furosemide and mannitol have been successful.

Artman M, Berth RC: Clonidine poisoning. *Am J Dis Child* 1983;**136**:171.

Banner W Jr et al: Failure of naloxone to reverse clonidine toxic effect. *Am J Dis Child* 1983;**137**:1170.

Bauman JH, Kimelblatt BJ: Cimetidine as an inhibitor of drug metabolism: Therapeutic implications and review of the literature. *Drug Intell Clin Pharm* 1982;**16**:380.

Freston JW: Cimetidine: Adverse reactions and patterns of use. *Ann Intern Med* 1982;**97**:728.

Roberts RK et al: Cimetidine-theophylline in patients with chronic obstructive airways disease. *Med J Aust* 1984;**140**:279.

Sedman AJ: Cimetidine-drug interactions. *Am J Med* 1984;**76**:109.

Yagupsky P, Gorodischer R: Massive clonidine ingestion with hypertension in a 9-month-old infant. *Pediatrics* 1983;**72**:500.

Table 24–3. Sympathetic and histamine blocking agents. (See p 353.)

Drug	Safe Dose	Toxic Effects
Atenolol	100 mg orally	Bradycardia, hypotension, dizziness, fatigue, nausea.
Azapetine (Ilidar)	1 mg/kg orally or IV	Nausea, vomiting.
Bretylium (Darenthin)	100 mg orally	Nasal congestion, muscular weakness, parotid pain, confusion, ventricular tachycardia and fibrillation.
Cimetidine (Tagamet)	300 mg orally or IV	Diarrhea, headache, fatigue, dizziness, muscle pain, rash, confusion, phytobezoar, delirium, psychosis, gynecomastia, elevated serum creatinine or liver enzymes, leukopenia, agranulocytosis, thrombocytopenia, erythema annulare centrifugum, ulcer perforation on withdrawal. Hepatitis and interstitial nephritis with renal failure have occurred.
Clonidine (Catapres)	0.1 mg orally	Bradycardia, drowsiness, gastrointestinal upset, possible hepatitis, heart failure, rash, coma, arrhythmia, hypotension, depressed respiration, apnea, increased sensitivity to alcohol. Hypertensive crisis on abrupt withdrawal.
Guanadrel (Hylorel) Guanethidine (Ismelin)	10 mg orally	Diarrhea, mydriasis, constipation, polyarteritis nodosa.
Labetolol (Normodyne)	0.4 g orally	Jaundice, tremor, hypotension, abdominal discomfort, fatigue, impotence, dyspnea, rash.
Methyldopa (Aldomet)	0.5 g orally	Fluid retention, fever, diarrhea, mental depression, hepatic toxicity, parkinsonism, arthralgia, leukopenia, hypertension, breast enlargement, amenorrhea, galactorrhea, pancreatitis, myocarditis, hemolytic anemia.
Metyrosine (Demser)	500 mg orally	Sedation, extrapyramidal signs, anxiety, psychosis, diarrhea.
Phenoxybenzamine (Dibenzyline)	10 mg orally	Nasal congestion, miosis, tachycardia, vertigo, indigestion, weakness, vasomotor collapse.
Phentolamine (Regitine)	100 mg orally, 5 mg IV	
Pindolol (Visken)	5 mg orally	Bradycardia, cardiac failure. 5 mg has caused bronchospasm.
Ranitidine (Zantac)	100 mg orally	Leukopenia, headache, nausea, possible liver and kidney damage, increased intraocular pressure.
Timolol (Blocadren)	10 mg orally	Bradycardia, hypotension, arrhythmias, headache, dizziness, disorientation, bronchospasm, gastrointestinal distress.
Tolazoline (Priscoline)	100 mg orally or IV	Pilomotor reactions, formication, tingling, chilliness, nausea, epigastric distress, severe cardiac pain.

BETA-SYMPATHETIC BLOCKING AGENTS: PROPRANOLOL, ATENOLOL, PINDOLOL, & OTHERS

Propranolol (Inderal) and other β-sympathetic blocking agents are used in a wide variety of conditions ranging from migraine to cardiac arrhythmias and narcotic withdrawal.

Initial doses of these drugs should not exceed the following: atenolol (Tenormin), 50 mg; metoprolol (Lopressor), 50 mg; Nadolol (Corgard), 40 mg; pindolol (Visken), 5 mg; propranolol (Inderal), 10 mg. Serious symptoms can occur after administration of 1 g of propranolol in adults or 10 mg/kg in children. Several fatalities have occurred.

The effects of propranolol are typical of this group of drugs: Propranolol reduces or blocks cardiac and bronchial response to β-sympathetic stimulation, produces a quinidinelike reduction in myocardial contractility, and has central nervous system effects. A metabolite, 4-hydroxypropranolol, has similar effects.

Clinical Findings

The principal manifestation of poisoning with these agents is hypotension.

A. Acute Poisoning: (From ingestion.) Overdoses cause dizziness, slow pulse, fall of blood pressure, hypoglycemia (in children), respiratory depression, convulsions, brochospasm, coma, catatonia, and delirium.

B. Chronic Poisoning: (From ingestion.) Continued administration of therapeutic doses has caused nausea and vomiting, diarrhea, constipation, insomnia, fatigue, alopecia, agranulocytosis, systemic lupus erythematosus (SLE) syndrome, pulmonary edema, pulmonary fibrosis, and thrombocytopenia. Myocardial infarction can occur after abrupt withdrawal.

C. Laboratory Findings: Electrocardiographic findings include intraventricular conduction defects including first-degree atrioventricular block, widened QRS complex, and absent P waves.

Treatment

A. Acute Poisoning:

1. Emergency measures–Maintain respiration, adequate airway, blood pressure, and blood glucose. Control convulsions with diazepam. Remove drug by ipecac emesis and gastric lavage with activated charcoal. Efforts to remove the drug are probably useless after 1 hour.

2. Antidote–Give isoproterenol, 1–4 μg/min by intravenous infusion, or glucagon, 50 μg/kg immediately followed by 50 μg/kg hourly by infusion. Atropine, 0.01–0.02 mg/kg, is sometimes useful to treat bradycardia. Maintenance of blood pressure may require trial of epinephrine, L-norepinephrine, dopamine, or dobutamine.

3. General measures–

a. Treat bronchospasm with intravenous aminophylline, 5 mg/kg as a loading dose, then 0.5–1 mg/kg/h to maintain serum aminophylline level just below 20 μg/mL.

b. Control convulsions with diazepam, 0.01 mg/kg intravenously over 10 minutes.

B. Chronic Poisoning: Discontinue use of the beta-blocking drug.

Prognosis

If blood pressure can be maintained for 24 hours, recovery is likely.

Dipalma JR: Beta-blocker drug interactions. *Am Fam Physician* (Sept) 1983;**28**:249.

Heath A: β-Adrenoceptor blocker toxicity: Clinical features and therapy. (Review.) *Am J Emerg Med* 1984;**2**:518.

Peterson CD et al: Glucagon therapy for β-blocker overdose. *Drug Intell Clin Pharm* 1984;**18**:394.

Weinstein RS: Recognition and management of poisoning with β-adrenergic blocking agents. *Ann Emerg Med* 1984;**13**:1123.

Weinstein RS et al: Beta blocker overdose with propranolol and with atenolol. *Ann Emerg Med* 1985;**14**:161.

ERGOT, ERGOTAMINE, & ERGONOVINE

Ergot is a fungus that grows on rye. The derivatives, including ergotamine, methysergide (Sansert), and dihydroergotamine, are used in the treatment of headaches; ergonovine and methylergonovine are used as uterine stimulants. Bromocriptine is used to suppress prolactin secretion. Rye flour is sometimes contaminated by the ergot fungus.

The fatal dose of ergot may be as low as 1 g. Fatalities from ergotamine or other purified derivatives have not been reported; presumably the fatal dose is high in relation to the therapeutic dose. However, a dose of 40 mg of ergotamine tartrate over a 5-day period has caused impending gangrene of all 4 extremities.

Ergot and its alkaloids stimulate smooth muscles of the arterioles, intestines, and uterus.

The pathologic findings include congestion and inflammatory changes in the gastrointestinal tract and kidneys. Gangrene of the fingers and toes may be present.

Clinical Findings

The principal manifestations of poisoning with these drugs are convulsions and gangrene.

A. Acute Poisoning: (From ingestion, injection, or application to mucous membranes.) Vomiting, diarrhea; dizziness; rise or fall of blood pressure; slow, weak pulse; dyspnea; convulsions; loss of consciousness. The dose necessary to produce abortion may cause fatal poisoning. Bromocriptine causes nausea, headache, dizziness, fatigue, hypertension, pulmonary infiltration, pleural effusion, and thickening of the pleura.

B. Chronic Poisoning: (From ingestion, injection, or application to mucous membranes.) Ergotism includes 2 types of manifestations, which may occur together or separately.

1. Those resulting from contraction of blood vessels and reduced circulation include numbness and coldness of the extremities, tingling, pain in the chest, heart valve lesions, alopecia, oliguria from reduced renal blood flow, and gangrene of the fingers and toes. Hypercoagulability has also been reported.

2. Those resulting from nervous system disturbances include vomiting, diarrhea, headache, tremors, contractions of the facial muscles, and convulsions. Additionally, methysergide has caused retroperitoneal or pleural fibrosis.

Prevention

Do not give over 3 mg of purified ergot derivatives (including ergotamine) daily; higher doses are likely to result in peripheral vascular disturbances.

Ergot preparations are contraindicated in pregnancy, obliterative vascular disease, hypertension, infections, and kidney or liver disease.

Treatment

A. Acute Poisoning:

1. **Emergency measures–**Remove drug by ipecac emesis followed by activated charcoal. Gastric lavage may be necessary (see pp 21–28).

2. **Antidote–**Give a vasodilator, such as tolazoline, 10–15 mg in 500 mL of 5% dextrose, by intravenous drip; control the rate of administration by monitoring pulse rate and blood pressure. Slow intravenous administration of sodium nitroprusside has been suggested for the treatment of ergot hypertension.

3. **General measures–**Treat convulsions with diazepam (see Table 4–3). Control hypercoagulability by the administration of heparin; maintain the blood clotting time at approximately 3 times normal. Treat hypotension (see p 66). Do not use vasopressors.

B. Chronic Poisoning: Discontinue the use of ergot preparations. Gangrene will require surgical amputation.

Prognosis

In acute poisoning from ergot, death may occur up to 1 week after poisoning. Complete recovery usually occurs in chronic poisoning if the use of ergot derivatives is discontinued prior to the appearance of gangrene.

Pandey SK, Haines CI: Accidental administration of ergometrine to newborn infant. *Br Med J* 1982;**285**:693.

Vermund SH et al: Accidental bromocriptine ingestion in childhood. *J Pediatr* 1984;**105**:838.

INTERACTIONS
(See p 17.)

Propranolol and other beta-blocking agents enhance the effects of quinidine, procainamide, antihypertensives, insulin, muscle relaxants, and sulfonylureas and possibly increase the serum level of lidocaine.

Levodopa can cause hypertension, especially in the presence of monoamine oxidase inhibitors. Levodopa also augments hypotensive effects of anesthetic agents. The action of levodopa is antagonize by pyridoxine and papaverine.

Methyldopa and guanethidine deplete catecholamines and increase the possibility of hypotension during anesthesia. Interaction of methyldopa and phenoxybenzamine can cause urinary incontinence.

Propantheline increases absorption of digoxin.

Neostigmine potentiates succinylcholine and antagonizes tubocurarine.

Parasympathetic block is enhanced by all of the following: atropine and congeners, antihistamines, tricyclic antidepressants, phenothiazines, and meperidine.

The pressor response from norepinephrine is increased by guanethidine, methyldopa, and tricyclic antidepressants; the pressor response from metaraminol, methoxamine, mephentermine, and phenylephrine is increased by guanethidine, monoamine oxidase inhibitors, and tricyclic antidepressants.

Methyldopa can cause severe hypertension with pargyline.

Atropinelike compounds delay absorption of drugs.

PHARMACOKINETICS & TOXIC CONCENTRATIONS
(See p 89.)

	pK_a	$t\frac{1}{2}$	V_d	% Binding	Toxic Concentration ($\mu g/mL$)
Albuterol	9.3, 10.3	2–4			
Amphetamine	9.9	10–30			
Atenolol	9.6	6–9	0.7	6–16	
Atropine	9.8	13–38		50	
Bethanidine		7–11	7		
Bretylium		4–17			
Bromocriptine		48	6	90–96	
Chlorphentermine	9.6	35–40			
Ephedrine		7			
Fenfluramine	9.9	13–30	12–16	34	
Guanethidine	9, 12	216–240			
Hyoscine		7		10	
Isoxsuprine	8.0, 9.8	1.25			
Levodopa	2.3–9.9	2.5			
Mazindol	8.5	33–55			
Metaproterenol	8.8, 11.8	1.5		10	
Methamphetamine	10.1				40
Methyldopa	2.2–12	1.75	0.29	< 20	
Metoclopramide	7.32	2–4	1.7–2.9		
Nadolol		9.6–14.2	1.4–3.4		
Phentermine	10.1	19–24			
Phenylpropanolamine		4			
Propantheline		9	1.5		
Propranolol	9.45	2–16	3.6, 4.6	90	
Pseudoephedrine		5–16			
Reserpine	6.1	46–168			
Terbutaline	10.1	3–4		25	

25 | Antiseptics

BORIC ACID & BORON DERIVATIVES

Boric acid (H_3BO_3) is a white compound that is soluble to the extent of 5% in water at 20 °C. Sodium borate, or borax ($Na_2B_4O_7 \cdot 10H_2O$), is a white compound that is soluble to the extent of 14% in water at 55 °C. Sodium perborate ($NaBO_3 \cdot 4H_2O$) is a white compound that is slightly soluble in cold water and decomposes in hot water. Boron oxide is used in industry. Pentaborane, decaborane, and diborane are used as propellants.

Boric acid was formerly used as an antiseptic and to make talcum powder flow freely. Sodium borate (borax) is used as a cleaning agent. Sodium perborate is used as a mouthwash and dentrifice.

The fatal dose of boric acid, sodium borate, or sodium perborate is 0.1–0.5 g/kg. The exposure limits for boron compounds are as follows: boron oxide, 10 mg/m³; anhydrous sodium borate, 1 mg/m³; sodium borate decahydrate, 5 mg/m³; sodium borate pentahydrate, 1 mg/m³; boron tribromide, 1 ppm; decarborane, 0.05 ppm; pentaborane, 0.005 ppm; diborane, 0.1 ppm.

Boric acid and borates are toxic to all cells. The effect on an organ is dependent on the concentration reached in that organ. Because the highest concentrations are reached during excretion, the kidneys are more seriously damaged than other organs. Renal excretion of toxic doses requires 1 week.

The pathologic findings in fatal cases are gastroenteritis, fatty degeneration of the liver and kidneys, cerebral edema, and congestion of all organs.

Clinical Findings

The principal manifestations of poisoning with these compounds are skin excoriations, fever, and anuria.

A. Acute Poisoning: (From ingestion, skin absorption, or absorption from mucous membranes.) Boron oxide dust is irritating to mucous membranes. Decaborane and pentaborane cause excitability and narcosis, which may be delayed up to 48 hours. Diborane is a pulmonary irritant. After ingestion of boric acid or borates, emesis usually occurs immediately, limiting toxicity of these substances. If they are retained, progressive development of the following occurs:

1. Vomiting and diarrhea of mucus and blood.

2. Erythroderma, followed by desquamation, excoriations, blistering, bullae, and sloughing of epidermis.

3. Lethargy.

4. Twitching of facial muscles and extremities, followed by convulsions.

5. Hyperpyrexia, jaundice, and kidney damage with oliguria or anuria.

6. Cyanosis, fall of blood pressure, collapse, coma, and death.

B. Chronic Poisoning: (From ingestion, skin absorption, or absorption from body cavities or mucous membranes.)

1. Prolonged absorption causes anorexia, weight loss, vomiting, mild diarrhea, skin rash, alopecia, convulsions, and anemia.

2. Local use of sodium perborate in high concentrations in the mouth may cause chemical burns, low resistance to trauma, and retraction of gums.

C. Laboratory Findings:

1. The urine contains protein, epithelial casts, and red blood cells.

2. One drop of urine acidified with hydrochloric acid and applied to turmeric paper produces a brownish-red color in the presence of boric acid or borate.

3. Blood urea nitrogen may be elevated.

4. Hepatic cell function may be impaired as revealed by appropriate tests (see p 75).

Prevention

Because deaths occur frequently following the improper use of boric acid powder or solution, and because this substance has no therapeutic function that cannot be served equally well by less toxic preparations, it should be removed from home and hospital.

Treatment

A. Acute Poisoning:

1. Emergency measures–

a. Establish airway and maintain respiration.

b. Remove boric acid from skin or mucous membranes by washing.

c. Remove poison by ipecac emesis followed by activated charcoal. Gastric lavage may be useful (see pp 21–28).

2. General measures–

a. Maintain urine output by giving liquids orally; if patient is vomiting, give 5% dextrose, 10–40 mL/kg intravenously daily, plus electrolyte replacement as necessary.

    b. Control convulsions by cautious administration of diazepam, 0.1 mg/kg intravenously (see Table 4–3).

    c. Remove boric acid or borates from the circulation by peritoneal dialysis or hemodialysis or by exchange transfusion in infants. Diuresis is hazardous if renal function is impaired.

    3. Special problems–Treat anuria (see p 72). Treat skin infection with organism-specific chemotherapy.

    B. Chronic Poisoning: Discontinue use of boric acid or borate products.

Prognosis

    In the past, more than 50% of infants with symptomatic boric acid poisoning died. This type of poisoning is now rare.

Hart RP et al: Neuropsychological function following mild exposure to pentaborane. *Am J Ind Med* 1984;**6**:37.

O'Sullivan K, Taylor M: Chronic boric acid poisoning in infants. *Arch Dis Child* 1983;**58**:737.

IODINE, IODOFORM, IODOCHLORHYDROXYQUIN, CHINIOFON, & IODIDES

    Iodine occurs as bluish-black plates that are soluble in alcohol but only slightly soluble (0.03%) in water. Tincture of iodine contains 2% iodine and 2.4% sodium iodide in alcohol; strong iodine solution contains 5% iodine and 10% potassium iodide in water. Iodine is precipitated by starch. The solubility of iodine is greatly increased in the presence of iodide. Iodoform, a slightly yellowish powder or crystalline material with a penetrating odor, is insoluble in water but soluble in alcohol. Iodochlorhydroxyquin, a brownish-yellow powder with a slight odor, is insoluble in water and alcohol. Sodium and potassium iodides are white crystals soluble in water.

    The fatal dose of iodine and iodoform is estimated to be 2 g. Fatalities have not been reported from iodochlorhydroxyquin or iodide poisoning. Organically bound iodine compounds such as iodinated glycerol, povidone-iodine, undecoylium chloride-iodine (Virac), iodoquinol (diiodohydroxyquin, Yodoxin), clioquinol, iodochlorhydroxyquin (Vioform), tetraglycine hydroperiodide (60% iodine), and chiniofon release iodine slowly and have a toxicity equivalent to about one-fifth of their iodine content. The exposure limit for iodine in air is 0.1 ppm; for iodoform, 0.6 ppm.

    Iodine acts directly on cells by precipitating proteins. The affected cells may be killed. The effects of iodine are thus similar to those produced by acid corrosives (see p 198). Iodoform in large doses depresses the central nervous system.

The pathologic findings are excoriation and corrosion of mucous membranes of the mouth, esophagus, and stomach. The kidneys show glomerular and tubular necrosis.

Clinical Findings

The principal manifestations of acute poisoning with these agents are vomiting, collapse, and coma.

A. Acute Poisoning:

1. Ingestion of iodine causes severe vomiting, frequent liquid stools, abdominal pain, thirst, metallic taste, shock, fever, anuria, delirium, stupor, and death in uremia. A patient who recovers from the acute stage may have esophageal stricture. Iodides may cause temporary enlargement of salivary glands or lymph glands.

2. Application of iodine to the skin may cause weeping, crusting, blistering, and fever. Individual susceptibility to such reactions is greatly varied; some will react after momentary contact with weak solutions, whereas others will not react after repeated contact with strong solutions.

3. Application of iodoform to skin or mucous membranes may cause vesiculation and oozing with intense itching, burning pain, tenderness, and irritability.

4. Injection of iodine compounds may cause sudden fatal collapse (anaphylaxis) as a result of hypersensitivity. Symptoms are dyspnea, cyanosis, fall of blood pressure, unconsciousness, and convulsions.

5. Ingestion of overdoses of organic iodine compounds causes nausea and vomiting and diarrhea. Respiratory distress, coma, and circulatory collapse have also been reported.

B. Chronic Poisoning:

1. Prolonged ingestion of iodine or iodine compounds leads to iodism, with erythema, conjunctivitis, stomatitis, acne, rhinorrhea, urticaria, parotitis, anorexia, weight loss, sleeplessness, and nervous symptoms. Myxedema can occur from prolonged administration of iodide.

2. Iodine and iodine compounds are potent sensitizers. For this reason, repeated contact may be followed by sensitivity dermatitis (see p 81), laryngeal edema, serum sickness with lymph node enlargement, and joint pain and swelling.

3. Clioquinol, iodoquinol, and other organic iodine compounds can cause nausea, vomiting, diarrhea, neurotoxicity, optic neuritis, peripheral neuropathy, and iodism.

C. Laboratory Findings:
Urine may contain protein, epithelial casts, and red blood cells.

Prevention

Patients should be tested for sensitivity to iodine or iodine compounds before these substances are used. A suitable test for drugs to be used on the skin is to place a drop of the solution on the skin and leave the area uncovered for 30 minutes. Any reaction contraindicates the further use of the drug in question. If injection of the drug is contemplated, a drop of the solution may be placed in the conjunctival sac and the presence of irritation noted after 30 minutes.

Treatment

A. Acute Poisoning:

1. Emergency measures–

a. Establish airway and maintain respiration.

b. Give milk; then absorb remaining iodine with starch solution made by adding 15 g of cornstarch or flour to 500 mL of water. Emesis and lavage are not indicated in the presence of esophageal injury.

c. Give milk orally every 15 minutes to relieve gastric irritation.

d. Treat anaphylaxis by giving epinephrine, 0.3–1 mL of 1:1000 solution subcutaneously or intramuscularly, to maintain pulse and blood pressure. Give positive-pressure artificial respiration. Give diphenhydramine (Benadryl), 50 mg slowly intravenously. Give hydrocortisone, 50 mg/h intravenously until symptoms abate.

e. After eye contact, wash thoroughly with saline.

2. Antidote–Sodium thiosulfate will immediately reduce iodine to iodide. Give 100 mL of 1% solution orally.

3. General measures–If urine output is reduced, regulate fluid and electrolyte intake (see p 72). Saline diuresis is useful if renal function is adequate.

4. Special problems–

a. Treat skin eruptions by applying mild astringent wet dressings (see p 83).

b. Treat esophageal stricture (see p 201).

B. Chronic Poisoning: Discontinue use of iodine or iodides. High sodium chloride intake will speed recovery. For iodism characterized by skin or mucous membrane reactions, give cortisone or equivalent corticosteroid, 25–100 mg every 6 hours orally until symptoms abate.

Prognosis

If the patient survives 48 hours after the ingestion of iodine, recovery is likely, although stricture of the esophagus may be a complication.

In sensitivity reactions following the injection of iodine compounds, survival is likely if the patient lives for 1 hour.

POTASSIUM PERMANGANATE

Potassium permanganate ($KMnO_4$) is a water-soluble, violet, crystalline compound used as a disinfectant and oxidizing agent. It has an undeserved reputation as an abortifacient when used in the vagina.

The fatal dose by ingestion is estimated to be 10 g.

Potassium permanganate acts by destroying cells of the mucous membranes by alkaline caustic action (see p 211).

Pathologic findings are necrosis, hemorrhage, and corrosion of the mucous membranes with which potassium permanganate has come in contact. The liver and kidneys show degenerative changes.

Clinical Findings

The principal manifestation of poisoning with potassium permanganate is corrosion.

A. Acute Poisoning:

1. Ingestion of solid or concentrated potassium permanganate causes brown discoloration and edema of the mucous membranes of the mouth and pharynx; cough, laryngeal edema, and stridor; necrosis of oral and pharyngeal mucosa; slow pulse; and shock with fall of blood pressure. If death is not immediate, jaundice and oliguria or anuria may appear.

2. Application of solid or concentrated potassium permanganate solution to the mucous membranes of the vagina or urethra causes severe burning, hemorrhages, and vascular collapse. Perforation of the vaginal wall may occur, resulting in peritonitis with fever and abdominal pain. Examination reveals a chemical burn that is stained brown.

B. Chronic Poisoning: (From ingestion or application to skin or mucous membranes.) Repeated use may lead to corrosive damage as described for acute poisoning. Repeated use of concentrations greater than 1:1000 on the skin may lead to a chemical burn.

Prevention

Patients should be warned of the dangers of using crystals or solutions of potassium permanganate. Possible errors in concentration make any use of potassium permanganate hazardous.

Treatment

A. Acute Poisoning:

1. **Emergency measures—**

a. Remove poison from mucous membranes by washing repeatedly with tap water. Give evaporated milk to inactivate ingested permanganate. Emesis and lavage are hazardous (see pp 21–28).

b. Treat shock (see p 66).

2. General measures–

a. Do esophagoscopy to determine extent of injury after ingestion.

b. Treat perforations surgically.

3. Special problems–Treat anuria (see p 72).

B. Chronic Poisoning: Discontinue use of potassium permanganate, and treat chemical burns.

Prognosis

Death may occur up to 1 month from the time of poisoning by potassium permanganate.

PHENOL & DERIVATIVES

Pure phenol (carbolic acid) is a white solid that liquefies (liquefied phenol) upon the addition of 5% water.

Creosotes (wood tar or coal tar) are mixtures of phenolic compounds and other compounds obtained by the destructive distillation of wood or coal.

A large number of phenol derivatives have been used in the past as antiseptics, disinfectants, caustics, germicides, surface anesthetics, antioxidants, and preservatives.

The antioxidants, di-tertiary-butyl-*p*-cresol (BHT, DBPD) and 4,4'-thio-bis(6-tertiary-butyl-*m*-cresol), have exposure limits of 10 mg/m³ and estimated fatal doses of 30 g. The fatal doses of other phenols are listed in Table 25–1. Even a weak phenolic compound such as tannic acid has caused fatalities when given rectally in excessive doses. For this reason, "universal antidote," which contains tannic acid, should never be used. To protect aquatic life, the level of pentachlorophenol in natural water should never exceed 3 μg/L.

Phenol denatures and precipitates cellular proteins and thus poisons all cells directly. In small amounts, it has a salicylatelike stimulating effect on the respiratory center. This causes respiratory alkalosis followed by acidosis, which results partly from uncompensated renal loss of base during the stage of alkalosis, partly from the acidic nature of the phenolic radical, and partly from derangements in carbohydrate metabolism. Methemoglobinemia may also occur, especially after administration of hydroquinone. The trichlorophenols and 2,4-dimethyl phenol may be carcinogens.

Pathologic findings in deaths from phenol or related compounds are necrosis of mucous membranes, cerebral edema, and degenerative changes in the liver and kidney. Bladder necrosis may also be present.

Table 25—1. Phenol and phenol derivatives.

	Exposure Limit	Fatal Dose (g or mL)
Amyl phenol		5
Benzyl chlorophenol		5
o-sec-Butyl phenol	5 ppm	10
Carvacrol		2
Catechol*	5 ppm	2
p-Chloro-m-cresol		5
Chlorophenols		5
Creosote (coal tar)		10
Cresol, o-, m-, or p-	5 ppm	2
Dichlorophene*		10
Gallic acid		20
Guaiacol		2
Hexachlorophene*		5
Hexylresorcinol†		5
Hydroquinone	2 mg/m³	2
Menthol		2
4-Methoxyphenol	5 mg/m³	10
Monobenzone (Benzylhydroquinone)		5
Naphthol (α or β)		5
Pentachlorophenol	0.5 mg/m³	1‡
Phenol	5 ppm	2
o-Phenyl phenol		10
Pyrogallol*		2
Resorcinol	10 mg/m³	2
Saponated solution of cresols		10
Tannic acid		20
Tetrachlorophenol		5
Thiocresol		5
Thymol		2
Wood tar		10

*May cause sensitivity dermatitis, photosensitivity, or stomatitis.
†Contraindicated in peptic ulcer.
‡Serum 46 μg/mL.

Clinical Findings

The principal manifestations of poisoning with these agents are vomiting, collapse, and coma.

A. Acute Poisoning: (From ingestion or application of phenolic compounds to skin or mucous membranes.) Local findings are painless blanching or erythema. Corrosion may occur. General findings are profuse sweating, intense thirst, nausea and vomiting, diarrhea, cyanosis from methemoglobinemia, hyperactivity, stupor, blood pressure fall, hyperpnea, abdominal pain, hemolysis, convulsions, coma, and pulmonary edema followed by pneumonia. If death from respiratory failure is not immediate, jaundice and oliguria or anuria may occur. Skin absorption of hexachlorophene can cause central nervous system damage, cerebral edema, and muscle contractions.

B. Chronic Poisoning: (From ingestion or absorption from skin or mucous membranes.) Repeated use may cause symptoms described for acute poisoning. Skin sensitivity reactions occur occasionally. Prolonged skin contact with β-naphthol may cause bladder tumors, hemolytic anemia, and lens opacities.

C. Laboratory Findings in Acute or Chronic Poisoning:

1. Test urine with a few drops of ferric chloride. A violet or blue color indicates the presence of a phenolic compound.

2. Urine contains red blood cells, protein, and casts.

3. The blood bicarbonate level may be below 20 meq/L. The urea nitrogen level is elevated. Methemoglobinemia may be present.

4. Hepatic cell function may be impaired as revealed by appropriate tests (see p 75).

Prevention

Phenol and derivatives must be stored safely. Phenolic ointments or solutions of derivatives such as hexachlorophene should not be used over large areas of the body.

Treatment

A. Acute Poisoning:

1. Emergency measures–

a. Establish airway and maintain respiration.

b. Ingestion–In the absence of corrosive injury, remove poison by ipecac emesis. Activated charcoal is also useful. Follow with 240 mL of milk. Gastric lavage and emesis are contraindicated in the presence of esophageal injury.

c. Surface contamination–Remove poison by washing skin or mucous membranes with large amounts of water for at least 15 minutes. Follow by repeated application of castor oil.

2. General measures–

a. If blood bicarbonate level is below 20 meq/L, treat as for salicylate poisoning (see p 298).

b. Control convulsions by cautious use of diazepam, 0.1 mg/kg slowly intravenously.

c. Treat methemoglobinemia (see p 78).

3. Special problems–Treat liver damage (see p 77). Treat anuria (see p 72).

B. Chronic Poisoning: Discontinue further use of phenol, and treat as for acute poisoning.

Prognosis

If the patient survives for 48 hours, recovery is likely.

Bowman CE et al: A fatal case of creosote poisoning. *Postgrad Med J* 1984;**60**:499.

Exon JH: A review of chlorinated phenols. *Vet Hum Toxicol* 1984;**26**:508.

Gray RE et al: Pentachlorophenol intoxication: Report of a fatal case, with comments on the clinical course and pathologic anatomy. *Arch Environ Health* 1985;**40**:161.

Wood S et al: Pentachlorophenol poisoning. *J Occup Med* 1983;**25**:527.

CATIONIC DETERGENTS

Cationic detergents are a group of organic compounds character-ized by the general formula

$$R_1 \underset{R_2}{\overset{R_3}{N^+}} R_4 \cdots\cdots X^-$$

where R_{1-4} represent alkyl or aryl substituents and X^- represents a halogen, such as bromide, iodide, or chloride. Cationic detergents are characterized by the fact that the hydrophobic part of the molecule

$$\left[R_1 \underset{R_2}{\overset{R_3}{N^+}} R_4 \right]$$

is a cation rather than an anion, as in ordinary soaps.

Cationic detergents such as benzethonium chloride (Phemerol), benzalkonium chloride (Zephiran), methylbenzethonium chloride (Diaparene), and cetylpyridinium chloride (Ceepryn) are used to destroy bacteria on skin, surgical instruments, cooking equipment, sickroom supplies, and diapers. Cationic detergents with 2 long-chain substituents are less toxic.

The fatal dose by ingestion is estimated to be 1–3 g. At least 3 fatalities have occurred from accidental ingestion.

Concentrated solutions of cationic detergents are readily absorbed and interfere with many cellular functions. Concentrations down to 1% are injurious to mucous membranes. Cationic detergents are rapidly inactivated by tissues and by ordinary soaps. After prolonged heating (eg, autoclaving or boiling), cationic detergents can break down to compounds capable of causing methemoglobinemia when they are absorbed by skin or mucous membranes.

The pathologic findings are not characteristic.

Clinical Findings

The principal manifestations of poisoning with these agents are vomiting, collapse, and coma.

The symptoms and signs from ingestion are nausea and vomiting, corrosive damage to the esophagus, collapse, hypotension, convulsions, coma, and death within 1–4 hours. Concentrations of 10% are corrosive to the esophagus and mucous membranes. Chronic poisoning has not been reported.

Prevention
Cationic detergent solutions should be stored in distinctive bottles (never in soft drink bottles) in a safe place.

Treatment
A. Emergency Measures:
1. Establish airway and maintain respiration.
2. Give milk or activated charcoal and remove by catharsis with Fleet's Phospho-Soda, 15–60 mL diluted 1:4 with water. Lavage and emesis are contraindicated in the presence of esophageal injury.

B. Antidote:
Ordinary soap is an effective antidote for unabsorbed cationic detergent. No antidote is known for the systemic effects following absorption.

C. General Measures:
Maintain respiration and treat convulsions (see Table 4–3). Treat hypotension by giving fluids or transfusions (see p 66). Dialysis and diuresis are not effective. Treat methemoglobinemia (see p 78).

Prognosis
If the patient survives for 48 hours, recovery is likely.

ZINC STEARATE

Zinc stearate is a white, water-insoluble powder that will readily absorb oils and odors. It is used as a powder to allay skin irritation, as an astringent, and as a mild local antiseptic. Zinc stearate is also used in the rubber industry, where the exposure limit is 10 mg/m^3. Pulmonary disease has occurred rarely during industrial exposure to zinc stearate.

The amount necessary to cause death in infants is unknown, but at least 30 deaths have occurred from inhalation of zinc stearate. In the lungs, zinc stearate acts as a chemical irritant, causing a progressive chemical pneumonitis.

The pathologic findings are pneumonia, pulmonary edema, and pulmonary granulomatosis.

Clinical Findings
The principal manifestations of zinc stearate poisoning are fever and respiratory difficulty.

A. Acute Poisoning: (From inhalation.) Fever, cough, difficult breathing, cyanosis, pulmonary edema, and evidence of pneumonia.

B. Chronic Poisoning: Repeated inhalation of zinc stearate leads to the findings described for acute poisoning.

C. X-Ray Findings: Examination of the chest reveals diffuse bronchial pneumonia.

Prevention

Zinc stearate should not be used in powders for application to the skin.

Treatment

A. Acute Poisoning: Discontinue use of zinc stearate. Treat pneumonia with organism-specific chemotherapy. Treat cyanosis with O_2 administration.

B. Chronic Poisoning: Treat as for acute poisoning.

Prognosis

Cases of zinc stearate pneumonitis have been almost uniformly fatal.

CHLORATES

Sodium chlorate ($NaClO_3$) and potassium chlorate ($KClO_3$) are frequent ingredients in mouthwashes and gargles and are also used in matches and weed killers. The heads of 20 large wooden matches contain 330 mg. The chlorates are water-soluble and act as strong oxidizing agents, forming explosive mixtures with organic material.

The fatal dose is about 15 g for adults and 2 g for children, but no fatalities have been reported in recent years. Chlorate ion is irritating to mucous membranes in concentrated solution; after absorption, it produces methemoglobinemia by virtue of its oxidizing properties. However, the chlorate is not reduced in the process but acts as a catalyst, so that a small amount of chlorate can produce a large amount of methemoglobin.

Pathologic findings in deaths from chlorate are gastrointestinal congestion and corrosion, kidney injury, liver damage, and chocolate color of the blood.

Clinical Findings

The principal manifestations of poisoning with these agents are vomiting and cyanosis.

A. Acute Poisoning: (From ingestion.) Nausea, vomiting, diarrhea, abdominal pain, hemolysis, cyanosis, anuria, confusion, convulsions.

B. Chronic Poisoning: (From ingestion.) Continued use in doses less than necessary to produce the symptoms described for acute poisoning may lead to loss of appetite and weight loss.

C. Laboratory Findings:

1. Methemoglobinemia, anemia of the hemolytic type, or elevation of serum potassium level.

2. Urine contains red blood cells, protein, casts, and hemoglobin products.

Prevention

Chlorates should never be taken internally. They should be replaced in mouthwashes and gargles by less harmful drugs.

Prevention

A. Acute Poisoning:

1. Emergency measures–Establish airway and maintain respiration. Remove ingested poison by ipecac emesis followed by activated charcoal. Airway-protected gastric lavage is necessary in patients with depressed respiration (see pp 21–28).

2. Antidote–Give sodium thiosulfate, 2–5 g in 200 mL of 5% sodium bicarbonate orally, to decompose chlorates. Methylene blue is not useful for reversing chlorate methemoglobinemia and may be hazardous. Ascorbic acid acts slowly (see p 78).

3. General measures–Give milk to relieve gastric irritation. Keep patient warm and quiet until cyanosis disappears. If urine output is adequate, force fluids to 2–4 L/d to remove chlorate. Remove chlorate by peritoneal dialysis or hemodialysis.

4. Special problems–Treat anuria (see p 72).

B. Chronic Poisoning: Discontinue use of drug and treat as for acute poisoning.

Prognosis

Death may occur up to 1 week after poisoning, but if symptoms are mild or absent after the first 12 hours, recovery is to be expected.

CHLORAMINE-T

Chloramine-T is a water-soluble compound containing about 12% available chlorine, which is released slowly on contact with water. In solid form it is used as a water purifier and in solution as a mouthwash.

The fatal dose may be as low as 0.5 g, although much larger doses have been ingested without adverse effects. At least 6 fatal cases of chloramine-T poisoning have occurred. It has been postulated that poisoning may occur through the conversion of chloramine-T to a cyanide derivative under certain circumstances.

The pathologic findings are not characteristic.

Clinical Findings

The principal manifestations of acute poisoning with chloramine-T are cyanosis and respiratory failure.

The symptoms and signs are cyanosis, collapse, frothing at the mouth, and respiratory failure within a few minutes after ingestion. Chronic poisoning has not been reported.

Prevention

Users of chloramine-T should be warned against ingesting the compound. It should be stored safely.

Treatment of Acute Poisoning:

A. Emergency Measures: Remove ingested chloramine-T by ipecac emesis followed by activated charcoal or evaporated milk. Airway-protected gastric lavage may be necessary in symptomatic patients (see pp 21–28).

B. Antidote: Give sodium nitrite and sodium thiosulfate as directed for cyanide poisoning (see p 254).

Prognosis

If the patient lives for 24 hours, recovery is likely.

SILVER & SILVER SALTS: SILVER NITRATE, SILVER PROTEINATES, & SILVER PICRATE

Silver nitrate is a water-soluble salt that precipitates with chloride to form insoluble and nontoxic silver chloride. It is used as a local styptic and antiseptic. The colloidal silver proteinates are used as antiseptics on skin and mucous membranes. Mild silver protein contains 19–23% silver; strong silver protein contains 7.5–8.5% silver. Silver picrate (Picragol) is used as 1% powder in kaolin, and in suppositories as an antiseptic on mucous membranes.

The fatal dose of silver nitrate may be as low as 2 g, although recovery has occurred following ingestion of larger doses. No fatalities have been reported in recent years. The silver proteinates and silver picrate have not produced fatal poisoning. The exposure limit for silver and its compounds is 0.01 mg/m^3.

Silver nitrate causes a local corrosive effect but is not likely to produce systemic effects because silver ion is precipitated by proteins and

Table 25–2. Miscellaneous antiseptics.
(For mercurial antiseptics, see p 238.)

Drug	Findings	Treatment
Acriflavine	Irritating or necrotizing on wounds; hypotension after absorption.	Discontinue.
Acrisorcin (Akrinol)	Blistering, vesicular eruptions, photodermatitis.	Discontinue.
Benzoic acid	Ingestion of 50 g causes gastric upset.	None.
Benzyl benzoate	Ingestion of 1 g/kg causes incoordination, excitement, convulsions.	Remove by gastric lavage.
Butamben picrate (Butesin picrate)	Exfoliative dermatitis with itching, burning, erythema, scaling.	Discontinue.
Carbamide peroxide (Debrox)	Irritation, pain.	Discontinue.
Chlorobutanol	Narcosis; kidney and liver damage.	Discontinue.
Chlorquinaldol (Sterosan)	Skin sensitivity reactions.	Discontinue.
Chrysarobin	Enteritis and renal damage after ingestion or skin absorption.	Discontinue.
Crotamiton (Eurax)	Burning in mouth. Lethal dose over 0.5 g/kg.	Wash skin and give fluids.
Hexetidine	Irritation of mucous membranes.	Discontinue.
Hydrogen peroxide, up to 90% solutions (exposure limit = 1 ppm)	Concentrated solutions (20–30%) of hydrogen peroxide are strong irritants to the skin or mucous membranes. 6% is a weak irritant; it releases 20 vol% O_2 on contact with skin or mucous membranes. When used as colonic lavage, hydrogen peroxide has caused gas embolism and gangrene of the intestine at concentrations down to 0.75%. **Treatment for ingestion:** Give water to dilute; use gastric tube to prevent increased pressure.	
Ichthammol	Nausea and diarrhea after ingestion.	Remove by gastric lavage.
Oxyquinoline sulfate	Gastrointestinal irritation. Lethal dose is 1 g/kg.	Remove by gastric lavage or emesis.
Parabens (p-hydroxybenzoic acid, alkyl esters)	Dermatitis.	Discontinue.
Phenacridane (Acrizane)	Irritation of mucous membranes.	Discontinue.
Proflavine	Irritating or necrotizing on wounds; hypotension after absorption.	Discontinue.
Salicylanilide	Skin irritation.	Discontinue.
Selenium sulfide (Selsun)	Diffuse hair loss, sensitivity reactions.	Discontinue.
Undecylenic acid and salts	Exudative dermatitis, nausea, fever, headache after ingestion. Lethal dose is 2 g/kg.	Discontinue.
Zinc pyridinethione	Gastrointestinal irritation.	Remove by gastric lavage or emesis.

chloride. Pathologic findings involve local corrosive damage to the gastrointestinal tract, and there may be degenerative changes in the kidneys and liver. Repeated use of silver in any form will eventually cause argyria. Excessive use of silver picrate may cause renal damage.

Clinical Findings

The principal manifestations of poisoning with these agents are blackening of mucous membranes, vomiting, and collapse.

A. Acute Poisoning: (From ingestion of silver nitrate.) Pain and burning in the mouth; blackening of the skin and mucous membranes, throat, and abdomen; salivation; vomiting of black material; diarrhea; anuria; collapse; shock; and death in convulsions or coma. Treatment of burns with silver nitrate has caused methemoglobinemia from absorption of nitrate ion.

B. Chronic Poisoning: (From application of silver compounds to skin or mucous membranes.) Repeated application or ingestion of silver nitrate or silver proteinates causes argyria, which is a permanent bluish-black discoloration of the skin, conjunctiva, and other mucous membranes. The discoloration first appears in areas most exposed to light, usually the conjunctiva. If silver is not immediately discontinued, the discoloration will spread over the entire body.

Prevention

Silver nitrate sticks should be stored safely. Silver proteinates should not be used repeatedly for the treatment of mucous membrane or skin diseases.

Treatment

A. Acute Poisoning:

1. Emergency measures–

a. Dilute ingested silver nitrate by giving water containing sodium chloride, 10 g/L, repeatedly to precipitate silver ion as silver chloride. Follow with catharsis using 30–60 mL of Fleet's Phospho-Soda diluted 1:4 in water containing 5 g of sodium chloride to precipitate and remove silver from the intestines.

b. Treat shock (see p 66).

c. Treat methemoglobinemia (See p 78).

2. General measures–Give milk to relieve gastric irritation. Give meperidine (Demerol), 100 mg, or codeine, 60 mg, to relieve pain.

B. Chronic Poisoning: No method is known that will bleach the pigmentation of argyria.

Prognosis

If treatment with sodium chloride can be started shortly after the ingestion of silver nitrate, recovery is likely.

The pigmentation of argyria is permanent.

References

Ito N et al: Carcinogenicity and modification of the carcinogenic response by BHA, BHT, and other antioxidants. *CRC Crit Rev Toxicol* 1985;**15**:109.

Cardiovascular Drugs | 26

DIGITALIS & DIGITALIS PREPARATIONS

Digitalis and cardiac glycosides are used for the treatment of heart failure.

Other digitalis preparations include deslanoside (Cedilanid-D), Digilanid, digoxin, gitalin (Gitaligin), and lanatoside C (Cedilanid), Squill and strophanthus have similar effects.

The fatal dose of digitalis or squill is approximately 2–3 g. All parts of the foxglove *(Digitalis purpurea, Digitalis lanata)* have similar toxicity. The dangerous dose of digitoxin is 3–5 mg. For other digitalis-like preparations, the fatal dose is 20–50 times the maintenance dose of the preparation. The fatal amount of the rodenticide scilliroside is 0.7 mg/kg.

Digitalis and the cardiac glycosides increase the force of contraction of the myocardium. In excessive doses they increase the irritability of the ventricular muscle, resulting first in extrasystoles, then in ventricular tachycardia, and eventually in ventricular fibrillation. Digitalis and digitalislike preparations also stimulate the central nervous system. Potassium loss by vomiting, diarrhea, or diuresis increases the toxicity.

Clinical Findings
The principal manifestations of digitalis poisoning are vomiting and irregular pulse.

A. Acute Poisoning: (From injection, ingestion, or diuresis in a fully digitalized patient.) Headache, nausea and vomiting, diarrhea, blurred vision, loss of visual acuity, delirium, slow or irregular pulse, fall of blood pressure, aberrant color vision, and death, usually from ventricular arrhythmias. In infants, cardiac arrhythmias are the most common manifestation of toxicity, and in children severe central nervous system depression sometimes occurs. Elderly patients are likely to have bizarre mental symptoms.

B. Chronic Poisoning: (From injection or ingestion.) The above symptoms will come on gradually if overdoses are taken. The occurrence of nausea and vomiting tends to limit dosage.

C. Laboratory Findings:
1. The ECG may show heart block, nodal tachycardia, atrial

tachycardia, premature ventricular contractions or ventricular extrasystoles, ventricular tachycardia, depressed ST segment, and lengthened PR interval.

2. Eosinophilia may be present.

3. Serum potassium is often elevated in acute overdose.

4. Toxic effects begin to occur at digoxin levels above 1.7 ng/mL and digitoxin levels above 25 ng/mL.

Prevention

Store digitalis safely. Reduce dosage of digitalis at the first sign of intoxication. Determine digitalis levels before giving large doses. Use extreme care in the administration of digitalis concomitantly with rauwolfia alkaloids such as reserpine. Rauwolfia apparently sensitizes the heart to the toxic effects of digitalis. The toxicity of digitalis is increased by potassium loss or calcium administration.

Treatment

A. Acute Poisoning:

1. Emergency measures–Establish airway and maintain respiration. Remove ingested drug by ipecac emesis followed by activated charcoal (see pp 21–28). Determine serum potassium and magnesium levels hourly. Monitor ECG. Be prepared for transvenous cardiac pacing. Do not give epinephrine or other stimulants—these may induce ventricular fibrillation.

2. Antidote–

a. For cardiac arrhythmias in the presence of hypokalemia, if renal function is normal, give potassium chloride, 5 g dissolved in fruit juice every hour orally, or 20 meq in 500 mL of 5% dextrose slowly intravenously at a rate not to exceed 0.4 meq/min, until the ECG shows improvement or reveals a potassium effect as indicated by peaking of the T wave. Administration of potassium should be stopped when the serum level rises to 5 meq/L. Do not use potassium in the presence of complete heart block due to digitalis.

b. To reduce an elevated potassium level, give Kayexalate, 20 g orally or by enema every 4 hours. Give 10 units of insulin while infusing 5% dextrose. Hemodialysis may be necessary to lower the potassium level.

c. For atrial and ventricular irregularities that do not respond to potassium therapy, give phenytoin, 0.5 mg/kg slowly intravenously at 1- to 2-hour intervals. The maximum dose should not exceed 10 mg/kg/24 h. Lidocaine, 1 mg/kg over 5 minutes, then 15–50 μg/kg/min to maintain normal rhythm, can be tried. Propranolol, quinidine, and procainamide are more hazardous.

d. Cholestyramine given orally reduces the half-life of digitoxin from 6 days to 4.5 days or prevents absorption of digitalis glycosides.

Phenytoin can also be given to speed the metabolism of digitalis glycosides.

e. Atropine, 0.01 mg/kg intravenously, can increase the heart rate in the presence of digitalis heart block.

f. The use of digoxin-specific antibody is now possible. Call the nearest regional poison center for information on its availability.

3. General measures—If renal function is impaired, enforce complete quiet and inactivity until signs of digitalis-induced ventricular abnormalities disappear from the ECG. If renal function is normal, give 2–3 L of fluids orally each 24 hours. Do not give diuretic agents in the presence of digitalis toxicity. Because of the large volume of distribution of digitalis drugs, hemodialysis and hemoperfusion are not warranted.

B. Chronic Poisoning: Discontinue the drug temporarily and then regulate dosage according to the needs of the patient.

Prognosis

Recovery is likely if the patient survives 24 hours.

Antman EM, Smith TW: Digitalis toxicity. *Annu Rev Med* 1985;**36**:357.

Bain RJI: Accidental digitalis poisoning due to drinking herbal tea. *Br Med J* 1985;**290**:1624.

Baud F et al: Time course of antidigoxin Fab fragment and plasma digitoxin concentrations in an acute digitalis intoxication. *J Toxicol Clin Toxicol* 1982;**19**:857.

Bigger JT Jr, Leahey EB Jr: Quinidine and digoxin: An important interaction. *Drugs* 1982;**24**:229.

Cohen L, Kitzes R: Magnesium sulfate and digitalis-toxic arrhythmias. *JAMA* 1983;**249**:2808.

Sonnenblick M et al: Correlation between manifestations of digoxin toxicity and serum digoxin, calcium, potassium, and magnesium concentrations and arterial pH. *Br Med J* 1983;**286**:1089.

Vincent J-L et al: Bretylium in severe ventricular arrhythmias associated with digitalis intoxication. *Am J Emerg Med* 1984;**2**:504.

Wenger TL et al: Treatment of 63 severely digitalis-toxic patients with digoxin-specific antibody fragments. *J Am Coll Cardiol* 1985;**5(5)**:118A.

QUINIDINE

Quinidine, a white water-soluble alkaloid obtained from cinchona bark, is used for the treatment of cardiac irregularities. The fatal dose of quinidine may be as low as 0.2 g as a result of hypersensitivity. The mortality rate from the use of quinidine in cardiac arrhythmias is 1%.

Quinidine depresses the metabolic activities of all cells, but its effect on the heart is most pronounced. Doses within the therapeutic range may cause slowing of conduction, prolonged refractory period, and even heart block. Larger doses may cause ventricular fibrillation.

The pathologic findings in acute fatalities are not characteristic. In some cases petechial hemorrhages may be seen throughout the body as a result of thrombocytopenia.

Clinical Findings

The principal manifestations of quinidine poisoning are fall of blood pressure and nausea.

A. Acute Poisoning: (From ingestion.) Overdoses and sometimes doses within the therapeutic range cause tinnitus, headache, nausea, diarrhea, dizziness, severe fall of blood pressure with disappearance of pulse, nystagmus, bradycardia, and respiratory failure.

B. Chronic Poisoning: (From ingestion.) Thrombocytopenic purpura may develop after a short course of quinidine. After recovery, single doses of 0.05–0.1 g will cause return of the purpuric manifestation. Drug fever, urticaria, exfoliation, and anaphylactoid reactions may also result.

C. Laboratory Findings:

1. In purpura from quinidine, the blood thrombocytes are diminished in number.

2. Electrocardiographic findings may include a notched T wave, T wave inversion, depression of the ST segment, widening of the QRS complex, lengthened QT interval, appearance of premature ventricular beats, lengthened PR interval, ventricular tachycardia, and ventricular fibrillation.

3. The blood level of quinidine in severe toxicity is 10 μg/mL.

Prevention

Store quinidine safely. Begin administration of quinidine gradually. Dosage should begin with a test dose of 0.1 g. If no reaction occurs, a second dose of 0.1 can be given after 2 hours. Maximum dosage should not exceed single doses of 0.2 g at intervals of not less than 1 hour. In some patients, fatal ventricular arrhythmias have occurred as late as 12 hours after the last dose of quinidine. Reduce dosage upon the appearance of therapeutic response or signs of toxicity as described above. Discontinue the administration of quinidine if the QRS complex widens by more than 25%. Do not give quinidine in the presence of complete heart block.

Treatment

A. Acute Poisoning:

1. Emergency measures–Establish airway and maintain respiration. Discontinue medication at the first sign of toxicity. Remove ingested overdoses of quinidine by ipecac emesis followed by activated charcoal (see pp 21–28). Raise blood pressure by intravenous saline, plasma, or blood transfusions (see p 66). Norepinephrine with electrocardiographic control can be used in the absence of arrhythmias. Treat ventricular arrhythmias with phenytoin (see p 378). Be prepared for transvenous cardiac pacing.

2. Antidote–Intravenous administration of sodium bicarbonate solution increases serum binding of quinidine and lowers the serum potassium level.

3. General measures–Normalize the serum potassium level (see p 378). As with digitalis overdoses, dialysis is useless.

B. Chronic Poisoning: Treat thrombocytopenic purpura by repeated small transfusions. Do not repeat administration of quinidine in such patients.

Prognosis

If the patient survives for 24 hours after acute poisoning, recovery is probable.

Alperin JB et al: Quinidine-induced thrombocytopenia with pulmonary hemorrhage. *Arch Intern Med* 1980;**140**:266.

Lesne M, Devos DM, Reynaert M: Enterogastric cycle and intoxication with hydroquinidine: A case report. *Clin Toxicol* 1981;**18**:659.

Summers WK et al: Does physostigmine reverse quinidine delirium? *West J Med* 1981;**135**:411.

Swerdlow CB et al: Safety and efficacy of intravenous quinidine. *Am J Med* 1983;**75**:36.

PROCAINAMIDE HYDROCHLORIDE

Procainamide is used for the treatment of cardiac irregularities. As little as 200 mg (2 mL of 10% solution) intravenously has caused death as a result of either hypersensitivity or rapid injection. At least 4 fatalities have been reported from procainamide poisoning.

The rapid administration of procainamide causes irregularities of ventricular contraction, including tachycardia or fibrillation. Agranulocytosis from procainamide is apparently a hypersensitivity reaction.

The pathologic finding in death from agranulocytosis is a lack of myeloid elements in the bone marrow. In sudden deaths following intravenous procainamide administration, the pathologic findings are not characteristic.

Clinical Findings

The principal manifestations of procainamide poisoning are irregular pulse and fall of blood pressure.

A. Acute Poisoning: (From injection.) Rapid intravenous administration of procainamide may cause the pulse to become suddenly irregular or disappear entirely, with collapse and fall of blood pressure and almost immediate onset of convulsions and death.

B. Chronic Poisoning: (From ingestion.) Continued use of procainamide has led to fever, chills, pruritus, urticaria, malaise, reversible lupus erythematosus-like syndrome including pericarditis but without central nervous system or renal involvement, and agranulocytosis.

C. Laboratory Findings:

1. In acute poisoning, the ECG reveals abnormalities of ventricular beat with ventricular extrasystoles.

2. In chronic poisoning, the blood count may reveal diminished or absent granulocytes.

Prevention

Do not give procainamide at a rate greater than 0.2 g/min intravenously. A complete blood count should be taken repeatedly when a patient develops an infectious illness during the administration of procainamide.

Treatment

A. Acute Poisoning:

1. Emergency measures–Treat cardiac arrest (see p 68) following intravenous injection of procainamide.

2. Special problems–Use epinephrine or norepinephrine with great caution. These may induce irregularities of ventricular contraction.

B. Chronic Poisoning:

1. Immediate measures–Discontinue use of the drug at the first sign of symptoms.

2. General measures–Treat agranulocytosis (see p 79).

Prognosis

If ventricular irregularity during the administration of procainamide does not progress to ventricular fibrillation, the patient will recover. At least 90% of patients with agranulocytosis from procainamide are likely to recover.

THIOCYANATES

Sodium thiocyanate (NaSCN) and potassium thiocyanate (KSCN) were formerly used for the treatment of hypertension but have been replaced.

The fatal serum level of thiocyanate is 20 mg/dL. More than 20 fatalities have been reported from thiocyanate poisoning.

Thiocyanates depress the metabolic activities of all cells, but effects are most noticeable on the brain and heart. The time required to reduce the blood level of thiocyanate by 50% is approximately 1 week if renal function is normal. In the presence of impaired renal function, excretion is even slower, and the possibility of toxic reactions is increased.

Pathologic findings include myocardial damage, focal brain damage, thyroid enlargement, and thrombophlebitis.

Clinical Findings

The principal manifestation of thiocyanate poisoning is psychotic behavior.

A. Acute Poisoning: (From ingestion.) Disorientation, weakness, low blood pressure, confusion, psychotic behavior, muscular spasms, convulsions, and death.

B. Chronic Poisoning: (From ingestion.) Prolonged use may cause dermatitis, hives, and abnormal bleeding. The thyroid may be enlarged.

C. Laboratory Findings: The blood thiocyanate level should never exceed 10 mg/dL.

Prevention

Thiocyanate should not be given therapeutically.

Treatment

A. Acute Poisoning:

1. Emergency measures–Remove ingested thiocyanate poison by gastric lavage or emesis (see pp 21–28).

2. General measures–

a. Give 2–4 L of fluid orally or intravenously daily in the presence of normal renal function to maintain adequate urine output.

b. Remove thiocyanate by peritoneal dialysis or by hemodialysis if necessary.

B. Chronic Poisoning: Discontinue the use of thiocyanate.

Prognosis

The patient may show temporary improvement when the administration of thiocyanate is discontinued. However, after several days of improvement, the patient may relapse and die as late as 2 weeks after the medication is stopped.

NITRITES & NITRATES

Nitroglycerin (glyceryl trinitrate), amyl nitrite, ethyl nitrite, sodium nitrite, mannitol hexanitrate, pentaerythritol tetranitrate, isosorbide dinitrate, and trolnitrite phosphate are used medically to dilate coronary vessels and to reduce blood pressure. Ethylene glycol nitrite and nitroglycerin are used to make dynamite. In some instances, nitrites such as bismuth subnitrate or nitrate from well water may be converted to nitrite by the action of intestinal bacteria. The nitrites then may cause nitrite poisoning. Nitrites are also used to preserve the color of meat in pickling or salting processes.

Fatal doses have been recorded as follows: ethyl nitrite, 4 g in a 3-year-old child, nitroglycerin, 2 g; sodium nitrite, 2 g. The allowable residue of nitrite in food is 0.01%. More than 10 ppm of nitrogen as nitrate in well water may induce methemoglobinemia in infants. The exposure limit for nitroglycerin, propylene glycol dinitrate, and ethylene glycol dinitrate in air is 0.05 ppm, but concentrations above 0.02 ppm may cause headache.

Nitrates and nitrites can interact with amines either alone or in biological systems to form nitrosamines, which are carcinogenic in animals and are suspected of being carcinogenic in humans (eg, N-nitrosodimethylamine; see p 144). These nitrosamines occur in surface water as a result of fertilizer contamination, in industrial cutting fluids, in plastics and plasticizers, in toiletries, and in pesticides.

The nitrites dilate blood vessels throughout the body by a direct relaxant effect on smooth muscles. Some nitrites will also cause methemoglobinemia.

The pathologic findings are chocolate-colored blood due to conversion of hemoglobin to methemoglobin and congestion of all organs.

Clinical Findings

The principal manifestations of poisoning with nitrites and nitrates are fall of blood pressure and cyanosis.

A. Acute Poisoning: (From ingestion, injection, inhalation, or absorption from skin or mucous membranes.) Headache, flushing of the skin, vomiting, dizziness, collapse, marked fall of blood pressure, cyanosis, convulsions, coma, and respiratory paralysis.

B. Chronic Poisoning: Repeated administration may lead to the above findings. Nitroglycerin workers show marked tolerance to repeated exposure, but since this tolerance disappears rapidly, a short absence from exposure may lead to severe poisoning from amounts that were previously safe.

C. Laboratory Findings: Determine blood methemoglobin level in presence of cyanosis. (Examination must be made quickly because methemoglobin disappears in standing blood.)

Prevention

Use water free of nitrates for preparing infant formulas. Curing salts containing nitrites must be used in quantities no greater than those allowable by the US Department of Agriculture. Such salts should not be used in other foods or as table salt.

Treatment

A. Acute Poisoning:

1. Emergency measures–Establish airway and maintain respiration. Remove ingested overdoses of nitrites by ipecac emesis followed by activated charcoal. Gastric lavage may be useful (see pp 21–28). Maintain blood pressure by fluid administration (see p 66). Remove poison from the skin by scrubbing with soap and water.

2. General measures–Treat methemoglobinemia over 30% with dyspnea by injection of methylene blue (see p 78).

B. Chronic Poisoning: Depending on the severity of the symptoms, treat as for acute poisoning.

Prognosis

If the blood pressure is maintained, recovery is likely.

Brunnemann KD et al: N-Nitrosamines: Environmental occurrence, in vitro formation, and metabolism. *J Toxicol Clin Toxicol* 1982;**19**:661.

Guss DA et al: Clinically significant methemoglobinemia from inhalation of isobutyl nitrite. *Am J Emerg Med* 1985;**3**:46.

Pedal I et al: Fatal nitrosamine poisoning. *Arch Toxicol* 1982;**50**:101.

Ten Brink WAG et al: Nitrite poisoning caused by food contaminated with cooling fluid. *J Toxicol Clin Toxicol* 1982;**19**:139.

ANTICOAGULANTS: DICUMAROL, ETHYL BISCOUMACETATE, HEPARIN, PHENINDIONE, WARFARIN, DIPHENADIONE, ACENOCOUMAROL

The various anticoagulant drugs are used medically to inhibit the clotting mechanism. Warfarin and a number of chemicals with similar action, including dicumarol (bishydroxycoumarin), pindone (2-pivaloyl-1,3-indandione, Pival), 2-isovaleryl-1,3-indandione (Valone), difenacoum, chlorophacinone, Bromadiolone, brodifacoum (Talon), coumatetryl (Racumin), and coumachlor, are also used as rodenticides. Warfarin is available commercially in 0.025% (250 mg/kg) and 0.5% concentrations for this use.

Single doses of these compounds are not dangerous. Fatalities have been recorded after the following repeated daily doses of anticoagulants: dicumarol, 100 mg; ethyl biscoumacetate (Tromexan), 0.6 g; phenindione (Danilone, Hedulin), 200 mg. The dangerous dosage of acenocoumarol, warfarin, phenprocoumon, cyclocoumarol, chlor-phenindione, and diphenadione is 10–100 mg daily. The exposure limit for warfarin and pindone is 0.1 mg/m³. The single-dose LD50 for bro-difacoum in rats is 0.67 mg/kg. The single dose of brodifacoum that would be dangerous in humans is unknown.

The coumarin and indandione anticoagulants inhibit formation in the liver of a number of clotting factors whose formation is dependent on vitamin K. These anticoagulants also increase capillary fragility. This effect is increased by repeated dosage. Heparin acts (by several as yet incompletely understood mechanisms) to prevent the conversion of prothrombin to thrombin and the action of thrombin on fibrinogen.

Numerous gross and microscopic hemorrhages are found at au-topsy.

Clinical Findings

The principal manifestation of poisoning with anticoagulants is bleeding.

A. Acute Poisoning: Hemoptysis, hematuria, bloody stools, hemorrhages in organs, widespread bruising, and bleeding into joint spaces.

B. Chronic Poisoning: Repeated use leads to findings as in acute poisoning. Necrosis of the skin is a rare complication. In addition to hemorrhagic effects, phenindione has caused jaundice, liver enlarge-ment, myocarditis, skin rash, agranulocytosis, vomiting, conjunctivi-tis, paralysis of ocular accommodation, steatorrhea, bloody diarrhea, orange staining of the urine, renal damage, and fever. Prolonged use of heparin has led to osteoporosis. Phenindione has caused severe renal and liver injuries, of which at least 5 cases have been fatal.

C. Laboratory Findings: The prothrombin concentration is low-ered after coumarin and indandione anticoagulants. The clotting time is prolonged after heparin. Gross or microscopic hematuria may be present. The white blood count may be decreased after pheninindione ad-ministration. The red blood count may be reduced. Hemoglobin levels should be determined and the presence of blood in the stools noted.

Prevention

Phenindione and other indandiones should be used with caution. Anticoagulant drugs are dangerous in blood dyscrasias; kidney, liver, or gastrointestinal diseases; hypertension; subacute infective endocardi-tis; and pregnancy. Administration of many other drugs increases the effect of anticoagulants.

The use of coumarin anticoagulants must be controlled by repeated reliable prothrombin determinations. Heparin dosage is controlled by clotting time determinations. These drugs should be used only under daily supervision by a physician.

Treatment

    A. Emergency Measures:

    1. Discontinue the drug at the first sign of bleeding or at the appearance of any skin rash.

    2. Give transfusions of fresh blood or plasma if hemorrhage is severe.

    B. Antidotes:

    1. For heparin overdosage, give protamine sulfate, 1% slowly intravenously. This drug will antagonize an equal weight of heparin.

    2. For overdosage of coumarin anticoagulants, give phytonadione (Mephyton), 0.1 mg/kg intramuscularly.

    C. General Measures: Absolute bed rest must be maintained to prevent further hemorrhages.

Prognosis

    Death may occur up to 2 weeks after discontinuing the drug. However, adequate therapy with vitamin K will bring the prothombin level back to normal in 24–48 hours.

Guay DRP, Richard A: Heparin-induced thrombocytopenia: Association with platelet aggregating factor and cross-sensitivity to bovine and porcine heparin. *Drug Intell Clin Pharm* 1984;**18**:398.

Jones EC, Growe GH, Naiman SC: Prolonged anticoagulation in rat poisoning. *JAMA* 1984;**252**:3005.

Lipton RA et al: Human ingestion of a "superwarfarin" rodenticide resulting in a prolonged anticoagulant effect. *JAMA* 1984;**252**:3004.

Serlin MJ, Breckenridge AM: Drug interactions with warfarin. *Drugs* 1983;**25**:610.

Van Der Weyden MB et al: Delayed-onset heparin-induced thrombocytopenia. A potentially malignant syndrome. *Med J Aust* 1983;**2**:132.

HYDRALAZINE

    Hydralazine (Apresoline) is a synthetic drug used for the treatment of hypertension.

    Deaths following hydralazine medication have been rare, but the incidence of serious reactions following continued administration is 10–20%. Pathologic findings in reactions to hydralazine include rheumatic nodules, collagenous necrosis of the skin, and proliferative and necrotizing involvement of the arterioles and arteries of the myocardium, kidney, spleen, jejunum, and ileum.

Clinical Findings

    The principal manifestations of hydralazine poisoning are fall of blood pressure and joint swelling.

A. Acute Poisoning: (From ingestion or injection.) Headache, severe hypotension, coronary insufficiency, and anuria.

B. Chronic Poisoning: (From ingestion.) Fever, headache, nausea and vomiting, fast pulse, anemia, blood dyscrasias, diffuse erythematous facial dermatitis, lymph gland enlargement, and splenomegaly, progressing to severe arthralgia simulating rheumatoid arthritis or disseminated lupus erythematosus. Joint involvement varies from vague generalized stiffness and aching to severe pain, swelling, and redness of one to several joints. Pericarditis with pleural effusion, polyneuritis, and activation of peptic ulcer have also been reported. Fatal intestinal bleeding has occurred as a result of vascular changes with accompanying ulcerations.

C. Laboratory Findings:

1. The urine may show protein or red blood cells.

2. The complete blood count may show microcytic or normocytic anemia, leukopenia, or lupus erythematosus cells.

3. Serum proteins may show an increase in the globulin fraction.

4. The ECG may show arrhythmias.

Prevention

Patients must be warned to discontinue the use of hydralazine upon the appearance of any reaction.

Treatment

A. Acute Poisoning:

1. **Emergency measures**–Establish airway and maintain respiration. Cautious reduction of dosage is indicated in severe hypotensive reactions. Overdoses should be removed by gastric lavage or emesis (see pp 21–28). Treat hypotension with fluids (see p 66). Vasopressors are hazardous. Dopamine, 5 μg/kg/min as an infusion to maintain blood pressure at 90 mm Hg and adequate renal perfusion, is safest.

2. **Special problems**–Treat anuria (see p 72).

B. Chronic Poisoning: Discontinue use. Give aspirin, 1–3 g daily, until symptoms regress.

Prognosis

If the patient lives for 24 hours after a severe hypotensive reaction, survival is likely. Complete recovery from rheumatoid reactions has always occurred.

Packer M et al: Deleterious effects of hydralazine in patients with pulmonary hypertension. *N Engl J Med* 1982;**306**:1326.

VERAPAMIL, NIFEDIPINE, & DILTIAZEM

Verapamil, nifedipine, and diltiazem block the reentry of calcium into muscle fibers and are used in the treatment of many conditions in which reduction of muscle contractility would be useful.

Toxicity occurs as a result of the expected actions of these drugs and by interactions with other drugs used at the same time.

Clinical Findings

The principal manifestations of overdose from these agents are bradycardia and hypotension.

A. Acute Poisoning: (From ingestion.) Bradycardia, hypotension, atrioventricular block, metabolic acidosis, and hyperglycemia.

B. Chronic Poisoning: (From ingestion.) Effects are as for acute poisoning plus gastrointestinal distress with nausea and constipation, skin rash, flushing, dependent edema, weakness, and dizziness. Of the 3 drugs, verapamil appears to be most likely to seriously weaken cardiac contractility, especially when used in combination with β-sympathetic blocking agents. Preexisting atrioventricular conduction abnormalities are enhanced by verapamil and diltiazem. Nifedipine is most likely to produce hypotension.

C. Laboratory Findings:

1. Hyperglycemia, hyperkalemia, elevated blood lactate level, reduced blood bicarbonate level, reduced arterial pH.

2. Verapamil and nifedipine increase digoxin blood levels.

3. Galactorrhea and prolactinemia with altered liver function have been noted after verapamil.

Prevention

Combination of these drugs with propranolol or other β-sympathetic blocking agents should be avoided, since it is more likely to produce serious hypotension.

Treatment

A. Emergency Measures: Remove ingested overdose with emesis followed by gastric lavage using activated charcoal (see p 21–28).

B. Antidote: Calcium chloride or calcium gluconate, 10–20 mg/kg as 10% solution diluted in normal saline, should be given intravenously over 30 minutes and repeated as necessary to control symptoms.

C. General Measures:

1. Atrioventricular block and bradycardia usually respond to atropine or isoproterenol. Intracardiac pacing may be necessary.

Table 26-1. Other cardiovascular drugs.

Drugs	Clinical Findings	Treatment
Carbonic anhydrase inhibitors: Acetazolamide Dichlorphenamide Ethoxzolamide Methazolamide (Neptazane)	Papular or erythematous skin eruptions, drowsiness, paresthesias, fatigue, nausea, acidosis, blood dyscrasias similar to those produced by sulfonamides (see p 396).	Discontinue.
Amiloride (Midamor)	Hyperkalemia, nausea, vomiting, diarrhea, abdominal pain, constipation, cough, impotence.	Discontinue.
Amisometradine (Rolicton)	Nausea, vomiting, diarrhea, headache.	Discontinue.
Ammonium chloride (Exposure limit, 10 mg/m³)	Nausea, vomiting, profound acidosis.	Discontinue; treat acidosis (see p 49).
Amrinone (Inocor)	Thrombocytopenia, arrhythmias, hypotension, nausea and vomiting, diarrhea, hepatotoxicity, pericarditis, pleuritis.	Discontinue.
Thiazide diuretics: Bendroflumethiazide (Naturetin) Benzthiazide (Exna) Chlorothiazide Chlorthalidone (Hygroton) Cyclothiazide (Anhydron) Flumethiazide (Ademol) Hydrochlorothiazide Hydroflumethiazide (Saluron) Indapamide (Lozol) Methylclothiazide (Enduron) Polythiazide (Renese) Trichlormethiazide	Chloride loss, potassium loss, lethargy, muscle cramps, acidosis, gastric upset, skin rash, salivary gland obstruction, psychosis, convulsions, hyperuricemia, leukopenia, jaundice, increased hepatic decompensation in hepatic cirrhosis, photosensitization, precipitation or aggravation of diabetes mellitus, ulceration of small intestine from combined therapy with potassium chloride, hypercalcemia, and, rarely, acute glomerulonephritis, pancreatitis, thrombocytopenic purpura, or agranulocytosis. Acute overdose may cause coma. Infants born of mothers receiving thiazide diuretics may show jaundice or thrombocytopenia. Severe pancreatitis has also occurred during pregnancy.	Discontinue. Determine serum sodium and potassium. Give sodium chloride or potassium chloride to replace measured deficits.
Bumetanide (Bumex)	Muscle cramps, dizziness, hypotension, headache, encephalopathy, ototoxicity.	Discontinue.
Captopril (Capoten)	Lymphadenopathy, proteinuria, renal failure, hemolytic anemia, pancytopenia.	Discontinue.
Clofibrate (Atromid-S) Gemfibrozil (Lopid)	Elevation of serum transaminase, nausea, vomiting, diarrhea, abdominal discomfort, headache, dizziness, fatigue, weakness, skin rash, and stomatitis. These drugs increase the risk of gallbladder disease and potentiate coumarin anticoagulants. Leukopenia, agranulocytosis, and Bromsulphalein retention have been reported.	Discontinue.

Table 26—1 (cont'd). Other cardiovascular drugs.

Drugs	Clinical Findings	Treatment
Dextran	Excessive bleeding, sensitivity reactions, hypertension.	Discontinue.
Diazoxide (Hyperstat)	Sodium and water retention, hyperglycemia, myocardial and cerebral ischemia, rash, hyperuricemia, arrhythmias, convulsions, shock, and mental depression; hypertension is rare.	Discontinue.
Dipyridamol (Persantine)	Headache, dizziness, nausea, flushing, weakness, syncope, gastrointestinal irritation, skin rash, exacerbation of chest pain.	Discontinue.
Disopyramide (Norpace)	Hypotension, cardiac decompensation, heart block, anticholinergic effects.	Discontinue.
Ethacrynic acid (Edecrin)	Hyperuricemia, anorexia, abdominal pain, nausea, vomiting, diarrhea, acute pancreatitis, jaundice, agranulocytosis, thrombocytopenia, deafness, ventricular fibrillation resulting from potassium loss.	Discontinue; give potassium chloride orally under laboratory control.
Furosemide (Lasix)	Skin rash, pruritus, paresthesia, deafness, blurring of vision, hypotension, tetany, dehydration, electrolyte loss, nausea, vomiting, diarrhea. Leukopenia, thrombocytopenia, and acute pancreatitis have occurred.	Discontinue. Give potassium chloride orally under laboratory control.
Ganglionic blocking agents: Chlorisondamine Hexamethonium Mecamylamine Pentolinium tartrate (Ansolysen) Trimethaphan	Prolonged fall in blood pressure, failure of renal function, myocardial infarction, intestinal obstruction, and urine retention. Tremor and psychosis only with mecamylamine.	Discontinue; treat low blood pressure.
Mannitol	Headache, nausea, vomiting, chills, dizziness, lethargy, confusion, chest pain, heart failure, pulmonary edema. Fatalities have occurred.	Discontinue.
Metolazone (Zaroxolyn)	Hypokalemia, natremia, hypochloremia, hyperuricemia, increased BUN, gastrointestinal upset, leukopenia, urticaria, palpitations, acute gout.	Discontinue.
Minoxidil (Loniten)	Sodium and water retention, hirsutism, pericardial effusion, Stevens-Johnson syndrome.	Discontinue.
Nitroprusside, sodium (Nipride) (See p 251.)	Severe hypotension, vomiting, apprehension, hyperventilation, tachycardia, muscular twitching, and reversible hypothyroidism.	Discontinue.
Pargyline (Eutonyl)	Hypotension, weakness, nausea, vomiting, headache, edema; pressor reactions with reserpine, cheese, beer, or wine; depressor response with amitriptyline, methyldopa, or monoamine oxidase inhibitors.	Reduce dosage. Treat pressor reactions with phentolamine (Table 24—3).
Polyamine-methylene resin (Resinat)	Gastric upset, fecal impaction, hypokalemia.	Discontinue.

Table 26—1 (cont'd). Other cardiovascular drugs.

Drugs	Clinical Findings	Treatment
Potassium chloride (coated tablets)	Ulceration, hemorrhage, obstruction, perforation of the small intestine, and cardiac arrest.	Discontinue.
Prazosin (Minipress)	Dizziness, headache, drowsiness, gastrointestinal disturbances, tachycardia, dyspnea, paresthesias, rash, dysuria, sweating.	Discontinue.
Probenecid (Benemid)	Nausea, skin rash; rarely, liver necrosis, nephrotic syndrome.	Discontinue.
Probucol (Lorelco)	Gastrointestinal disturbances, sweating, sensitivity reactions, dizziness, faintness, anemia, altered liver enzymes.	Discontinue.
Quinethazone (Hydromox)	Gastrointestinal upset, skin rash, weakness, dizziness.	Discontinue.
Rauwolfia preparations: Alseroxylon (Rauwiloid) Deserpidine (Harmonyl) Rescinnamine (Moderil) Reserpine (Serpasil) Syrosingopine (Singoserp)	Diarrhea, nasal stuffiness, anginal pain, extrasystoles, edema, congestive failure, thrombocytopenia, tremors, muscular stiffness, severe hypotension in conjunction with general anesthetic administration, emotional depression.	Discontinue.
Sodium azide	0.1 mg/kg can cause hypotension.	Reduce dosage.
Sodium morrhuate Sodium psylliate Sodium tetradecyl-sulfate	Injection causes pain, sensitivity reactions, sloughing, pulmonary embolism, paraplegia.	Occlude vein prior to injection. Treat symptoms.
Streptokinase-streptodornase (Varidase)	Fever, kidney damage, vascular collapse, localized bleeding, sensitivity reactions.	Discontinue.
Tocainide (Tonocard)	Blood dyscrasias, pulmonary fibrosis.	Discontinue.
Triamterene (Dyrenium)	Gastrointestinal upset, dry mouth, weakness, tachycardia, hypotension, hyperkalemia, hypokalemia, rise in BUN, leukopenia.	Reduce dosage.
Urokinase	Hemorrhage, hypersensitivity reactions, fever.	Discontinue.

2. Treat hypotension by placing the patient in the supine position and giving intravenous fluids. Pressor agents should be used cautiously; dopamine is possibly the safest.

3. Insulin administration may be necessary.

Prognosis

Survival for 24 hours has been followed by complete recovery.

Coaldrake LA: Verapamil overdose. *Anesth Intensive Care* (May) 1984;**12**:174.

Jacob AS et al: Fatal ventricular fibrillation following verapamil in Wolff-Parkinson-White syndrome with atrial fibrillation. *Ann Emerg Med* 1985;**14**:159.

Lewis JG: Adverse reactions to calcium antagonists. *Drugs* 1983;**25**:196.

Morris DL, Goldschlager N: Calcium infusion for reversal of adverse effects of intravenous verapamil. *JAMA* 1983;**249**:3212.

Schiffl H et al: Clinical features and management of nifedipine overdosage in a patient with renal insufficiency. *J Toxicol Clin Toxicol* 1984;**22**:387.

INTERACTIONS
(See p 17.)

Coumarin anticoagulants enhance the effects of clofibrate and thyroid hormone. Anabolic steroids, clofibrate, glucagon, phenylbutazone, chloramphenicol, phenyramidol, quinidine, chloral hydrate, tetracyclines, allopurinol, ethacrynic acid, disulfiram, sulfonamides, and thyroid drugs enhance the effects of coumarin anticoagulants by displacing them from protein binding.

Probenecid and carinamide reduce clearance of penicillins, dapsone, indomethacin, sulfinpyrazone, and *p*-aminosalicyclic acid.

In the presence of elevated potassium, digitalized patients given succinylcholine have ventricular arrhythmias.

Antihypertensives enhance the effects of central nervous system depressants, anesthetics, diuretics, monoamine oxidase inhibitors, and tranquilizers.

Quinidine enhances the effects of muscle relaxants.

Antidepressant or antihypertensive drugs (except thiazide diuretics) have increased adverse effects when they are combined with pargyline.

The risk of toxicity from digitalis glycosides is increased by administration of sympathomimetics, reserpine, succinylcholine, or calcium and potassium loss induced by diuretics, carbenoxolone, amphotericin B, corticosteroids, or laxative abuse.

Furosemide can cause tachycardia, hypertension, flush, and sweating in the presence of chloral hydrate.

Salicylates enhance the risk of bleeding when heparin is given.

Thiazide diuretics enhance potassium loss and increase the effect of curare drugs but have no effect on succinylcholine.

Reserpines deplete catecholamines, with resulting hypotension during anesthesia. Patients are then more sensitive to vasopressors.

Hydralazine potentiates anesthetic agents, makes hypotension more likely during anesthesia, and reduces pressor response to drugs.

Quinidine and procainamide increase susceptibility to curare.

Anticoagulants increase susceptibility to bleeding following injection procedures or intratracheal intubation.

Cyclopropane, halothane and other anesthetic agents, neostigmine, atropine, and d-tubocurarine trigger arrhythmias in digitalized patients.

PHARMACOKINETICS & TOXIC CONCENTRATIONS
(See p 89.)

	pK_a	$t_{1/2}$ (hours)	V_d (L/kg)	% Binding	Toxic Concentration ($\mu g/mL$)
Acetazolamide	7.2	2.4—5.8		90—95	
Chlorothiazide	6.7, 9.5	0.75—2		20—80	
Clofibrate	2.95	8—54*	0.09	95—98	
Clonidine	8.25	6—23		20	
Diazoxide	8.74	21—36		90—93	
Dicumarol	5.7	7—100		95	
Digitoxin		96—144	40.9	90—97	0.025
Digoxin		3—40	5.3, 16*	20—23	0.0017
Disopyramide	9.6	5	0.6—1.3	35—95	4†
Ethacrynic acid	3.5	0.5—1			
Ethyl biscoumacetate	3.1	3.1	2—3.5		90
Furosemide	3.8	1—3.5	0.1	95—97	
Heparin		1—2	0.06	0	
Hydralazine	7.1	2—7.8	0.45	87	
Hydrochlorothiazide		2—15			
Isosorbide dinitrate		0.3			
Lanatoside C		33—36		23—25	
Mannitol		1.5			
Nitroglycerin		0.3			
Nitroprusside		150			
Phenindione		5—10			
Probenecid	3.4	4—12	0.12—0.18	83—94	
Procainamide	9.2	2.2—4	1.7—2.2	15	12
Quinidine	4.3, 8.4	3—16	2.1—2.6	73—96	10
Reserpine		50—100			
Spironolactone		13—24		98	
Thiocyanate					120
Triamterene	6.2	2		67	
Verapamil		3—7		6.5	90
Warfarin	5.05	15—70	0.1	97	

*For children.
†Fatal.

References

Cooper RA: Captopril-associated neutropenia. *Arch Intern Med* 1983;**143**:659.

Currie P et al: Paranoid psychosis induced by tocainide. *Br Med J* 1984;**288**:606.

Edmonds OP, Bourne MS: Sodium azide poisoning in five laboratory technicians. *Br J Ind Med* 1982;**39**:308.

Johnson JE, Wright LF: Thiazide-induced hyponatremia. *South Med J* 1983;**76**:1363.

Mandal SK, Datta SK: Nodal bradycardia induced by tocainide. *Postgrad Med J* 1983;**59**:262.

Maronde RF et al: Response of thiazide-induced hypokalemia to amiloride. *JAMA* 1983;**249**:237.

Nappi J et al: Severe hypoglycemia associated with disopyramide. *West J Med* 1982;**138**:95.

Ryngestad PK, Dale O: Self-poisoning with prazosin. *Acta Med Scand* 1983;**213**:157.

Sheehan J, White A: Diuretic-associated hypomagnesaemia. *Br Med J* 1982;**285**:1157.

Stapleton JT et al: Hypoglycemic coma due to disopyramide toxicity. *South Med J* 1983;**76**:1453.

27 | Anti-infective Drugs

SULFONAMIDES

Fatalities have occurred following therapeutic doses of almost all sulfonamides.

Sulfonamide compounds or their acetyl derivatives frequently precipitate in the kidney tubules or the ureters, causing renal damage and blocking the secretion of urine. The sulfonamides may affect the function of the bone marrow, liver, or heart by as yet unknown mechanisms. Some reactions are on the basis of hypersensitivity (Stevens-Johnson syndrome). Hemolytic anemia following the administration of sulfonamide apparently occurs, at least in some cases, on the basis of a deficiency of glucose-6-phosphate dehydrogenase activity in erythrocytes.

The pathologic findings are crystalline deposits in the kidney tubules, calices, and ureters. In deaths from sulfonamides, necrotic or inflammatory lesions may be found in the liver, heart, kidneys, bone marrow, or other organs. The bone marrow may be lacking in myeloid

Table 27—1. Sulfonamide and sulfone derivatives.

Diaminodiphenylsulfone (DDS, dapsone, Avlosulfon)*†	Sulfamerazine‡
Mafenide (Sulfamylon)	Sulfamethizole (Thiosulfil)
Phthalylsulfathiazole (Sulfathalidine)	Sulfamethoxazole (Gantanol)
Solapsone (Sulphetrone)*	Sulfamethoxypyridazine
Succinylsulfathiazole (Sulfasuxidine)	Sulfanilamide*
Sulfabenzamide	Sulfanilamidomethoxypyrimidine (sulfameter)
Sulfacetamide (Sulamyd)	Sulfasalazine (Azulfidine)‡
Sulfachloropyridazine (Sonilyn)	Sulfathiazole§
Sulfacytine (Renoquid)	Sulfisomidine (Elkosin)
Sulfadiazine‡	Sulfisoxazole (Gantrisin)
Sulfadimethoxine (Madribon)	Sulfoxone (Diasone)*§
Sulfaethidole (Sul-Spansion)	

*Causes methemoglobinemia (in addition to clinical findings listed on p 397).
†Also causes restlessness and coma.
‡Agranulocytosis has been reported in at least 7 cases.
§Incidence of hematuria is highest with these sulfonamides.

elements or may be completely aplastic. The liver may show degenerative changes.

Clinical Findings

The principal manifestation of sulfonamide poisoning is hematuria.

A. Acute Poisoning: (From ingestion or injection.) Gastrointestinal irritation, maculopapular erythematous skin eruptions, fever, mental and visual disturbances, sensitivity reactions, urticaria, hematuria, pain on urination, oliguria or anuria with azotemia, agranulocytosis, hemolytic anemia, thrombocytopenia, purpura, conjunctival injection, bullous lesions of the skin, petechiae, jaundice, and increased erythema or injury from sunlight beginning days or weeks after institution of therapy. Such reactions are more frequent after repeated courses of therapy. In addition, sulfasalazine has caused irreversible neuromuscular and central nervous system changes and fibrosing alveolitis. Long-acting sulfonamides, including sulfadimethoxine (Madribon), sulfanilamidomethoxypyrimidine (sulfameter), and sulfamethoxypyridazine and its acetyl and phenylazodiamino pyridine derivatives (eg, Kynex, Kynex acetyl, Azo Kynex, Midicel, Midicel acetyl), have caused at least 116 cases of a syndrome characterized by exudative, erythematous skin eruption; fever; and visceral lesions including pneumonitis, myocarditis, or nephritis (Stevens-Johnson syndrome). Approximately 25% of these cases have been fatal. Peripheral neuropathy has occurred from long-term dapsone therapy. The combination of trimethoprim and sulfamethoxazole (co-trimoxazole, Bactrim, Septra) has caused anemia, reduction in renal function, thrombocytopenia, nausea and vomiting, diarrhea, mental depression, confusion, facial swelling, headache, bone marrow depression, and liver impairment.

B. Chronic Poisoning: Findings are the same as those described for acute poisoning.

C. Laboratory Findings:

1. The complete blood count may reveal thrombocytopenia and diminution or absence of leukocytes. The red blood cell count may also be diminished.

2. The urine may contain crystals, red blood cells, and protein.

3. Blood sulfonamide levels above 10 mg/dL are considered toxic.

4. In jaundice from sulfonamide administration, hepatic cell damage is revealed by appropriate tests (see p 75).

Prevention

Do not prescribe sulfonamides unnecessarily. Use the minimum doses necessary to cure the disease. Discontinue long-acting sulfonamides immediately if skin rash occurs.

Renal complications can be minimized if the urine is kept slightly alkaline with sodium bicarbonate, 5–15 g daily, and if the 24-hour urine volume is maintained above 1 L with oral fluids to 2 L daily. Blood sulfonamide levels should be determined frequently if maximum doses are being given.

Treatment

A. Acute Poisoning:

1. Emergency measures–Discontinue use at the first sign of skin rash or other untoward reaction. Remove swallowed overdoses by gastric lavage or emesis (see pp 21–28).

2. General measures–If renal function is normal, force fluids to 4 L daily to speed excretion of sulfonamides.

3. Special problems–Hemodialysis is useful if renal function is depressed. Treat agranulocytosis (see p 79). Treat aplastic anemia by repeated blood transfusions. Methemoglobinemia from sulfonamides does not appear to respond to methylene blue administration. Treat disturbed central nervous system function as for depressant drugs (see p 319).

B. Chronic Poisoning: Treat as for acute poisoning.

Prognosis

Renal function may return after 2 weeks of anuria. Agranulocytosis from sulfonamides responds to treatment in 50–75% of cases.

Berlin G et al: Acute dapsone intoxication: A case treated with continuous infusion of methylene blue, forced diuresis and plasma exchange. *J Toxicol Clin Toxicol* 1984;**22:**537.

Fligner CF et al: Hyperosmolality induced by propylene glycol: A complication of silver sulfadiazine therapy. *JAMA* 1985;**253:**1606.

Gordin FM: Adverse reactions to trimethoprim-sulfamethoxazole in patients with acquired immunodeficiency syndrome. *Ann Intern Med* 1984;**100:**495.

Neuvonen PJ et al: Acute dapsone intoxication: Clinical findings and effect of oral charcoal and haemodialysis on dapsone elimination. *Acta Med Scand* 1983;**214:**215.

Wheelan KR et al: Multiple hematologic abnormalities associated with sulfasalazine. *Ann Intern Med* 1982;**97:**726.

ANTIBIOTICS

Most of the deaths that occur as a result of administration of antibiotics are due to hypersensitivity reactions or overgrowth of resistant organisms. It is possible that some fatalities following the injection of insoluble antibiotics have been due to intravenous injection. More than 30 fatalities from aplastic anemia have been reported in patients who had previously taken chloramphenicol.

The pathologic findings in sudden death from hypersensitivity reactions after the injection of antibiotics are constriction of the bronchioles, distention of the lungs, pulmonary edema, congestion of the viscera, and hemorrhages in the lungs. Findings in deaths from overgrowth of resistant organisms are dependent upon the type of organism.

Clinical Findings

A. Acute Poisoning: (From injection, ingestion, or application to mucous membranes.) The following occur most commonly following parenteral administration of penicillin or streptomycin, less often following administration of other antibiotics: Pallor, cyanosis, wheezing, collapse, frothy sputum, pulmonary edema, and death in respiratory failure may occur within seconds to minutes after injection of an antibiotic or its application to mucous membranes. Delayed reactions may consist of fever, skin eruptions, and pharyngeal or laryngeal edema. Oral administration, especially of penicillin, can also cause anaphylactoid reactions characterized by nausea and vomiting, abdominal pain and cramping, localized edema, cyanosis, respiratory distress, convulsions, severe chest pain, and death in respiratory failure.

B. Chronic Poisoning: (From repeated injection, ingestion, or application to mucous membranes.) The most common untoward reaction to the administration of antibiotics is the overgrowth of organisms not affected by the antibiotic agent, which can occur even after the parenteral injection of antibiotics. In some cases these organisms elaborate toxins that cause severe vomiting, diarrhea, and circulatory collapse. The following antibiotics have additional specific effects:

1. Penicillins–Urticaria, fever, rash, peripheral neuritis, wheezing, pruritus, flushing of skin, neutropenia, and fall of blood pressure occur variably after either intermittent or continuous use. Rapid intravenous administration of potassium penicillin can cause cardiac arrhythmia and cardiac arrest. Liver necrosis and hemolytic anemia resulting from anaphylactic reaction have also occurred. Ampicillin has caused reversible impairment of liver function and diarrhea. Methicillin has caused renal damage. Dicloxacillin has caused gastrointestinal upset, skin rash, and possible hepatic dysfunction. Carbenicillin and ampicillin have caused leukopenia. Bacampicillin and amoxicillin are similar to ampicillin. Benzyl penicilloyl polylysine, used as a skin test antigen for penicillin sensitivity, has caused severe sensitivity reactions and does not reveal all penicillin-sensitive individuals.

2. Tetracyclines–Chlortetracycline (Aureomycin), oxytetracycline (Terramycin), tetracycline (Tetracyn), doxycycline (Vibramycin), demeclocycline (Declomycin), minocycline (Minocin), and methacycline (Rondomycin) can cause nausea, anorexia, diarrhea, perianal itching, skin eruptions, fever, toxemia, rising blood urea nitrogen, psychotic reactions, anaphylaxis, and collapse from overgrowth of intestinal organisms. Increased intracranial pressure with bulging of fontanels has occurred in infants. A syndrome resembling lupus erythematosus can occur. Chlortetracycline and tetracycline have caused fatal liver damage after large oral or intravenous doses. A similar response is possible with other tetracyclines. It is believed that blood levels for tetracycline that exceed 16 μg/mL of serum contribute to the development of liver damage. The daily oral dose should not exceed 2 g/d. When left standing, tetracyclines decompose into more toxic products that cause renal damage with polyuria, acidosis, and loss of protein, glucose, amino acids, and potassium. For this reason, a tetracycline should not be used later than the expiration date shown on the package. Tetracycline present during odontogenesis causes hypoplasia and discoloration of teeth; this can occur in utero or during childhood. Unless no alternative exists, tetracyclines should not be given for long or indefinite periods to children under 8 years of age. Demeclocycline has caused increased sensitivity to sunlight and reversible diabetes insipidus. Methacycline can cause a parasympathomimetic response.

3. Aminoglycosides–Streptomycin, vancomycin (Vancocin), kanamycin (Kantrex), spectinomycin (Trobicin), capreomycin (Capastat), amikacin (Amikin), gentamicin (Garamycin), netilmicin (Netromycin), and tobramycin (Nebcin) can cause paresthesias, lassitude, dizziness, headaches, blurring of vision, fever, and eighth nerve injury with tinnitus, deafness, loss of sense of balance, renal damage, neuromuscular blockade, and vertigo after parenteral injection. Hearing loss, which may be permanent, occurs most frequently after dihydrostreptomycin, vancomycin, capreomycin, or tobramycin; infants are especially susceptible. Severe central nervous system and respiratory depression has occurred in infants given streptomycin. Respiratory and cardiac arrest has followed intravenously administered kanamycin. Spectinomycin also causes urticaria, nausea, fever, sleeplessness, and decrease in hemoglobin. Skin rash has occurred after topical application of aminoglycosides. Because these drugs are excreted almost entirely by glomerular filtration, periodic evaluation of renal function is essential.

4. Chloramphenicol (Chloromycetin)–Nausea and vomiting, diarrhea, mucous membrane lesions, toxemia, hepatitis, and collapse from overgrowth of intestinal organisms; aplastic anemia or agranulocytosis occurs sufficiently often to require blood counts once weekly. Aplastic anemia is believed to result from an idiosyncratic response to excessive blood levels of chloramphenicol. Optic and peripheral neuritis has occurred in conjunction with chloramphenicol therapy. A sudden onset of vomiting, diarrhea, and irreversible cardiovascular collapse has occurred in premature and newborn infants given more than 25 mg/kg/d. Newborn infants are deficient in the hepatic conjugating enzyme system that ordinarily detoxifies chloramphenicol. Caution should be used in the administration of chloramphenicol to any patient with liver or kidney injury.

5. Polymyxins–Bacitracin, polymyxin B, and colistin (Coly-Mycin) can cause paresthesias and acute renal damage with proteinuria, nitrogen retention, and oliguria or anuria following injection of these antibiotics. Polymyxin B also causes dizziness, weakness, paresthesias, and severe fall of blood pressure from histamine release. These signs of toxicity from polymyxin B are much more frequent at doses greater than 2.5 mg/kg/d. Colistimethate has also caused leukopenia, neurotoxicity, dizziness, slurred speech, apnea, and fever.

6. Cycloserine (Seromycin)–Headache, dizziness, lethargy, polyneuritis, psychotic behavior, and convulsions are especially frequent with doses over 0.5 g/d.

7. Neomycin and viomycin (Viocin)–Loss of hearing, vestibular damage, skin eruptions, steatorrhea, and kidney damage with proteinuria, edema, and electrolyte disturbances. Large injected doses of neomycin cause respiratory arrest and paralysis of voluntary muscles.

8. Novobiocin–Skin rash, urticaria, fever, liver injury with jaundice, hemolysis, and reversible leukopenia in 7–20% of patients.

9. Erythromycin–Nausea and vomiting, diarrhea, prostration, skin rash. Jaundice as a result of intrahepatic cholestasis has occurred after administration of erythromycin estolate (Ilosone).

10. Nystatin (Mycostatin)–Nausea and vomiting, diarrhea, skin rash.

11. Amphotericin B (Fungizone)–Therapeutic doses produce fever, anorexia, pain at the injection site, and, if administration is prolonged, gradual reduction of renal function as shown by increased blood urea nitrogen and nonprotein nitrogen.

12. Oleandomycin (Matromycin) and troleandomycin (Cyclamycin)–Skin rash, diarrhea. Liver damage with jaundice has occurred after troleandomycin administration.

13. Griseofulvin (Fulvicin)–Urticaria, nausea, diarrhea, headaches, confusion, dizziness, photosensitivity, renal damage, porphyria, and temporary leukopenia have occurred. Griseofulvin markedly potentiates the toxicity of colchicine in experimental animals.

14. Lincomycin (Lincocin) and clindamycin (Cleocin)–Nausea and vomiting, severe inflammation of the colon with diarrhea, skin and mucous membrane reactions, impairment of liver function with jaundice, and reversible leukopenia.

15. Cephalosporins–Cephalothin (Keflin) has caused skin rash, intense tissue irritation with pain on injection, fever, meningitis, renal failure, thrombocytopenia, and reversible leukopenia. Cephaloglycin (Kafocin) and cefalexin (Keflex) have caused vomiting and diarrhea, dermatitis, itching, dizziness, and malaise. Toxic psychosis has occurred when these drugs were used in combination with other drugs. Cephaloridine (Loridine) has caused urticaria, skin rash (or itching without skin rash), rise in eosinophil count, drug fever, leukopenia, and tubular necrosis after doses above 4 g daily. Cephradine (Anspor), cephapirin (Cefadyl), and cefazolin (Ancef) have caused drug fever, skin rash, elevation of SGOT and other liver enzymes, and eosinophilia. Cefadroxil (Duricef), cefamandole (Mandole), cefoxitin (Mefoxin), cefotaxime (Claforan), and cefaclor (Ceclor) have caused gastrointestinal disturbances, hypersensitivity reactions, neutropenia, rise in liver enzymes, and a rise in blood urea nitrogen. Cefonicid (Monocid), ceforanide (Precef), ceftizoxime (Cefizox), cefoperazone (Cefobid), and cefuroxime (Zinacef) have caused pain on injection, skin rash, itching, eosinophilia, diarrhea, vomiting, and possible alterations in liver and kidney function. Reduced hemoglobin can occur, especially with cefuroxime.

    16. Candicidin (Candeptin)—Rarely, irritation or sensitization of the skin.

    17. Paromomycin (Humatin)—Gastrointestinal disturbances with doses over 3 g daily.

    18. Rifampin (Rimactane)—Gastrointestinal upset, mental effects, exacerbation of previous liver dysfunction, neurologic disturbances, thrombocytopenia and other blood dyscrasias, and renal damage.

    C. Laboratory Findings:

    1. A complete blood count may reveal a decrease in red blood cells, white blood cells, or thrombocytes.

    2. Bacitracin and polymyxin B sulfate may cause proteinuria, hematuria, and increase in blood urea nitrogen.

    3. Administration of amphotericin B, bacitracin, and polymyxin B must be discontinued if blood urea nitrogen rises above 20 mg/dL.

Prevention

    Patients must be carefully questioned concerning previous drug reactions, including rashes, asthma, or local swelling, prior to any injection. Most patients who are susceptible to severe penicillin reactions can be identified beforehand by placing 1 drop of a penicillin preparation (1000 units/mL) on the inner forearm and making a deep scratch in the skin through the drop. If a wheal appears immediately, 1:1000 epinephrine is applied to the scratch and 0.25 mL is given subcutaneously. A tourniquet is applied above the site of the scratch. For patients showing a wheal reaction to the penicillin scratch test, alternative therapy should be used.

Treatment
    A. Acute Poisoning:

1. Emergency measures for treatment of severe sensitivity reactions (anaphylaxis)–

a. Give 1 mL of 1:1000 epinephrine intramuscularly. If no response is obtained, give 1 mL of 1:10,000 epinephrine slowly intravenously.

b. Give positive-pressure artificial respiration.

c. Give diphenhydramine (Benadryl), 50 mg slowly intravenously. Give dexamethasone, 1 mg/kg intravenously every 6 hours until symptoms abate.

2. Antidote–

a. Penicillinase (Neutrapen) will reverse delayed penicillin reactions but is not useful in anaphylaxis. Penicillinase is itself capable of causing serious anaphylactic reactions.

b. Respiratory paralysis from neomycin can be antagonized by intravenous administration of 2–10 mL of 10% calcium gluconate.

B. Chronic Poisoning:

1. Immediate measures–Discontinue drug if there is any untoward change in the patient's condition, and evaluate the possibility of drug reaction.

2. General measures–

a. Treat gastrointestinal distress from oral antibiotics by giving milk every 3 hours alternating with bismuth subcarbonate, 5 g every 3 hours.

b. Treat toxemia from overgrowth of intestinal organisms with an appropriate chemotherapeutic agent after determining the type and sensitivity of the organism. Treat circulatory collapse (see p 66). Stop antibiotics if possible.

3. Special problems–Treat aplastic anemia by repeated blood transfusions. Treat anuria (see p 72).

Prognosis

Anaphylactic reactions to antibiotics are frequently fatal. At least 75% of patients with idiosyncratic type aplastic anemia from chloramphenicol have died.

Ackerman BH et al: Aminoglycoside therapy. *Postgrad Med* (Feb) 1984;**75**:177.
Amendola MA: Doxycycline-induced esophagitis. *JAMA* 1985;**253**:1009.
Beeley L: Allergy to penicillin. *Br Med J* 1984;**288**:511.
Freundlich M et al: Management of chloramphenicol intoxication in infancy by charcoal hemoperfusion. *J Pediatr* 1983;**103**:485.
Fripp R et al: Cardiac function and acute chloramphenicol toxicity. *J Pediatr* 1983;**103**:487.
Johnson JT et al: Aminoglycoside ototoxicity: An update with implications for all drug therapies. *Postgrad Med* (April) 1985;**77**:131.
Wong P et al: Acute rifampin overdose: A pharmacokinetic study and review of the literature. *J Pediatr* 1984;**104**:781.

IPECAC & EMETINE

Ipecac is used as an emetic in the syrup form, never in the fluidextract form; the fluidextract is 14 times as concentrated as the syrup, and 10 mL is hazardous. Emetine, the alkaloid from ipecac (the roots and rhizomes of *Cephaelis ipecacuanha*), is used in the treatment of amebiasis.

The fatal dose of emetine is approximately 1 g. The fatal dose of ipecac cannot be stated, since vomiting prevents estimation of the amount taken.

Emetine weakens cardiac contraction by direct action on the myocardium. The effect is cumulative over a period of 1 month or longer.

The pathologic findings are gastrointestinal congestion and degenerative changes in the kidneys, heart, and liver.

Clinical Findings

The principal manifestations of poisoning with these drugs are fall of blood pressure and vomiting.

A. Acute Poisoning: (From ingestion or injection of emetine or ingestion of ipecac.) Therapeutic doses of emetine sometimes cause nausea and vomiting, fatigue, dyspnea, tachycardia, low blood pressure, collapse, unconsciousness, and death from heart failure. Ingestion of ipecac fluidextract has caused convulsions and coma as well as esophageal damage with stricture. Doses of emetine above the therapeutic ranges almost always produce toxic effects; syrup of ipecac ordinarily causes only vomiting. If vomiting persists for more than 2–3 hours after ipecac administration, a search for its cause must be made.

B. Chronic Poisoning: The effect of emetine is cumulative over a period of weeks. Cardiomyopathy has occurred from repeated use of syrup of ipecac.

C. Laboratory Findings: The ECG reveals depressed T waves and arrhythmias. The urine may contain protein. Leukocytosis is common, and the extent of liver damage should be determined (see p 75).

Prevention

Repeated courses of emetine should be avoided. The incidence of myocardial damage is greatly increased when the total dose is over 1 g. Patients should be kept at bed rest during the administration of emetine, and activity should be restricted for several weeks afterward. No more than 30 mL of syrup of ipecac should be used to induce emesis.

Treatment

A. Acute Poisoning:

1. Emergency measures–Delay absorption of ingested

fluidextract of ipecac by giving activated charcoal, and then remove by gastric lavage (see pp 21–28).

2. General measures–The patient should be kept at complete bed rest until recovery is assured. Cautious digitalization may be helpful for myocardial weakness. Replace fluid loss with 5% dextrose in normal saline.

B. Chronic Poisoning: Treat as for acute poisoning.

Prognosis

Complete recovery after symptomatic myocardial damage from emetine is not likely. Patients with myocardial damage indicated only by electrocardiographic changes may recover completely in 6 months to 1 year.

QUININE, QUINACRINE, & CHLOROQUINE

Quinine, quinacrine (mepacrine, Atabrine), chloroquine, and hydroxychloroquine (Plaquenil) are used in the treatment of malaria and for other medical purposes. Quinine is also used (to the extent of 30 mg/500 mL) as the bitter flavoring agent in many tonic drinks. This amount is sufficient to cause severe sensitivity reactions. The fatal dose of any of these drugs can be less than 20 mg/kg in children under age 2 years. At least 3 such fatalities occurred due to chloroquine, in one instance after 1 or 2 tablets. These drugs depress functions in all cells and especially in the heart. The kidneys, liver, and nervous system may also be affected.

The pathologic findings are degenerative changes in the liver, kidneys, brain, and optic nerve.

Clinical Findings

The principal manifestations of poisoning with these agents are vomiting and fall of blood pressure.

A. Acute Poisoning: (From ingestion.) Progressive tinnitus, blurring of vision, weakness, fall of blood pressure, hemoglobinuria, oliguria, and cardiac irregularities. Injection or ingestion of large doses causes sudden onset of cardiac depression. Convulsions and respiratory arrest also occur. Severe sensitivity reactions occur, especially to quinine. These reactions are characterized by edema, erythema, vesiculation, weeping, and bullae and may occur with doses as small as 30 mg. Laryngeal edema and systemic reactions—including headache, fever, dyspnea, nausea, and diarrhea—also occur.

B. Chronic Poisoning:

1. Repeated ingestion of quinine in large doses causes visual loss associated with bilateral dilated pupils, pallor of optic disks, narrowing

Table 27—2. Chemotherapy: Miscellaneous agents.

Drug	Clinical Findings and Contraindications	Treatment
Acyclovir (Zovirax)	Local reactions, transient increase in BUN, encephalopathy, rash, nausea, vomiting, abdominal pain, thrombocytosis, thrombo-cytopenia, leukopenia.	Discontinue use.
Amantadine (Symmetrel)	Insomnia, dizziness, ataxia, psychosis, and other CNS signs. Do not use in children. Nonfatal convulsions at 0.5 g/kg.	Discontinue use.
p-Aminosalicylic acid (PAS)	Fever, pruritus, erythematous macular or bullous eruptions, acidosis, hypokalemia, crystalluria, nausea, vomiting, anorexia, hepatic necrosis, diarrhea, leukocytosis, laryngeal edema, hemolytic anemia, met-hemoglobinemia, thrombocytopenia, leuko-penia, thyroid suppression.	Reduce dosage or discontinue drug.
Amodiaquine (Camoquin)	Nausea, vomiting, diarrhea, salivation, clum-siness, convulsions, hepatitis, agranulocyto-sis.	Reduce dosage or discontinue drug.
Aspidium	Vomiting, diarrhea, visual disturbances, con-vulsions, death in respiratory failure.	Remove poison, treat symptoms.
Bephenium (Alcopar)	Nausea, vomiting, possible fall of blood pressure. Treat ill patients only in hospital.	Control electro-lytes.
Bismuth sodium triglycollamate (Bistrimate)	Gastroenteritis, jaundice, exfoliative derma-titis.	Treat as for arse-nic (see p 223).
Bismuth subcarbo-nate Bismuth subnitrate Bismuth subsalicy-late	Exposure 4 weeks to 30 years can cause tem-porary encephalopathy with mental deterio-ration and epileptiform convulsions.	Discontinue use.
Bithionol (Lorothidol)	Vomiting, diarrhea, dizziness, headache, der-matitis.	Treat overdoses as for phenol (see p 368).
Carbarsone	Nausea and vomiting. Rarely, optic neuritis and hepatitis.	Reduce dosage or discontinue drug; give dimercaprol (see p 84).
Chaulmoogra oil	Gastric upset, hepatic and renal damage, hemolysis.	Discontinue use.
Chenopodium	Vomiting, diarrhea, blindness, deafness, con-vulsions, coma. Do not use.	
Chloroguanide (Guanatol)	Nausea, hematuria, anorexia, proteinuria, anuria.	Reduce dosage or discontinue drug.
Ciclopirox (Loprox)	Itching and burning.	Discontinue use.
Cinoxacin (Cinobac)	Nausea, vomiting, diarrhea, headache, dizzi-ness, tinnitus, rash, itching.	Discontinue use.
Clotrimazole (Lotrimin)	Irritation to blistering of skin.	Discontinue use.

Table 27—2 (cont'd). Chemotherapy: Miscellaneous agents.

Drug	Clinical Findings and Contraindications	Treatment
Crotamiton (Eurax)	Irritant, sensitizer.	Discontinue use.
Diethylcarbamazine (Hetrazan)	Fever, headache, lassitude, leukocytosis, nausea, vomiting, skin rash.	Reduce dosage. Administer cortisone.
Dithiazanine (Delvex)	Nausea, vomiting, diarrhea, abdominal pain. Deaths have also occurred, apparently from sensitivity reactions, with hypotension, acidosis, and coma. Use cautiously in debilitated patients or those with renal or other disease.	Discontinue drug or reduce dosage.
Econazole (Spectazole)	Burning, itching, redness.	Discontinue use.
Ethambutol (Myambutol)	Reversible decrease in visual acuity, anaphylactoid reactions, headache, malaise, anorexia, fever, skin rash, joint pain, numbness and tingling of the extremities, increase in serum uric acid, transient impairment of liver function, toxic epidermal necrolysis.	Reduce dosage or discontinue drug.
Ethionamide (Trecator)	Nausea, diarrhea, skin rash, peripheral neuropathy, toxic psychosis, and liver damage. Injury to the fetus has occurred in experimental animals.	Discontinue use.
Flucytosine (Ancobon)	Gastrointestinal upset, blood dyscrasias, elevation of hepatic enzymes and BUN, CNS disturbances.	Discontinue use.
Furan derivatives: Furazolidone (Furoxone) Nitrofurantoin (Furadantin) Nitrofurazone (Furacin)	Nausea and vomiting, maculopapular erythematous eruption, anemia, jaundice, bleeding, acute polyneuritis which may be irreversible, pulmonary infiltration, leukopenia, cerebellar dysfunction, and circulatory collapse. Nitrofurantoin has caused hemolytic anemia of the naphthalene type (see p 194).	Use cautiously in presence of renal function impairment. Discontinue if necessary.
Gentian violet	Methemoglobinemia after large doses. Cardiovascular collapse and death in respiratory failure from large doses orally. Nausea, vomiting, kidney irritation.	Reduce dosage or discontinue drug.
Haloprogin (Halotex)	Reactions include irritation, burning, vesicle formation, and exacerbation of preexisting lesions.	Discontinue use.
Hydroxystilbamidine	Transitory fall in blood pressure, rapid pulse, dizziness, nausea, vomiting. Kidney injury from old solutions.	Use only fresh solutions.
Idoxuridine (Herplex)	Irritation from topical application.	Discontinue use.
Ketoconazole (Nizoral)	Nausea, vomiting, pruritus, abdominal pain, CNS effects, hepatitis.	Discontinue use.
Lucanthone (Miracil D, Nilodin)	Gastric upset, CNS symptoms with twitchings.	Discontinue drug or reduce dosage.

Table 27–2 (cont'd). Chemotherapy: Miscellaneous agents.

Drug	Clinical Findings and Contraindications	Treatment
Mandelic acid	Gastric irritation, nausea, renal irritation, acidosis.	Discontinue use.
Mebendazole (Vermox)	Contraindicated in pregnancy. Causes abdominal pain and diarrhea in massive worm infestations.	Discontinue use.
Methenamine	Skin rash, kidney and bladder irritation, hematuria, nausea, vomiting.	Discontinue use.
Metronidazole (Flagyl)	Nausea, diarrhea, skin rash, dizziness, drowsiness, headache, leukopenia, sensitivity to alcohol. Carcinogenic in rodents. Do not use in early pregnancy.	Discontinue use.
Miconazole (Monistat)	Phlebitis, mucous membrane irritation, rash, diarrhea, anorexia, thrombocytopenia.	Discontinue use.
Moxalactam (Moxam)	Hypersensitivity, neutropenia, leukopenia, anemia, thrombocytopenia, nausea, vomiting, possible liver or kidney impairment.	Discontinue use.
Nalidixic acid (NegGram)	Nausea, vomiting, skin eruptions, exacerbation of epilepsy, hyperglycemia, photosensitivity reactions.	Discontinue drug or reduce dosage.
Oxamniquine (Vansil)	Dizziness, headache, gastrointestinal distress, convulsions, fever, proteinuria, rash.	Discontinue use.
Oxolinic acid (Utibid)	Nausea, vomiting, restlessness, hallucinations, convulsions.	Discontinue use.
Oxophenarsine hydrochloride (Mapharsen)	Severe fall of blood pressure. For other findings, see Arsenic, p 221.	See p 223.
Pamaquine naphthoate Pentaquine phosphate Primaquine diphosphate	Hemolytic anemia, postural hypotension, methemoglobinemia, gastric distress, weakness.	Reduce dosage or discontinue drug.
Pelletierine tannate	Dizziness, visual disturbances, headache, weakness, vomiting and diarrhea, muscular cramps progressing to twitching, convulsions, and paralysis.	Reduce dosage or discontinue drug.
Pentamidine Propamidine	Fall of blood pressure, convulsions, kidney and liver damage. Protect solutions of pentamidine from light in order to prevent formation of hepatotoxic compounds.	Discontinue drug or reduce dosage.
Phenarsone sulfoxylate (Aldarsone)	Severe fall of blood pressure. For other findings, see Arsenic, p 221.	See p 223.
Phenazopyridine (Pyridium)	Methemoglobinemia, hemolytic reactions. Unsafe in presence of kidney or liver disease.	Discontinue use.
Piperazine* (Antepar, etc)	Urticaria, vomiting, blurred vision, weakness, and convulsions in doses above 1 g/kg.	Gastric lavage.

*Exposure limit, 5 mg/m^3.

Table 27–2 (cont'd). Chemotherapy: Miscellaneous agents.

Drug	Clinical Findings and Contraindications	Treatment
Praziquantel (Biltricide)	Dizziness, drowsiness, headache, malaise, gastrointestinal distress, liver function impairment.	Discontinue use.
Pyrantel pamoate (Antiminth)	Anorexia, nausea, vomiting, cramps, abdominal cramps, diarrhea, possible liver injury, headache, drowsiness, ataxia, skin rash.	Discontinue use.
Pyrazinamide	Hepatic damage, gout, gastric upset, fever.	Discontinue drug or reduce dosage.
Pyrimethamine (Daraprim)	Anemia, leukopenia, thrombocytopenia.	Discontinue use.
Pyrvinium (Povan)	Nausea and vomiting, kidney and liver injury after prolonged use.	Discontinue drug or reduce dosage.
Santonin	Vomiting, diarrhea, yellow vision, convulsions, death. Do not use.	
Silver sulfadiazine (Silvadene)	Itching, burning, sulfonamide toxicity, leukopenia, possible renal impairment.	Discontinue use; see p 398.
Stibamine glucoside (Neostam) Stibocaptate (Astiban) Stibophen (Fuadin)	Vomiting, diarrhea, fall in blood pressure, respiratory depression, sensitivity reactions, liver damage. Contraindicated in liver, kidney, or pulmonary disease.	Reduce dosage or discontinue use.
Stilbamidine isethionate and hydroxystilbamidine	Transitory fall in blood pressure, rapid pulse, dizziness, nausea, vomiting. Trigeminal nerve damage, liver or kidney damage from old solutions. Not used in liver or kidney disease.	Use only fresh solutions.
Suramin (Naphuride)	Kidney and liver damage, hemolysis, fever.	Discontinue use or reduce dosage.
Thiabendazole (Mintezol)	Vomiting, nausea, dizziness, anorexia, abdominal pain, constipation or diarrhea, headache, skin eruptions, CNS depression, and, rarely, crystalluria.	Discontinue use or reduce dosage.
Thiosemicarbazone	Liver damage, skin eruptions, anemia, leukopenia.	Reduce dosage or discontinue use.
Tolnaftate (Tinactin)	Mild irritation and, rarely, sensitization.	Discontinue use.
Trifluridine (Viroptic)	Increased intraocular pressure, corneal damage.	Discontinue use.
Trimethoprim (Proloprim)	Itching, rash, gastrointestinal distress, anemia, leukopenia, thrombocytopenia, methemoglobinemia, possible renal impairment.	Discontinue use.
Vidarabine (Vira-A)	Gastrointestinal disturbances, tremor, confusion, psychosis, ataxia, anemia, leukopenia, thrombocytopenia, elevated liver enzymes and bilirubin, corneal changes, sensitivity reactions.	Discontinue use.

of retinal vessels, and papilledema. Late findings include constriction of visual fields.

2. Quinacrine causes headache, hepatitis, aplastic anemia, psychosis, and jaundice.

3. Chloroquine causes diarrhea, nausea, headache, deafness, dizziness, porphyria, muscular weakness, blurred vision from corneal lesions, lens opacities, and retinal damage, including macular degeneration. Retinal damage is usually irreversible. Fetal injury has also been reported.

C. Laboratory Findings: The urine may contain red blood cells, protein, and casts. The pseudoisochromatic color vision plate (Hardy-Rand-Rittler) can be used as a screening test for the early detection of retinopathy.

Treatment

A. Acute Poisoning:

1. Emergency measures–Maintain respiration. Remove swallowed drug by gastric lavage or emesis (see pp 21–28). Treat blood pressure fall by injection of norepinephrine. Treat cardiac arrhythmias (see pp 378–382).

2. General measures–If urine secretion is adequate, give 2–4 L of fluids daily to promote renal excretion. Acidify urine with 0.5 g of ascorbic acid every 4 hours. Exchange transfusion may be useful.

3. Special problems–Treat anuria (see p 72).

B. Chronic Poisoning: No treatment appears to be effective for quinine amblyopia.

Prognosis

If the patient lives for 48 hours, recovery is likely. Retinal damage from quinine or chloroquine is likely to be permanent, but other adverse effects are reversible.

Boland ME et al: Complications of quinine poisoning. *Lancet* 1985;**1**:384.

Heath A et al: Resin hemoperfusion in chloroquine poisoning. *J Toxicol Clin Toxicol* 1982;**19**:1067.

Morgan MDL et al: The treatment of quinine poisoning with charcoal hemoperfusion. *Postgrad Med J* 1983;**59**:365.

ISONIAZID

Isoniazid (INH) is used in the treatment of tuberculosis, and patients are often given a supply adequate for several months.

At least some of its toxicity results from relative pyridoxine deficiency induced by isoniazid. Long-term treatment carries a risk of liver damage, especially in patients over 50 years of age.

Pathologic findings in deaths from isoniazid include liver damage with multilobular necrosis.

Clinical Findings

The principal manifestation of acute isoniazid poisoning is convulsions.

A. Acute Poisoning: (From ingestion.) Nausea and vomiting, disorientation, lethargy, psychotic behavior, increased reflexes, acidosis, restlessness, muscle twitching, urinary retention, convulsions, coma, cardiorespiratory depression. Hemolysis may occur in patients with glucose 6-phosphate dehydrogenase deficiency.

B. Chronic Poisoning: (From ingestion.) Peripheral neuropathy and jaundice occur often with long-term administration. The risk of liver damage increases with age.

C. Laboratory Findings:

1. Hyperglycemia, reduced blood bicarbonate level, reduced arterial pH.

2. Abnormal liver function tests.

Prevention

Isoniazid should only be dispensed in child-resistant containers. The daily dose should not exceed 10 mg/kg or a total of 300 mg. Each 100 mg of isoniazid should be supplemented with 10 mg of pyridoxine. Patients on long-term therapy should have monthly SGOT determinations and should be warned to see the physician at the first sign of liver toxicity.

Treatment

A. Acute Poisoning:

1. Emergency measures–Remove ingested isoniazid with emesis or gastric lavage using activated charcoal (see p 21–28).

2. Antidote–Give pyridoxine, 5 g intravenously, to control convulsions; repeat as necessary. The amount of pyridoxine given should at least equal the amount of isoniazid ingested.

3. General measures–

a. Control convulsions with diazepam or phenytoin (see p 53).

b. Dialysis or hemoperfusion is probably not useful.

B. Chronic Poisoning:

1. Treat liver damage (see p 77).

2. Give pyridoxine, 5 g daily.

Prognosis

Patients who survive for 24 hours after acute overdoses will recover completely. In patients who were receiving long-term isoniazid therapy that was discontinued when SGOT levels reached 5 times normal, liver damage was not irreversible.

Brown A: Acute isoniazid intoxication: Reversal of CNS symptoms with large doses of pyridoxine. *Pediatr Pharmacol* 1984;**4**:199.

O'Brien RJ et al: Hepatotoxicity from isoniazid and rifampin among children treated for tuberculosis. *Pediatrics* 1983;**72**:491.

Pellock JM et al: Pyridoxine deficiency in children treated with isoniazid. *Chest* 1985;**87**:658.

Rubin DH et al: Chronic isoniazid poisoning. *Clin Pediatr* 1983;**22**:518.

Wason S et al: Single high-dose pyridoxine treatment for isoniazid overdose. *JAMA* 1981;**246**:1102.

Yarbrough BE, Wood JP: Isoniazid overdose treated with high-dose pyridoxine. *Ann Emerg Med* 1983;**12**:303.

INTERACTIONS
(See p 17.)

Allopurinol increases the risk of ampicillin rash.

Tetracyclines increase renal toxicity of methoxyflurane.

Furosemide and ethacrynic acid increase nephrotoxicity of cephalosporins and ototoxicity of aminoglycosides. Aminoglycosides enhance nephrotoxicity of cephalosporins.

Sulfisoxazole potentiates thiopental. Sulfonamides potentiate the effects of warfarin, tolbutamide, chlorpropamide, and phenytoin by displacement from protein binding sites. Sulfonamides displace bilirubin from plasma protein binding and drive it into tissues, with increased brain injury in newborn infants (kernicterus).

Quinacrine displaces pamaquine from tissue binding sites and increases pamaquine plasma levels up to 5-fold.

Combination of p-aminosalicylate and salicylates gives a mutual increase of toxicity.

Ethanol increases the toxicity of cycloserine.

Aminoglycosides can induce prolonged hypotension during anesthesia.

PHARMACOKINETICS & TOXIC CONCENTRATIONS
(See p 89.)

	pK_a	$t_{1/2}$	V_d	% Binding
Amantidine		9–15		
Amikacin		2–3	0.2–0.3	10
Amoxicillin		1	0.2	17
Amphotericin B		24	4	90
Ampicillin	2.5, 7.2	1–1.5, 2*	0.39	23
Benzylpenicillin	2.8	0.5	0.3	65
Carbenicillin	3.3	1–1.5	0.17	50
Cefalexin	2.5, 7.3	0.5–1	0.23	15
Cefazolin		1.75–2	0.14	84
Cephaloridine		1–1.5	0.23	20
Cephalothin	2.5	0.5–1	0.26	50
Cephapirin		0.6	0.14	44–50
Cephradine	2.6, 7.3	0.7	0.29	10
Chloramphenicol		2.1–8.3	1.4	25–60
Chloroquine	8.4, 10.8	72		55
Clindamycin	7.45	2–4	0.5,* 1.14	94
Cloxacillin	2.7	0.5	0.34	95
Colistimethate		3–8	0.54	50
Dapsone	1.2	17–21		72–80
Dicloxacillin	2.7	0.5	0.29	98
Doxycycline		12–20		
Erythromycin	8.8	1.4	0.57	73
Ethambutol		4–6		
Floxacillin	2.7	0.8		95
Flucytosine		3–8		
Fusidic acid	5.35	4.8–16.5	0.08–0.24	97
Gentamicin†	8.2	2.3	0.28, 0.56*	70–80
Griseofulvin		22		
Isoniazid	3.5	0.5–1.5‡	0.9	
Kanamycin	7.2	1.5–3.2	0.19, 0.8*	0–3
Lincomycin	7.6	4.6–5.6	0.49	72
Methenamine		2–6		
Methicillin	2.8	0.5	0.9	37
Metronidazole		6–14		
Nafcillin	2.7	0.5	0.63	90
Nalidixic acid	6.7	1.1–2.5	0.26–0.45	93–97
Neomycin		3		
Nitrofurantoin	7.2	0.3–0.6		25–60
Oxacillin	2.9	0.5	0.41	94
Penicillin G		0.5		
Phenoxymethylpenicillin	2.7	0.5	0.73	79
Polymyxin B		4.4		
Pyrimethamine	7.2	96		

*For children.
†The toxic concentration for gentamicin is 10 μg/mL; for tetracycline, 16 μg/mL.
‡Slow acetylators, 2–4.

	pK$_a$	t½	V$_d$	% Binding
Quinacrine	7.7, 10.3	120		90
Quinine	4.3, 8.4	8.5		90
Rifampin		1.5–5		
Spectinomycin		1.7		
Streptomycin		2–3	0.26	20–30
Sulfamethoxazole	5.7	8–11	0.17	62
Sulfasalazine	0.6–11	6–10		99
Sulfisoxazole		5–7		
Tetracycline†	7.7	9–11	2.5–4	
Tobramycin		2–3	0.31	70–80
Trimethoprim		6–17		
Vancomycin		6–8		

†The toxic concentration for gentamicin is 10 µg/mL; for tetracycline, 16 µg/mL.

References

Adverse reactions to Fansidar and updated recommendations for its use in the prevention of malaria. *MMWR* 1984;**33:**713.

Bailes J et al: Encephalopathy with metronidazole in a child. *Am J Dis Child* 1983;**137:**290.

Basinger MA et al: Antidotes for acute bismuth intoxication. *J Toxicol Clin Toxicol* 1983;**20:**159.

Derbes SJ: Trimethoprim-induced aseptic meningitis. *JAMA* 1984;**252:**2865.

Meisel S: Severe bleeding diathesis associated with moxalactam administration. *Drug Intell Clin Pharm* 1984;**18:**721.

Penn RG, Griffin JP: Adverse reactions to nitrofurantoin in the United Kingdom, Sweden, and Holland. *Br Med J* 1982;**284:**1440.

Sartori M, Pratt CM, Young JB: Torsade de Pointe: Malignant cardiac arrhythmia induced by amantadine poisoning. *Am J Med* 1984;**77:**388.

Selby CD et al: Fatal multisystemic toxicity associated with prophylaxis with pyrimethamine and sulfadoxine (Fansidar). *Br Med J* 1985;**290:**113.

Shann F: Co-trimoxazole toxicity. *Lancet* 1984;**2:**1477.

Stimulants, Antidepressants, & Psychotomimetic Agents | 28

MONOAMINE OXIDASE INHIBITORS: IPRONIAZID & RELATED DRUGS

Tranylcypromine (Parnate) and phenelzine (Nardil) are used in the treatment of depression. Pargyline (Eutonyl) is used in the treatment of hypertension. Iproniazid, isocarboxazid, pheniprazine, and nialamide are no longer marketed in the USA because of toxicity.

Deaths have occurred with single doses of 25–100 mg/kg, and as little as 50 mg/d has caused fatal liver necrosis. The incidence of symptomatic liver damage from iproniazid has been about 0.1%. Following the ingestion of large doses, the immediate effects result from central nervous system stimulation, whereas the most serious delayed effect is jaundice from acute liver necrosis.

These compounds are all monoamine oxidase inhibitors (MAOI), and they greatly potentiate the action of compounds such as sympathomimetic amines, barbiturates, meperidine, aminopyrine, and possibly morphine.

Clinical Findings

The principal manifestations of poisoning are stimulation and jaundice.

A. Acute Poisoning: Overdose causes dry mouth, ataxia, stupor, excitement, rise or fall of blood pressure, fever, tachycardia, precordial pain, acidosis, and convulsions. Death occurs from respiratory and circulatory failure.

B. Chronic Poisoning: Repeated administration of any of these drugs causes dizziness, weakness, ataxia, hallucinations, mania, psychopathologic behavior, hyperirritability, constipation, dry mouth, urine retention, and excessive rise or fall of blood pressure. Iproniazid and pheniprazine may cause liver injury at any time during drug therapy. Symptoms begin with nausea and lethargy; rapid progression of liver damage is indicated by intractable vomiting. Pheniprazine has caused impaired vision from bilateral optic tract lesions. Combinations of these drugs or these drugs combined with others such as imipramine

(Tofranil) or opium derivatives have been more likely to cause extreme reactions, including fatal hyperpyrexia. Tranylcypromine, phenelzine, and related drugs have caused severe hypertension following the ingestion of cheese, beer, and wine, which contain sympathomimetic amines, and drugs such as meperidine and amphetamine.

C. Laboratory Findings: Hepatic cell injury is indicated by appropriate tests (see p 75).

Prevention

Drugs with a significant record of hepatic damage should not be used over prolonged periods without close supervision. Avoid administration of these drugs with imipramine or other stimulant drugs.

Treatment

A. Emergency Measures:

1. Remove ingested drugs by gastric lavage and emesis (see pp 21–28).

2. If respiration is depressed, give artificial respiration.

3. Maintain blood pressure (see p 66).

4. Control convulsions by cautious administration of diazepam slowly intravenously (see Table 4–3). Use drugs cautiously to prevent possible hyperreactions. *Do not give stimulants or pressor amines.* Blockade with propranolol has been suggested.

B. General Measures: Discontinue drug at the first appearance of jaundice. Treat liver damage (see p 77). Dialysis is reported to be effective. Pyridoxine, 200 mg slowly intravenously, has been suggested. Control of acidosis may require sodium bicarbonate, up to 3 meq/kg/h.

Prognosis

The fatality rate in acute poisoning has been 1%. About 25% of patients with severe liver damage have died.

Linden CH, Rumach BH, Strehlke C: Monoamine oxidase inhibitor overdose. *Ann Emerg Med* 1984;**13**:1137.
Smookler S, Bermudez AJ: Hypertensive crisis resulting from an MAO inhibitor and over-the-counter appetite suppressant. *Ann Emerg Med* 1982;**11**:482.

CAFFEINE & THEOPHYLLINE

Caffeine, theophylline, and the derivatives dyphylline and pentoxifylline (Trental) are used for the treatment of shock, asthma, and heart disease and as diuretics.

Fatalities have resulted from 0.1 g of aminophylline (theophylline ethylenediamine) intravenously, 25–100 mg/kg by rectal suppository, or as little as 8.4 mg/kg orally in a child. At least 4 deaths have followed the repeated use of aminophylline rectal suppositories in children. Fatalities from caffeine, 183–250 mg/kg, have been reported.

Injection of aminophylline in hypersensitive subjects causes immediate vasomotor collapse and death. Rapid intravenous injection of aminophylline apparently causes cardiac inhibition.

In large doses, aminophylline depresses the central nervous system, whereas caffeine stimulates it.

The pathologic findings are not characteristic.

Clinical Findings

The principal manifestations of poisoning with these drugs are collapse and blood pressure fall.

A. Acute Poisoning: Intravenous administration of aminophylline is sometimes followed by sudden collapse and death within 1–2 minutes. Oral theophylline can cause vomiting, coma, hyperreflexia, ventricular arrhythmias including fibrillation, hypotension, convulsions, and respiratory arrest. Repeated rectal administration of aminophylline to infants may cause severe vomiting, collapse and death. Doses of caffeine up to 10 g orally have caused gastric irritation, vomiting, and convulsions; complete recovery occurred in 6 hours.

B. Chronic Poisoning: Repeated doses of caffeine or theophylline and its salts orally, intravenously, or rectally may cause restlessness, epigastric pain, headache, nausea and vomiting, fever, agitation, tachycardia, arrhythmias, hyperventilation, convulsions, and respiratory failure. Caffeine withdrawal may cause headache.

C. Laboratory Findings: Urinalysis may reveal proteinuria.

Prevention

Test the sensitivity of the patient to intravenous aminophylline by giving 0.1 mL intravenously and waiting 1 minute. The rate of injection should not exceed 4 mg/kg every 12 hours, especially in infants. The serum concentration of theophylline should not exceed 20 μg/mL.

Treatment

A. Emergency Measures:

1. Remove ingested drugs by emesis or gastric lavage using activated charcoal whether or not vomiting has occurred (see pp 21–28).

2. Give O_2 by pressure mask.

3. Maintain blood pressure by administration of fluids. Norepinephrine is the safest pressor drug. Other pressor agents may induce cardiac arrhythmias.

4. Remove rectally administered aminophylline by enema.

B. General Measures: Control convulsions by intravenous administration of diazepam (see Table 4–3). Treat dehydration by administration of normal saline or 5% dextrose in water. Charcoal hemoperfusion removes these drugs more effectively than does peritoneal dialysis; the effectiveness of peritoneal dialysis can be increased by adding red blood cells to the dialysate.

Prognosis

About 50% of patients with convulsions after theophylline administration have died. Convulsions after caffeine are less likely to be fatal.

Clancy RR et al: Neonatal theophylline neurotoxicity. *Clin Pediatr* 1985;**24:**168.

Gal P et al: Oral activated charcoal to enhance theophylline elimination in an acute overdose. *JAMA* 1984;**251:**3130.

Greenberg A et al: Severe theophylline toxicity: Role of conservative measures, antiarrhythmic agents, and charcoal hemoperfusion. *Am J Med* 1984;**76:**854.

Levine JH et al: Multifocal atrial tachycardia: A toxic effect of theophylline. *Lancet* 1985;**1:**12.

Parish RA et al: Interaction of theophylline with erythromycin base in a patient with seizure activity. *Pediatrics* 1983;**72:**828.

Park GD et al: Use of hemoperfusion for theophylline intoxication. *Am J Med* 1983;**74:**961.

Powell JR et al: Inhibition of theophylline clearance by cimetidine but not ranitidine. *Arch Intern Med* 1984;**144:**484.

Shaul PW et al: Caffeine toxicity as a cause of acute psychosis in anorexia nervosa. *J Pediatr* 1984;**105:**493.

Woo OF et al: Benefit of hemoperfusion in acute theophylline intoxication. *J Toxicol Clin Toxicol* 1984;**22:**411.

STRYCHNINE

Strychnine is an important component of various tonics and cathartic pills and is used as a rodenticide. Castrix, which has been used as a rodenticide, is as toxic as strychnine and has similar effects. Derivatives of strychnine and related compounds, such as N-oxystrychnic acid and brucine, have been used as stimulants.

The fatal dose of strychnine is 15–30 mg. The exposure limit for strychnine is 0.15 mg/m^3.

Strychnine causes greatly increased reflex excitability in the spinal cord; this results in a loss of the normal inhibition of spread of motor cell stimulation, so that all muscles contract simultaneously.

Rigor mortis sets in almost immediately after death. Other pathologic findings are not characteristic.

Clinical Findings

The principal manifestation of acute strychnine poisoning is convulsions. Doses less than necessary to cause acute poisoning are without toxic effect.

A. Acute Poisoning: After ingestion, strychnine and related compounds and derivatives cause first an increase in deep reflexes followed by noticeable stiffening at the knees, especially when going up and down stairs; single extensor spasms then involve the arms and legs. As poisoning progresses, spasms increase in severity and frequency until the patient is in almost continuous opisthotonos. Any sound or movement will elicit a spasm. Death is from respiratory failure.

B. Laboratory Findings: Strychnine can be identified in gastric washings or vomitus by appropriate tests. Arterial pH and serum potassium concentrations should be determined.

Prevention

Strychnine rodent baits are extremely dangerous. The use of strychnine in remedies should be discontinued.

Treatment

A. Emergency Measures: Give artificial respiration with O_2 during convulsions. After convulsions and hyperactivity are controlled, remove strychnine by gastric lavage using activated charcoal (see pp 21–28).

B. General Measures: If symptoms have begun, avoid any manipulation such as gastric lavage or emesis. Enforce absolute quiet and absence of stimuli. Control convulsions by the administration of succinylcholine (see Table 4–3). Give diazepam, 0.05–0.1 mg/kg slowly intravenously, and repeat every 30 minutes as necessary. Phenytoin may also be useful. Saline diuresis has been suggested. Administration of 100–200 mmol of sodium bicarbonate and 100–200 mmol of potassium may be necessary to control acidosis and hypokalemia.

Prognosis

If the patient lives for 24 hours, recovery is probable.

Decker WJ et al: Two deaths resulting from apparent parenteral injection of strychnine. *Vet Hum Toxicol* 1982;**24**:161.

CAMPHOR

Camphor is used in certain moth-damage preventives and in camphorated oil as a respiratory aid and stimulant. The fatal dose of camphor is approximately 1 g for a 1-year-old child. This amount of camphor is contained in 5 mL of camphorated oil or 20 mL of Vicks Vaporub. At least 12 fatal cases of camphor poisoning have occurred. The exposure limit for camphor is 2 ppm. Camphor causes convulsions by stimulating the cells of the cerebral cortex.

The pathologic findings include congestion and edematous changes in the gastrointestinal tract, kidneys, and brain.

Clinical Findings

The principal manifestation of acute camphor poisoning is convulsions.

After ingestion, symptoms are burning in the mouth and throat, epigastric pain, thirst, nausea and vomiting, feeling of tension, dizziness, irrational behavior, unconsciousness, rigidity, rapid pulse, slow respiration, twitching of facial muscles, muscular spasms, and generalized convulsions. Poisoning has also occurred after intramuscular injection.

Treatment

A. Emergency Measures: Establish airway and maintain respiration. After convulsions are controlled, remove swallowed poison by airway-protected gastric lavage followed by 30–60 mL of Fleet's Phospho-Soda diluted 1:4 in water (see pp 21–28).

B. General Measures: Control convulsions with diazepam or succinylcholine (see Table 4–3).

Prognosis

If the patient lives for 24 hours, recovery will probably occur.

PICROTOXIN, PENTYLENETETRAZOL, & NIKETHAMIDE

Picrotoxin is a nonnitrogenous compound of known structure obtained from cocculus indicus (fish berries), the berry of *Anamirta cocculus,* an East Indian plant. Poisoning has occurred from adulteration of beverages with cocculus indicus.

Nikethamide (Coramine) and pentylenetetrazol (Metrazol) are synthetic chemicals. Pentylenetetrazol is no longer available in the USA.

The fatal convulsive dose of picrotoxin may be as low as 20 mg. The fatal dose of cocculus indicus (fish berries) may be as low as 0.5 g. In the treatment of drug-induced coma in which the convulsive threshold is raised, doses of picrotoxin over 300 mg in 24 hours are likely to induce severe toxic manifestations other than convulsions. The fatal dose of pentylenetetrazole may be as low as 1 g. The maximum dose should be limited to 6 g in 24 hours. The fatal dose of nikethamide has not been established.

Picrotoxin, pentylenetetrazol, and nikethamide stimulate the spinal cord, medulla, and cerebral cortex. The action persists with picrotoxin for 12–24 hours; with pentylenetetrazol, from 5 minutes to 3 hours; with nikethamide, from 5 to 60 minutes.

The pathologic findings in fatal cases consist of congestion of all organs.

Clinical Findings

The principal manifestation of acute poisoning is convulsions. Chronic poisoning has not been reported.

Serious poisoning from therapeutic administration has only occurred after injection. Picrotoxin in fish berries can be absorbed after ingestion. Symptoms and signs include nausea and vomiting, increased respiration, headache, twitching, convulsions, and coma. The stimulant effect of picrotoxin begins about 20 minutes after injection, reaches a maximum in about 1 hour, and persists for 6–24 hours. Stimulation following the use of pentylenetetrazol and nikethamide begins almost immediately after injection; the maximum effect is reached in 5–10 minutes and persists up to 3 hours.

When picrotoxin, pentylenetetrazol, or nikethamide is used in the treatment of drug-induced coma, the dose necessary to produce stimulation is greatly increased. For this reason, the large amount given to awaken the patient may cause undesirable toxic effects such as hyperthermia, cardiac irregularities, anuria, cerebral injury, pulmonary edema, and liver injury. These effects have occurred most frequently after administration of picrotoxin, but they also occur after use of pentylenetetrazol and nikethamide.

Convulsions occurring during the use of these stimulants in the treatment of drug-induced coma may be followed by severe central nervous system depression.

Prevention

Sale of cocculus indicus (fish berries) should be strictly controlled. Picrotoxin, pentylenetetrazol, and nikethamide are too dangerous to be used therapeutically.

Treatment

A. Emergency Measures:

1. Establish airway and maintain respiration.

2. Delay absorption of ingested poison by giving activated charcoal; then remove by gastric lavage (see pp 21–28).

3. Slow absorption of poison injected intramuscularly or subcutaneously by application of ice packs and tourniquet (see p 28).

B. General Measures:

1. Treat convulsions. Give diazepam, 2–10 mg intravenously at a rate not greater than 1 mg/min. Other anticonvulsants can also be tried (see Table 4–3).

2. Treat hyperthermia by application of wet towels.
3. Treat anuria (see p 72).
4. Treat pulmonary edema (see p 65).

Prognosis

Convulsions occurring during picrotoxin, pentylenetetrazol, or nikethamide treatment of drug-induced depression are followed by additive depression, frequently with fatal outcome. Hyperthermia and cardiac arrhythmias occurring during picrotoxin, pentylenetetrazol, or nikethamide therapy are also frequently fatal.

POLYCYCLIC ANTIDEPRESSANTS: AMITRIPTYLINE, IMIPRAMINE, & RELATED DRUGS

Amitriptyline (Elavil), imipramine (Tofranil), desipramine (Norpramin, Pertofrane), protriptyline (Vivactil), doxepin (Sinequan), cyclobenzaprine (Flexeril), trimipramine (Surmontil), and nortriptyline (Aventyl) are related drugs used as antidepressants.

Deaths have occurred following doses of imipramine of 5 g in adults, as little as 250 mg in a 2-year-old child, and 500–750 mg in a 16-year-old child. In a 1-year-old child, 1 g of amitriptyline was fatal, and 1.5 g of desipramine was fatal in a 4-year-old child. In general, doses over 30 mg/kg are dangerous to life.

These compounds block parasympathetic responses, and their effects are potentiated by monoamine oxidase inhibitors (see p 415).

Clinical Findings

The principal manifestations of poisoning with these drugs are central nervous system stimulation and cardiac arrhythmias.

A. Acute Poisoning: Overdoses cause coma, hypothermia, clonic movements or convulsions, fall of blood pressure, respiration depression, mydriasis, and disturbances of cardiac rhythm and conduction. These cardiac disturbances can include sinus tachycardia, cardiac ischemia, multifocal extrasystoles, wandering pacemaker, and various degrees of atrioventricular or intraventricular block. Ventricular fibrillation immediately precedes death and may occur after apparent recovery.

B. Chronic Poisoning: Dryness of the mouth, drowsiness, blurred vision, skin eruptions, excitement, excessive sweating, constipation, urine retention, hypotension, tachycardia, increased intraocular pressure, jaundice with acute liver necrosis, tremors, cardiac arrhythmias, paresthesias, confusion, restlessness, abdominal pain, anxiety, and ataxia. Lethargy, convulsions, activation of schizophrenic symptoms, leukopenia, and purpura have occurred rarely. Renal damage has been reported after imipramine, and pulmonary consolidation has been reported after amitriptyline. Abrupt withdrawal can precipitate psychosis.

C. Laboratory Findings: The ECG may reveal atrioventricular or intraventricular block, prolonged PR and QT intervals, widened QRS complex, flat or inverted T wave, supraventricular or ventricular tachycardia, and ventricular fibrillation or asystole.

Prevention

These drugs should not be used in conjunction with monoamine oxidase inhibitors (see p 415) or other drugs. If a change from one type of drug to another is contemplated, at least 2 weeks must elapse between the administration of the 2 drugs.

Treatment

A. Emergency Measures: (Observe all patients with a history of ingestion for 6 hours.)

1. Establish airway and maintain respiration. Monitor ECG until the patient is free of arrhythmia for 24 hours.

2. Remove ingested drug by gastric lavage after giving activated charcoal (see pp 21–28).

3. Maintain blood pressure by giving fluid (see p 66). Transfusion of whole blood, up to 20 mL/kg in the first 2 hours, may be necessary to maintain blood pressure. Avoid vasoconstrictor agents.

Table 28—1. Miscellaneous stimulants and antidepressants.

Drug	Clinical Findings	Treatment
Amiphenazole	Convulsions.	Reduce dosage.
Amoxapine (Asendin)	Anxiety, insomnia, confusion, nausea, atrial flutter.	Reduce dosage.
Doxapram (Dopram)	Clonus, muscle spasticity, hyperpyrexia, carpopedal spasm, seizures, hypertension, nausea, vomiting.	Discontinue use.
Ethamivan (Emivan)	Sneezing, generalized pruritus, muscular twitching, excitation, restlessness.	Reduce dosage or discontinue drug.
Flurothyl (Indoklon)	Memory loss, fractures, prolonged apnea, small cardiac infarcts, or cardiac arrhythmias.	Reduce dosage.
Histamine	Headache, fall of blood pressure, nausea, abdominal pain, asthma.	Give diphenhydramine, 50 mg IM.
Maprotiline (Ludiomil)	Hyperirritability, convulsions, anticholinergic effects, confusion, arrhythmias, heart block.	Reduce dosage.
Trazodone (Desyrel)	Drowsiness, dizziness, gastrointestinal distress, bradycardia, hypotension, arrhythmias, possible liver impairment.	Discontinue use.

4. Control convulsions by giving diazepam, 0.05–1.0 mg/kg slowly intravenously. Diazepam is currently preferred for initial management of convulsions. Succinylcholine administration with control of respiration may be necessary.

5. Control arrhythmias by giving phenytoin, 0.5 mg/kg/min intravenously up to a total of 5 mg/kg. Administration of sodium bicarbonate, 2–3 meq/kg, in glucose solution to keep the serum pH above 7.40–7.45 may also be effective against arrhythmias. The use of physostigmine, quinidine, procainamide, disopyramide, corticosteroids, propranolol, or atropine can be hazardous. Ventricular pacing may be necessary.

B. General Measures: Osmotic diuresis and dialysis are not effective. Treat cardiac arrest (see p 69).

Prognosis

Patients have died as late as 72 hours after ingestion of an overdose.

Callaham M et al: Epidemiology of fatal tricyclic antidepressant ingestion: Implications for management. *Ann Emerg Med* 1985;**14**:1.

Hodes D: Sodium bicarbonate and hyperventilation in treating an infant with severe overdose of tricyclic antidepressant. *Br Med J* 1984;**288**:1800.

Hulten B-A, Heath A: Clinical aspects of tricyclic antidepressant poisoning. *Acta Med Scand* 1983;**213**:275.

Linden CH: Cyclobenzaprine overdosage. *J Toxicol Clin Toxicol* 1983;**20**:281.

Lum BKB et al: Experimental studies on the effects of physostigmine and of isoproterenol on the toxicity produced by tricyclic antidepressant agents. *J Toxicol Clin Toxicol* 1982;**19**:51.

Pentel PR et al: Hemoperfusion for imipramine overdose: Elimination of active metabolites. *J Toxicol Clin Toxicol* 1982;**19**:239.

Rudorfer MV: Cardiovascular changes and plasma drug levels after amitriptyline overdose. *J Toxicol Clin Toxicol* 1982;**19**:67.

PHENCYCLIDINE

Phencyclidine (PCP) has become one of the most common street drugs. It occurs under a variety of street names or is misrepresented as other psychotomimetic agents.

The fatal dose is about 1 mg/kg in adults. Children are more susceptible. Several deaths have occurred.

Phencyclidine is related to the anesthetic agent ketamine and, like ketamine, has both excitatory and depressant effects. Symptoms may persist for several days, with a cyclic course resulting from excretion of the drug into the stomach and reabsorption from the intestine.

Pathologic findings are not contributory.

Clinical Findings

The principal manifestations of serious phencyclidine poisoning are psychosis, convulsions, and respiratory depression.

A. Acute Poisoning: Doses under 5 mg in adults cause hyperactivity, rigidity, peripheral anesthesia, nystagmus, incoordination, and wild movements. Doses of 5–10 mg cause stupor or coma, fever, muscle rigidity, and salivation. Doses over 10 mg cause, in addition, hypertension, convulsions, decreased or absent reflexes, laryngeal stridor, respiratory depression, hyperthermia, and sweating. Acute rhabdomyolysis may occur.

B. Laboratory Findings: The EEG reveals a slowed delta rhythm and rhythmic to dysrrhythmic theta activity at doses above 10 mg. Fatalities have occurred at drug blood levels above 2 $\mu g/mL$. Renal shutdown may occur as a result of myoglobin release.

Treatment

A. Emergency Measures: In the presence of respiratory difficulty, intubate the trachea and maintain respiration. Remove the drug by gastric lavage and administration of a saline cathartic (30 mL of Fleet's Phospho-Soda diluted to 200 mL). Activated charcoal is useful.

B. General Measures:

1. Monitor vital signs, prevent injuries, restrict sensory input, and maintain gastric suction except for 1 hour after each administration of oral drugs.

2. In patients with coma, convulsions, or respiratory depression, maintain respiration. Control convulsions by giving diazepam, 2–5 mg slowly intravenously. Repeat every 30 minutes as necessary.

3. In the presence of myoglobinuria, maintain urine volume with intravenous fluids and mannitol. Alkalinization of the urine with sodium bicarbonate will minimize deposition of myoglobin in the kidney.

Prognosis

Patients ordinarily recover consciousness in 24–48 hours, but a week may be necessary for complete recovery.

Aniline O, Pitts FN Jr: Phencyclidine (PCP): A review and perspectives. *CRC Crit Rev Toxicol* 1982;**10**:145.

Budd RD, Lindstrom DM: Characteristics of victims of PCP-related deaths in Los Angeles County. *J Toxicol Clin Toxicol* 1982;**19**:997.

Giannini AJ et al: Comparison of chlorpromazine, haloperidol, and pimozide in the treatment of phencyclidine psychosis. *J Toxicol Clin Toxicol* 1984;**22**:573.

Patel R: Acute uric acid nephropathy: A complication of phencyclidine intoxication. *Postgrad Med J* 1982;**58**:783.

PSYCHOTOMIMETIC AGENTS

Psychotomimetic agents can be classified as follows:

(1) LSD (lysergic acid diethylamide): Semisynthetic, from ergot.

(2) DMT (dimethyltryptamine): Synthetic and from a South American plant *(Piptadenia peregrina)*.

(3) DET (diethyltryptamine): Synthetic.

(4) "STP," DOM (2,5-dimethoxy-4-methylamphetamine): Synthetic.

(5) MDA (methylene dioxyamphetamine): Synthetic.

(6) MDMA, Ecstasy (3,4-methylene dioxymethamphetamine): Synthetic.

(7) Psilocybin and psilocin: Derivatives of 4-hydroxytryptamine. Synthetic; also from a mushroom *(Psilocybe mexicana)*.

(8) Bufotenine (dimethyl serotonin): Synthetic; also from *Piptadenia peregrina, Amanita muscaria,* and the skin of a toad *(Bufo marinus)*.

(9) Ibogaine: From the plant *Tabernanthe iboga*.

(10) Harmine and harmaline: From plants *(Peganum harmala* and *Banisteria caapi)*.

(11) Ditran: Synthetic.

(12) Marihuana: From the plant *Cannabis sativa*.

(13) Mescal (peyote): From the plant *Lophophora williamsii*. Contains mescaline; also available in synthetic form.

(See also Amphetamine, p 347.)

Clinical Findings

Manifestations requiring medical intervention are hyperexcitability, uncontrollability, ataxia, hypertension or hypotension, convulsions, coma, and prolonged psychotic states. In addition, LSD causes mydriasis, tremor, exaggerated reflexes, fever, psychopathic personality disorders, increased homicidal or suicidal risk, and prolonged mental dissociation.

Treatment

Give diazepam, 0.1 mg/kg orally, to control excitement or convulsions. Treat coma as for barbiturate poisoning.

Burns RS et al: The clinical syndrome of striatal dopamine deficiency: Parkinsonism induced by 1-methyl-4-phenyl-1,2,3,6-tetrahydropyridine (MPTP). *N Engl J Med* 1985;**312**:1418.

Carney MWP et al: Psychosis after *Cannabis* abuse. *Br Med J* 1984;**288**:1047.

Mercieca J, Brown EA: Acute renal failure due to rhabdomyolysis associated with use of a straitjacket in lysergide intoxication. *Br Med J* 1984;**288**:1949.

Urine testing for detection of marihuana: An advisory. *MMWR* 1983;**32**:469.

INTERACTIONS
(See p 17.)

The risk of paralytic ileus and central nervous system depression from tricyclic antidepressants is increased by ethanol.

Blood levels of and possible toxicity from tricyclic antidepressants are also increased by the use of aspirin, chloramphenicol, haloperidol, chlorpromazine, perphenazine, and diazepam.

The risk of cardiac arrhythmias from tricyclic antidepressants is increased by the presence of levodopa, guanethidine, bethanidine, and debrisoquine and by prior administration of thyroid hormone. The effect of nortriptyline is enhanced by hydrocortisone and perphenazine. Amitriptyline increases absorption of coumarin anticoagulants.

Tricyclic antidepressants are atropinelike and quinidinelike and potentiate hypotensive effects of quinidine and other hypotensive agents. Tricyclics alter catecholamine levels in the brain and interact dangerously with monoamine oxidase inhibitors.

If given with tricyclic antidepressants, meperidine, or furazolidone, monoamine oxidase inhibitors cause agitation, tremor, pyrexia, and coma.

Monoamine oxidase inhibitors can potentiate anesthetic and pressor agents.

In the presence of monoamine oxidase inhibitors or isoniazid, tyramine in beer, wine, cheese, and other fermented foods can cause hypertension. Monoamine oxidase inhibitors enhance the effects of hypoglycemic drugs.

PHARMACOKINETICS & TOXIC CONCENTRATIONS
(See p 89.)

	pK_a	$t_{1/2}$	V_d	% Binding	Toxic Concentration ($\mu g/mL$)
Amitriptyline	9.4	32–40		83–96	1
Caffeine		3			100*
Desipramine	9.5	12–54	22–59	73–92	1
Imipramine	9.5	8–16	20–40	75–95	1
Nortriptyline	9.7	15–90	20–57	90–94	1
Phencyclidine	8.6–9.4	48–168			0.02
Theophylline	8.75	3–7	0.33, 0.74†	15	20

*Fatal.
†For children.

References

Bergman RN et al: Cardiac toxicity associated with acute maprotiline self-poisoning. *Am J Emerg Med* 1984;**2**:144.

Curtis RA et al: Fatal maprotiline intoxication. *Drug Intell Clin Pharm* 1984;**18**:716.

Damlouji NF, Ferguson JM: Trazodone-induced delirium in bulimic patients. *Am J Psychiatry* 1984;**141**:434.

Knudsen K, Heath A: Effects of self-poisoning with maprotiline. *Br Med J* 1984;**288**:601.

Kulig K et al: Amoxapine overdose: Coma and seizures without cardiotoxic effects. *JAMA* 1982;**248**:1092.

Lesar T et al: Trazodone overdose. *Ann Emerg Med* 1983;**12**:221.

Litovitz TL, Troutman WG: Amoxapine overdose. *JAMA* 1983;**250**:1069.

Irritants & Rubefacients | 29

CANTHARIDIN

Cantharidin, the most important active principle of *Cantharis vesicatoria* (Spanish fly), is used as a skin irritant or vesicant and has an undeserved reputation as an aphrodisiac. The fatal dose may be as small as 10 mg. Cantharidin is an extremely potent irritant to all cells and tissues. The pathologic findings are necrosis of the esophageal and gastric mucosa and intense congestion of the genitourinary tract, with free blood in the renal pelves, ureters, and bladder. The cells of the renal tubules are damaged. Hemorrhagic changes are also found in the ovaries.

Clinical Findings
The principal manifestations of cantharidin poisoning are vomiting and collapse.

A. Acute Poisoning: (From ingestion or application to skin or mucous membranes.) Severe irritation of skin or mucous membranes with formation of bullae, abdominal pain, nausea, diarrhea, vomiting of blood, severe fall of blood pressure, hematuria, uremia, coma, and death in respiratory failure.

B. Chronic Poisoning: Repeated small amounts may cause the findings described for acute poisoning.

C. Laboratory Findings: Microscopic or gross hematuria, erythrocytosis, leukocytosis, and hemoglobinemia.

Prevention
As cantharidin has no use that cannot be achieved by less dangerous substances, it should not be prescribed or sold for any purpose.

Treatment
Remove swallowed poison by gastric lavage or emesis with activated charcoal (see p 21–28). Treat cardiovascular collapse and shock by blood transfusions and intravenous administration of saline (see p 66). Prevent renal damage by maintaining maximal diuresis with intravenous fluids, mannitol, and diuretics.

Prognosis

If the patient is asymptomatic at the end of 72 hours, recovery is likely. Death may occur, however, up to 1 week after poisoning.

METAL SALTS: ALUMINUM, COPPER, TIN, NICKEL, & ZINC SALTS

Salts of metals are used as astringents, deodorants, and antiseptics. The salts most used are copper sulfate ($CuSO_4$), zinc sulfate ($ZnSO_4$), aluminum acetate ($[CH_3COO]_3Al$), aluminum subacetate ($[CH_3COO]_2AlOH$), stannous chloride ($SnCl_2$), nickel ammonium sulfate ($NiSO_4[NH_4]_2SO_4$), potassium alum ($KAl[SO_4]_2$), aluminum chloride ($AlCl_3$), and ammonium alum ($NH_4Al[SO_4]_2$). Soluble salts with similar toxicities are formed by the action of acids on galvanized or copper-lined utensils. These salts are all water-soluble. Their precipitating effect on proteins forms the basis of their astringent and antiseptic effects. Zinc oxide, which is insoluble, has no acute toxicity. The exposure limit for these salts is 2 mg/m³.

Fatalities have been reported following the ingestion of 10 g of zinc or copper sulfate. No fatalities from aluminum salts have been reported in recent years, but excessive aluminum loading can occur as a result of dialysis, intravenous therapy, or administration of aluminum hydroxide in the presence of renal impairment.

The pathologic findings in deaths from astringent salts include hemorrhagic gastroenteritis and kidney and liver damage.

Clinical Findings

The principal manifestations of poisoning with metal salts are vomiting and collapse.

A. Acute Poisoning: (From ingestion.) Burning pain in the mouth and throat, vomiting, water or bloody diarrhea, tenesmus, retching, hemolysis, hematuria, anuria, liver damage with jaundice, hypotension, collapse, and convulsions. Hyperglycemia has been reported after a dose of zinc sulfate from which the patient subsequently died.

B. Chronic Poisoning: Repeated application of solutions to the skin may cause erythematous, papular, and granulomatous reactions in susceptible individuals. Lotions containing zirconium are especially likely to produce granulomatous reactions; the amount that must enter the skin to produce such a reaction is extremely small. Copper poisoning has occurred from the application of copper sulfate to extensive areas of burned skin. Inhalation of copper-containing sprays is reported to be associated with an increased incidence of lung cancer and—possibly—hepatic injury. Symptoms of aluminum poisoning include encephalopathy, weakness, osteomalacia, and elevated serum calcium level. Excessive intake of zinc is reported to affect immune responses. Excessive zinc absorption from toys is reported to cause refractory anemia.

C. Laboratory Findings:

1. Urinalysis may reveal hematuria and proteinuria. Urine volume may be reduced.

2. Blood urea nitrogen and creatinine levels are elevated in the presence of renal damage.

Prevention

Solutions of astringent salts should be stored safely.

Treatment

A. Emergency Measures: Dilute the poison immediately with water or milk and remove by gastric lavage unless the patient is already vomiting.

B. Antidote: For copper and zinc poisoning, give calcium disodium edetate orally and intravenously (see p 85). Penicillamine is also effective in copper poisoning (see p 87).

C. General Measures:

1. Treat hypotension (see p 66).

2. To relieve irritation, give milk or starch drinks made by dissolving 10 g of cornstarch or flour in 1 L of water.

3. Replace fluids lost by vomiting or diarrhea with 5% dextrose in saline.

4. Keep the patient warm and quiet.

5. Relieve pain by giving meperidine or morphine in adequate dose.

D. Special Problems: Treat anuria (see p 72) and liver damage (see p 77).

Prognosis

The patient is likely to recover if symptoms are mild after the first 6 hours. In severe poisoning, death may occur up to 1 week after ingestion.

Andreoli SP et al: Aluminum intoxication from aluminum-containing phosphate binders in children with azotemia not undergoing dialysis. *N Engl J Med* 1984;**310**:1079.

Charhon SA et al: Serum aluminium concentration and aluminium deposits in bone in patients receiving haemodialysis. *Br Med J* 1985;**290**:1613.

Illness associated with elevated levels of zinc in fruit punch—New Mexico *MMWR* 1983;**32**:257.

Jantsch W, Kulig K, Rumack BH: Massive copper sulfate ingestion resulting in hepatotoxicity. *J Toxicol Clin Toxicol* 1984;**22**:585.

Madias NE, Levey AS: Metabolic alkalosis due to absorption of "nonabsorbable" antacids. *Am J Med* 1983;**74**:155.

Sedman AB et al: Encephalopathy in childhood secondary to aluminum toxicity. *J Pediatr* 1984;**105**:836.

VOLATILE OILS

Volatile or essential oils are colorless liquids consisting of mixtures of saturated or unsaturated cyclic hydrocarbons, ethers, alcohols, esters, and ketones. Natural oil of bitter almonds contains 4% hydrogen cyanide, and artificial oil of bitter almonds contains mandelonitrile (see Table 16–1). These liquids all evaporate readily at room temperature. Volatile oils or the plants containing them—turpentine, citronella, sassafras, anise, cinnamon, apiol, pepper, clove, pine, absinthe, pennyroyal, savin, rue, tansy, and eucalyptus—are used as skin irritants. Some volatile oils or the plants from which they are derived have undeserved reputations as abortifacients. The plants contain 1–5% of volatile oil.

Ingestion of 15 g of a volatile oil such as turpentine has caused death, although many patients have survived ingestion of much larger doses with minimal symptoms. The exposure limit for turpentine is 100 ppm.

The poisonous effect of volatile oils is to some extent related to volatility, since the less volatile substances are more slowly absorbed. For example, pine oil, the less volatile residue after the removal of turpentine, is about one-fifth as poisonous as turpentine. The effects of the less volatile and poorly absorbed volatile oils resemble those of kerosene, and systemic effects are far less pronounced than the local effects resulting from aspiration.

Volatile oils irritate all tissues intensely.

The pathologic findings in fatalities from ingestion of volatile oils include renal degenerative changes and intense congestion and edema in the lungs, brain, and gastric mucosa.

Clinical Findings

The principal manifestations of acute poisoning with the volatile oils are vomiting and circulatory collapse. Aspiration causes a pneumonitis like that due to kerosene.

A. Symptoms and Signs: Symptoms from ingestion are abdominal burning, nausea and vomiting, diarrhea, dysuria, hematuria, unconsciousness, shallow respiration, and convulsions. Inhalation causes dizziness; rapid, shallow breathing; tachycardia; bronchial irritation; and unconsciousness or convulsions. Anuria, pulmonary edema, and bronchial pneumonia may complicate recovery after either type of exposure. An amount of volatile oil capable of inducing abortion is likely also to produce irreversible renal damage.

B. Chronic Poisoning: No cumulative effects have been reported.

C. Laboratory Findings: The urine may contain hemoglobin, red blood cells, protein, casts, and reduced sugar. Anemia may be present.

Prevention

Medications containing turpentine or other volatile oils must be labeled *for external use only;* after use, any remaining medication should be discarded.

A mask capable of absorbing organic vapors may be used for short periods if atmospheres containing high concentrations of volatile oils must be entered.

Treatment

A. Emergency Measures:

1. Give 120–240 mL of milk; then remove by gastric lavage or emesis, taking care to prevent aspiration (see pp 21–28). Follow these procedures by administering 30–60 mL of Fleet's Phospho-Soda diluted 1:4 in water.

2. Give artificial respiration if necessary.

B. General Measures:

1. Give milk, 250 mL, as necessary to allay gastric irritation.

2. Give atropine, 1 mg, to decrease bronchial secretions.

3. If kidney function is normal, give fluids to 3–4 L daily to maintain maximum urinary output after the danger from pulmonary edema has passed (after the first 24 hours).

4. Keep the patient warm and quiet.

C. Special Problems: Treat pulmonary edema (see p 65) and anuria (see p 72). Control convulsions (see Table 4–3).

Prognosis

If the patient lives for 48 hours, complete recovery is likely; laboratory evidence of renal damage may persist for several months.

ACONITE

Aconite consists of the dried tuberous root of *Aconitum napellus* (monkshood). The most active principle, aconitine, is an alkaloid.

Tincture of aconite is used in liniments as a skin irritant. Monkshood or aconite *(Aconitum columbianum* or *A napellus)* has caused poisoning when eaten in a salad or when mistaken for radishes. Larkspur

(*Delphinium* species) has similar toxicity and contains a number of alkaloids, including delphinine and aconitine. All parts of the plants are poisonous.

The fatal dose of aconite may be as small as 1 g of the plant, 5 mL of the tincture, or 2 mg of aconitine. Fatalities have been rare in recent years.

Aconite contains the alkaloid aconitine, which stimulates and then depresses myocardium, smooth muscles, skeletal muscles, central nervous system, and peripheral nerves.

Clinical Findings

The principal manifestations of aconite poisoning are low blood pressure and slow respirations.

A. Acute Poisoning: (From ingestion or absorption through the skin.) Nausea and vomiting; burning followed by numbness and tingling of the mouth, throat, and hands; blurred vision; slow, weak pulse; fall of blood pressure; chest pain; shallow respiration; convulsions; and death due to respiratory failure or ventricular fibrillation. In one case, cardiac infarction was apparently related to excessive application of aconite liniment over 2 weeks.

B. Chronic Poisoning: Repeated application or ingestion causes symptoms described for acute poisoning.

C. Laboratory Findings: The ECG may reveal changes associated with myocardial infarction.

Prevention

Any use of tincture of aconite as a liniment should be avoided. Children should be warned against eating wild plants that may be aconite.

Treatment

A. Emergency Measures: Delay absorption of ingested aconite

Table 29–1. Miscellaneous irritants.*

Irritant	Clinical Findings
Arnica	Irritating to skin and mucous membranes.
Capsicum	Ingestion of more than 30 mg causes vomiting, diarrhea, and pain on urination. Drowsiness and coma can occur.
Cashew nut oil	Blisters skin, causes vomiting and diarrhea.
Cocillana	Vomiting, diarrhea, collapse, headache, and rhinorrhea.
Oil of mustard	Blistering and corrosion of skin or gastrointestinal tract. A single drop in the eye has caused blindness.

*Treatment: For ingestion, gastric lavage; for skin contamination, wash in running water for at least 15 minutes, then apply wet dressings (see p 83).

by giving activated charcoal, then remove by gastric lavage (see pp 21–28). Give artificial respiration or O_2 as necessary.

B. General Measures: Keep the patient warm and quiet. Digitalization may counteract cardiac depression. Treat convulsions (see p 51). Manage cardiac arrhythmias (see p 378–382).

Prognosis

Survival for 24 hours is usually followed by recovery.

Monsereenuso RNY et al: Capsaicin: A literature survey. *CRC Crit Rev Toxicol* 1982;**10**:321.

30 | Cathartics

MAGNESIUM SULFATE & OTHER MAGNESIUM SALTS

Magnesium sulfate ($MgSO_4$) is a water-soluble salt that is used orally as a cathartic and intravenously as an anticonvulsant and antihypertensive agent in managing toxemia.

The fatal dose of absorbed magnesium ion is approximately 30 mg/kg, an amount that would raise the serum magnesium to the lethal level of 13–15 meq/L. The fatal dose by oral or rectal administration has been as low as 30 g in the presence of inadequate renal function. Fatalities are rare.

Elevated serum levels of magnesium depress or paralyze nerves and muscles. This action is antagonized by calcium. Systemic effects are ordinarily absent after ingestion of magnesium sulfate, since the normal kidney is able to remove magnesium ion more rapidly than it can be absorbed from the gastrointestinal tract. However, if renal function is impaired, dangerous serum magnesium levels may be reached.

Pathologic findings in poisoning with magnesium salts are hemorrhagic gastroenteritis and congestion of the lungs.

Clinical Findings

The principal manifestations of acute poisoning with magnesium salts are watery diarrhea and respiratory failure.

A. Acute Poisoning: Ingestion of a large quantity of a concentrated solution of magnesium sulfate will cause gastrointestinal irritation, vomiting, abdominal pain, watery or bloody diarrhea, tenesmus, and collapse.

Rectal administration of magnesium sulfate has caused flushing, thirst, coma, respiratory depression, flaccid paralysis, fall of blood pressure, and death. Intravenous administration causes these same symptoms depending on the rapidity of the injection. Symptoms of restlessness, flushing, and slight fall of blood pressure begin at serum magnesium levels of 4 meq/L and progress to coma, flaccid paralysis, and failure of respiration at serum magnesium levels of 13–15 meq/L.

B. Chronic Poisoning: Long-term use of magnesium-containing antacid (Gelusil) has caused renal failure from precipitation of magnesium ammonium phosphate in the kidney.

C. Laboratory Findings: Serum magnesium levels should be determined if magnesium poisoning is suspected. Levels above 4 meq/L indicate dangerous retention of magnesium.

Prevention

Do not give concentrated magnesium sulfate solutions orally or by enema. Intravenous magnesium sulfate must be given cautiously and with continuous supervision, since the therapeutic margin is small and respiratory paralysis may occur suddenly.

Treatment

A. Emergency Measures: Establish airway and maintain respiration. Dilute orally or rectally administered magnesium sulfate by giving tap water. Give artificial respiration if necessary.

B. Antidote: Give calcium gluconate, 1 mL of 10% solution per kilogram, slowly intravenously up to a total of 10 mL.

C. General Measures: Keep the patient warm. If renal function is normal, give adequate fluids to allow the removal of magnesium ion. If renal function is impaired, dialysis may be necessary to reduce serum magnesium.

Prognosis

The patient will recover if the initial effect is survived.

Garcia-Webb P et al: Hypermagnesaemia and hypophosphataemia after ingestion of magnesium sulphate. *Br Med J* 1984;**288**:759.

CROTON OIL, COLOCYNTH, PODOPHYLLUM, ELATERIN, BRYONIA, & GAMBOGE

Croton oil is a nonvolatile oil obtained from the seeds of *Croton tiglium*. The oil contains about 10% of a resin that is responsible for the effects of the oil. The active principles of colocynth (from *Citrullus colocynthis*), bryonia (from *Bryonia alba*), and elaterin (from the fruit of *Ecballium elaterium*) are mixtures of alkaloids, resins, and glycosides. Podophyllum resin (from *Podophyllum peltatum*, mayapple) and gamboge (from *Garcinia hanburyi*) are gum resins.

These drugs are all extremely potent irritants and cathartics. The fatal dose of any may be as low as 1 mL or 1 g, but fatalities have not been reported in recent years.

The resinous principles are irritating to all cells and tissues and can be dangerous even when applied to the intact skin.

The pathologic findings in fatalities from these drugs include congestion and degenerative changes in the gastrointestinal tract, liver, kidneys, and brain.

Clinical Findings

The principal manifestations of acute poisoning are vomiting, diarrhea, and collapse. Chronic poisoning does not occur.

A. Symptoms and Signs: (From ingestion or application to the skin.) Burning pain in the mouth and stomach, tenesmus, vomiting, watery or bloody diarrhea, pallor, collapse, fall of blood pressure, tachycardia, coma, and death.

B. Laboratory Findings: Gross or occult blood in the stools; proteinuria and gross or microscopic hematuria.

Table 30–1. Miscellaneous cathartics.*

Drugs	Clinical Findings or Effects
Mineral oil, liquid petrolatum	Dissolves and prevents the absorption of vitamin A from the intestinal contents; deposition of mineral oil can be found in the lymph glands of chronic users, but a deleterious effect from this deposition has not been noted. Aspiration, with subsequent pulmonary infiltration, has also occurred. Use of mineral oil nose drops has led to pulmonary deposition of mineral oil.
Aloe Aloin	Purging, gastrointestinal distress, collapse, blood in the stools.
Senna Cascara sagrada	Purging, collapse, blood in the stools.
Phenolphthalein	Two types of reactions have been reported rarely, characterized by (1) purging, collapse, and fall of blood pressure, or (2) an erythematous, itching skin rash that may progress to persistent ulceration.
Castor oil (ricinoleic ester)	Self-limited irritation of small intestine.
Bisacodyl (Dulcolax) Danthron (Danthro-Lax) Oxyphenisatin (Lavema) Casanthranol	Abdominal cramps, skin rash, prolonged diarrhea. Oxyphenisatin has caused liver damage.
Dehydrocholic acid (Atrocholin)	Sensitivity reactions.
Etulos Karaya Magnocyl Methylcellulose Polycarbophil Psyllium hydrophilic mucilloid (Metamucil) Sterculia gum	If insufficient water is taken, these drugs might cause intestinal obstruction.
Sodium sulfate	Purging, fluid loss, blood in stools, fall of blood pressure, hypernatremia.
Sodium phosphate	See p 211.

*Treatment: Reduce dosage or discontinue use. Treat shock (see p 66).

Prevention

All of these irritant resinous cathartics are too dangerous for medicinal use and should be abandoned.

Treatment of Acute Poisoning

A. Emergency Measures:

1. Delay absorption and reduce gastrointestinal irritation by giving tap water, milk, or liquid petrolatum. Remove by gastric lavage or emesis (see pp 21–28). These measures are of little use after symptoms occur.

2. Treat shock (see p 66).

B. General Measures:

1. Give milk, 250 mL, or liquid petrolatum, 30 mL, every hour to relieve gastrointestinal irritation.

2. Maintain hydration by giving fluids orally or intravenously.

3. Relieve pain with meperidine (Demerol), 100 mg subcutaneously as necessary.

4. Give atropine, 1 mg every 4 hours, to reduce gastrointestinal secretions.

Prognosis

Recovery is likely if the patient lives for 48 hours.

Cassidy DE et al: Podophyllum toxicity: A report of a fatal case and review of the literature. *J Toxicol Clin Toxicol* 1982;**19**:35.

References

Forbes DA et al: Laxative abuse and secretory diarrhoea. *Arch Dis Child* 1985;**60**:58.

31 | Endocrine Drugs

ANTITHYROID DRUGS
(See also Iodides, p 362.)

Methimazole (Tapazole), methylthiouracil, carbimazole, iothiouracil (Itrumil), and propylthiouracil are used in the treatment of hyperthyroidism. They act by interfering with the formation of thyroxine by the thyroid gland.

An accurate estimate of the number of fatalities from antithyroid drugs is not possible, but several deaths have been reported from their side effects. The incidence of leukopenia or agranulocytosis from these drugs may be 0.5–1% of users, but over 90% of these recover.

The antithyroid drugs may depress formation of granulocytes in the bone marrow, apparently as a hypersensitivity reaction.

Pathologic findings in deaths from antithyroid drugs include ulcerations in the pharynx and gastrointestinal tract, bronchial pneumonia, and aplasia of the bone marrow.

Clinical Findings

The principal manifestations of antithyroid drug poisoning are skin rash and leukopenia. Acute poisoning has not been reported.

A. Symptoms and Signs: (From ingestion.) Adverse reactions usually appear in the first few weeks of therapy and may consist of skin rash, urticaria, joint pains, fever, sore throat, anorexia, malaise, and agranulocytosis. Toxic neuropathy has been reported in one case after methimazole therapy had been continued for 40 days. The patient suddenly developed difficulty in walking, which progressed rapidly to left foot drop, absent knee and ankle reflexes, and inability to stand. Hypoprothrombinemia with purpura has been reported during propylthiouracil therapy, and hepatic injury has been reported during methimazole and propylthiouracil therapy.

B. Laboratory Findings: A complete blood count (cbc) reveals decrease or absence of granulocytes.

Prevention

Patients being started on antithyroid drug therapy should receive a weekly complete blood count for the first month, since the incidence of agranulocytosis or leukopenia appears to be highest in the first few weeks. After this period, patients should be warned to discontinue antithyroid drugs and report for examination upon the appearance of fever, sore throat, purpura, malaise, loss of appetite, or other illness.

Treatment
A. General Measures:
1. Give organism-specific chemotherapy to control intercurrent infections during agranulocytosis.

2. Good oral hygiene should be maintained.

3. Exposure to infectious diseases should be avoided during the period of leukopenia or agranulocytosis.

B. Special Problems: Treat toxic neuropathy by physiotherapy.

Prognosis
Only about 1–5% of patients developing leukopenia or agranulocytosis from antithyroid drugs have died.

In one patient having a toxic neuropathy during methimazole therapy, leg weakness persisted for over a year.

Cooper DS et al: Agranulocytosis associated with antithyroid drugs. *Ann Intern Med* 1983;98:26.

CORTICOSTEROIDS:
ADRENAL CORTEX HORMONES & SUBSTITUTES

Cortisone, hydrocortisone, desoxycorticosterone acetate, fludrocortisone, prednisolone, prednisone, triamcinolone, methylprednisolone, other synthetic substitutes, and corticotropin (the adrenal-stimulating hormone of the pituitary) are used in replacement therapy for adrenal insufficiency and in the treatment of many other diseases. Glycyrrhizin, the active principle of licorice, acts in a manner similar to cortisone.

Fatalities following administration of the adrenal hormones or corticotropin are rare and have occurred as complications of existing disease. Anaphylaxis has followed injection of corticotropin.

These hormones cause salt and water retention, electrolyte imbalance, increase in blood volume, negative nitrogen balance, and decrease in resistance to microorganisms.

Pathologic findings in deaths following cortisone, hydrocortisone, or corticotropin administration have not indicated specific organ damage.

Table 31—1. Miscellaneous drugs used for endocrine effects.*

Drug	Clinical Findings
Acetohexamide (Dymelor)	Hypoglycemia, vomiting, headache, diarrhea, intolerance to alcohol, paresthesias, skin rash, and, rarely, jaundice, leukopenia, and alteration in liver function tests.
Aminoglutethimide (Cytandren)	Skin rash, nausea, anemia, pancytopenia.
Androgens and anabolic steroids:	
Danazol, dromostanolone, fluoxymesterone, methandrostenolone, nandrolone, oxymetholone, stanozolol	Abnormal liver function tests, salt and water retention, and masculinization, particularly of the female fetus.
Methyltestosterone (Metandren)	Jaundice from bile stasis, enlarged liver, fatal biliary cirrhosis.
Calcitonin (Calcimar)	Nausea, vomiting, sensitivity reactions, local inflammation, and facial flushing.
Chlorpropamide (Diabinese)	Prolonged hypoglycemia, nausea, vomiting, intolerance to alcohol, and, rarely, severe liver damage, exfoliative dermatitis, granulocytopenia, photosensitivity, pulmonary eosinophilic infiltration, and thrombocytopenia.
Clomiphene (Clomid)	Hot flashes, abdominal discomfort, nausea, vomiting, nervous tension and insomnia, headache, and dizziness. Contraindicated in liver disease.
Contraceptives, oral: Dimethisterone–ethinyl estradiol Ethynodiol–ethinyl estradiol Ethynodiol–mestranol Norethindrone–ethinyl estradiol Norethindrone-mestranol Norethynodrel-mestranol Norgestrel-ethinyl estradiol	Nausea, vomiting, fluid retention, jaundice, menstrual irregularities. Thrombophlebitis with episodes of thromboembolic disease, as well as fatal embolism and eye changes (including papilledema, paralysis of eye muscles, and temporary diminution of vision), has occurred in rare cases.
Cosyntropin (Cortrosyn)	Hypersensitivity.
Dinoprost, dinoprostone	Vomiting, bronchospasm, hypotension, chest pain, abdominal cramps.
Desmopressin, lypressin	Mucous membrane irritation, headache, dyspnea, fluid retention.
Estrogens: Chlorotrianisene, dienestrol, diethylstilbestrol, estradiol, estrone, conjugated estrogens, estropipate	Headache, nausea and vomiting, and excessive vaginal bleeding; breasts enlarged from inhalation during manufacture or application to skin as hormone cream. Genital abnormalities in male offspring and genital cancer in female offspring of mothers exposed to diethylstilbestrol during pregnancy. Chlorotrianisene has caused alteration in corneal curvature.
Glipizide (Glucotrol) Gliburide (Diabeta)	Nausea, vomiting, diarrhea, constipation, hypoglycemia, jaundice, increased BUN, rash, thrombocytopenia, leukopenia.

*Treatment: Reduce dosage or discontinue. Give glucose for insulin, acetohexamide, chlorpropamide, or tolbutamide overdose. In thyroid overdose, lower body temperature to normal and maintain fluid balance. Digitalize if necessary.

Table 31—1 (cont'd). Miscellaneous drugs used for endocrine effects.*

Drug	Clinical Findings
Glucagon	Nausea, vomiting, hypotensive reaction or other sensitivity reaction.
Gonadorelin (Factrel)	Headache, nausea, abdominal discomfort, flushing, local swelling and pain, possible hypersensitivity reactions.
Hydroxyprogesterone (Delalutin)	Edema, exacerbation of epilepsy, migraine, asthma.
Insulin	Hypoglycemia, anaphylaxis.
Lututrin (Lutrexin)	Sedation.
Metyrapone (Metopirone)	Severe adrenal insufficiency.
Norethindrone (Norlutate)	Jaundice and death from liver damage have occurred. Masculinization can be irreversible in the female fetus.
Oxytocin	Uterine rupture, fetal damage.
Phenformin (DBI)	Metallic taste, nausea, loss of appetite, diarrhea, weakness, abdominal cramps, ketonuria, and acidosis that may be irreversible.
Potassium perchlorate	Fatal aplastic anemia has occurred in at least 4 patients.
Progesterone	Porphyria, masculinization of the female fetus.
Prostaglandin E_1 (Alprostadil)	Apnea, bradycardia, fever, convulsions, hypothermia, diarrhea.
Secretin	Hypersensitivity reactions, fainting.
Somatotropin	Pain and swelling at injection site, lipodystrophy, muscle pain, headache, hypercalciuria.
Spironolactone (Aldactone)	Drowsiness, confusion, rash, gynecomastia, and impotence.
Tamoxifen (Nolvadex)	Menopause induction, hypercalcemia, edema. Teratogenic.
Testolactone (Teslac)	Rash, hypertension, edema, gastrointestinal distress.
Thrombin (Thrombinar)	Hypersensitivity reactions.
Thyroid preparations: 　Dextrothyroxine 　(Choloxin)	Increased metabolism, cardiac arrhythmia, myocardial infarction. Potentiates the effect of the coumarin anticoagulants.
Levothyroxine 　Liothyronine	Tachycardia, headache, excessive sweating.
Thyroid	Ingestion of desiccated thyroid, 0.3 g/kg, has caused fever, tachycardia, hypertension, hyperactivity, and cardiovascular collapse. Recovery followed.
Thyrotropin	Headache, fever, tachycardia, gastrointestinal distress, hypersensitivity reactions.
Tolazamide (Tolinase)	Hypoglycemia, nausea and vomiting, skin eruptions, weakness, fatigue, dizziness, and, rarely, leukopenia.
Tolbutamide (Orinase)	Hypoglycemia, nausea and vomiting, weakness, intolerance to alcohol, skin eruptions, and, rarely, leukopenia, thrombocytopenia, thyroid suppression, hyperlipemia, or gastrointestinal bleeding from ulceration.
Yohimbine (Yocon)	Edema, elevated blood pressure, irritability, tremors, sweating, nausea and vomiting, dizziness.

*Treatment: Reduce dosage or discontinue. Give glucose for insulin, acetohexamide, chlorpropamide, or tolbutamide overdose. In thyroid overdose, lower body temperature to normal and maintain fluid balance. Digitalize if necessary.

Clinical Findings

The principal manifestations of poisoning with these drugs are hypertension and edema.

A. Acute Poisoning: (From injection of corticotropin.) Anaphylaxis with prostration, rigor, weak pulse, loss of consciousness, and death. Other acute reactions have not developed, although aggravation of peptic ulcer, edema, hypokalemia, or infection may occur.

B. Chronic Poisoning: Hypertension; edema; nervousness; sleeplessness; skin eruptions; depression; cataracts; amenorrhea; alkalosis; euphoria; decrease in pain sensation; psychosis; weakness; deafness; convulsions; hirsutism in women; intestinal perforation in ulcerative colitis; activation of peptic ulcer with bleeding or perforation; modification of immune responses with activation of a tuberculous, fungal, or other infection; increase in severity of diabetes; thrombotic episodes; hypokalemia with muscular weakness progressing to muscle degeneration; acute pancreatitis; rupture of the Achilles tendon; osteoporosis; aseptic bone necrosis; pseudotumor cerebri; and cardiac conduction defect. Repeated intra-articular injection has caused destruction of the joint. Abrupt withdrawal of adrenal cortex hormones may cause symptoms of adrenal cortex deficiency: hypotension, coma, weakness, and tremors. Death from steroid therapy ordinarily results from either acute adrenal insufficiency or gastric ulcer with hemorrhage or perforation.

Application of corticosteroids to the eye causes an increase in intraocular pressure.

Application of corticosteroids to the skin can cause atrophic changes in the skin, secondary infections, burning, itching, irritation, dryness, folliculitis, hypertrichosis, acne, and pigmentation. Absorption can cause pituitary suppression and potassium depletion.

C. Laboratory Findings: Serum electrolyte studies may indicate hypernatremic, hypokalemic alkalosis.

Prevention

Use minimal effective doses of corticosteroids or corticotropin. Decrease dosage or discontinue the drug at the first sign of toxicity. If prolonged therapy is needed, serum sodium and potassium levels should be monitored to prevent severe electrolyte imbalance. Restriction of sodium intake and administration of supplementary potassium may be necessary. In treating children, increase the dosage gradually.

Treatment

A. Acute Poisoning (Anaphylaxis Due to Corticotropin):

1. Emergency measures—Give epinephrine, 1 mg of 1:1000 solution subcutaneously. Give positive pressure artificial respiration. Give aminophylline, 0.5 g slowly intravenously.

2. General measures–Keep the patient warm and quiet.

B. Chronic Poisoning:

1. Immediate measures–Reduce dosage of cortisone or related compounds to minimal maintenance dose at the first sign of toxicity.

2. General measures–Intestinal perforation will require surgical closure. Treat convulsions (see p 51).

Observe caution in the systemic administration of steroids during bacterial or viral infections. Do not use steroids on the eye in such cases.

Prognosis

Recovery is likely if the patient survives for 24 hours.

INTERACTIONS
(See p 17.)

The hypoglycemic effect of the sulfonylureas (tolbutamide, chlorpropamide) may be increased by ethanol, dicumarol, sulfafenazole, oxyphenbutazone, aspirin, phenylbutazone, and chloramphenicol.

The following drugs reduce the effectiveness of hypoglycemic agents: thiazide diuretics, diazoxide, corticosteroids, oral contraceptives, frusemide, and ethacrynic acid.

Anabolic steroids potentiate vitamin K.

The effect of insulin may be increased by ethanol, propranolol, levodopa, and monoamine oxidase inhibitors.

Phenytoin increases the effects of thyroid drugs.

Methandrostenolone enhances plasma levels of oxyphenbutazone.

One week of adrenal steroid administration can impair pituitary adrenal control for 9–10 months, with resulting marked hypotension during anesthesia or other procedures.

PHARMACOKINETICS
(See p 89.)

	pK$_a$	t½	V$_d$	% Binding
Acetohexamide		3.5—11		
Chlorpropamide	4.8	24—42	0.09—0.27	88—96
Cortisone		0.5—2		
Dexamethasone		3—4.5		77
Fludrocortisone		0.5	70—79	
Glibenclamide	5.3	10—16	0.3	99
Glibornuride		5—12	0.25	97
Glipizide		3—7	0.16	92—99
Hydrocortisone		1.5—2		>90
Insulin		2	0.66	
Levothyroxine		150		
Liothyronine		35—60		>99
Methimazole		6—7		
Methylprednisolone		3.5	1.5	
Phenformin		11		19
Prednisolone		2.5—3		90
Propylthiouracil	7.8	2—4		
Thyroxine		80—180		>99
Tolazamide	3.1, 5.7	7		
Tolbutamide	5.3	4—10	0.14	95—97
Triamcinolone		>5		

References

Campbell IW, Ratcliffe JG: Suicidal insulin overdose managed by excision of the insulin injection site. *Br Med J* 1982;**285**:408.

Chan CF et al: Hydrocortisone-induced anaphylaxis. *Med J Aust* 1984;**141**:444.

Harris NZ et al: Breast cancer in relation to patterns of oral contraceptive use. *Am J Epidemiol* 1982;**116**:643.

Lehrner LM, Weir MR: Acute ingestions of thyroid hormones. *Pediatrics* 1984;**287**:313.

Litovitz TL, White JD: Levothyroxine ingestions in children. *Am J Emerg Med* 1985;**3**:297.

Newton RW et al: Adrenocortical suppression in workers employed in manufacturing synthetic glucocorticosteroids. *Br J Ind Med* 1982;**39**:179.

Perry PJ et al: Prednisolone psychosis: Clinical observations. *Drug Intell Clin Pharm* 1984;**18**:603.

Statczynski JS, Haskell RJ: Duration of hypoglycemia and need for intravenous glucose following intentional overdoses of insulin. *Ann Emerg Med* 1984;**13**:505.

Miscellaneous Therapeutic & Diagnostic Agents | 32

DISULFIRAM & THIOCARBAMATES

Disulfiram (Antabuse) is used in the treatment of alcoholism. It is thought that this drug interferes with the enzymatic breakdown of ethanol at the acetaldehyde level and allows acetaldehyde to accumulate. Another possible explanation is that the toxicity of disulfiram is much greater in the presence of ethanol because ethanol alters the body's ability to detoxify disulfiram. Severe toxic reactions occur at blood acetaldehyde levels greater than 0.5 mg/dL. Fatalities may occur at blood ethanol levels of 1 mg/mL (0.1%) after the ingestion of as little as 0.5–1 g of disulfiram. At least 6 such fatalities have been reported. No fatalities have been reported from the ingestion of disulfiram without the ingestion of ethanol. Disulfiram is not known to increase the toxicity of isopropyl alcohol. Animal experiments indicate that ingestion by an adult of 30 g of disulfiram as a single dose would produce serious toxic effects.

A large number of thiocarbamates and dithiocarbamates (Table 32–1) are used in agriculture and veterinary medicine. These agents probably have toxic effects similar to disulfiram, although poisoning has not been reported. The exposure limit for ferbam is 10 mg/m³; for disulfiram, 2 mg/m³; and for thiram, 5 mg/m³.

Disulfiram is absorbed slowly, reaching a peak level 24 hours after a single dose. The excretion is slow, since only about 50% of the drug in the body is excreted in 1 week. Thus, a severe reaction to ethanol may occur several weeks after discontinuation of disulfiram.

The effects of disulfiram on the body have not been studied extensively. Slight effects on the central nervous system have been noted after ordinary doses, but the mechanism of their production is unknown.

The pathologic findings in deaths from disulfiram-ethanol reactions are not characteristic.

Clinical Findings

The principal manifestations of ethanol ingestion while under

Table 32-1. Thiocarbamates and dithiocarbamates.

	Exposure Limit (mg/m³)	LD50 (mg/kg)
Avadex, diallate		395
Avadex BW, triallate, Far-Go		1,675
Benthiocarb, Saturn, Bolero		560
Butylate, Sutan		4,650
Cycloate, Ro-Neet, hexylthiocarbam		3,160
Drepamon		10,000+
Eptam, EPTC		1,650
Eradicane		2,000+
Ferbam	10	17,000
Maneb		6,750
Metam, Vapam, Sistan, carbam		820
Metiram, Polyram		10,000+
Nabam		400
Pebulate, Tillam		1,120
Propineb, Antracol		8,000
Thiram	5	780
Vegadex, Sulfallate		850
Urbacid, Monzet		100
Vernam, Vernolate		1,625
Zineb		5,200
Ziram		1,400

treatment with disulfiram are fall of blood pressure and hyperventilation.

A. Acute Poisoning:

1. From ingestion of ethanol in any form or inhalation of ethanol while under treatment with disulfiram–As little as 10 mL of ethanol can be dangerous.

a. Mild symptoms–Flushing, sweating, tachycardia, breathlessness, hyperventilation, fall in blood pressure, nausea and vomiting, and drowsiness.

b. Severe symptoms–Severe blood pressure fall, cardiac arrhythmias, air hunger, and chest pain or cardiac infarction.

2. From ingestion of disulfiram, carbamate, or thiocarbamates without ethanol–Central nervous system depression, headache, rash, optic or peripheral neuropathy, psychotic behavior. Corrosive injury to mucous membranes is possible. Skin exposure to Vegadex (2-chloroallyl diethyl dithiocarbamate) has caused pain on washing hands in hot or cold water for up to 48 hours. Some of these agents cause convulsions in animals.

B. Chronic Poisoning: (From ingestion of disulfiram or thiocarbamates.) Fatigue, weakness, impotence, and headache may occur, but these symptoms disappear with continued use. Toxic psychosis, hepatitis, and central nervous system depression have been reported.

C. Laboratory Findings: Blood ethanol levels above 50 mg/dL (0.05%) are extremely dangerous during the administration of disulfiram. Determine SGOT levels before and during use of disulfiram to monitor liver function.

Prevention

The dose of disulfiram should not exceed 0.5 g daily.

Disulfiram-ethanol reactions are extremely dangerous in the presence of heart disease, diabetes mellitus, pregnancy, arteriosclerosis, or hyperthyroidism. Disulfiram should not be given to patients with cirrhosis of the liver or nephritis or to patients taking paraldehyde. Test drinks of ethanol for a patient under disulfiram therapy should not exceed 10 mL.

Do not begin disulfiram therapy until the patient has abstained from drinking ethanol for at least 24 hours.

Treatment

A. Acute Poisoning: Give artificial respiration and O_2, and maintain blood pressure (see p 66). Ascorbic acid administration has been reported to ameliorate disulfiram-ethanol reactions; the suggested dose is 0.1–1 g.

B. Chronic Poisoning: Mild symptoms tend to disappear on continued use. Mental symptoms may require discontinuance of disulfiram therapy.

Prognosis

In a patient receiving disulfiram therapy, sudden death may occur up to 24 hours after ingesting ethanol.

IRON SALTS

Iron for the treatment of anemia is in either the ferrous (Fe^{2+}) or the ferric (Fe^{3+}) form. Ferric iron is not absorbed as such but must be converted to ferrous iron for absorption.

The dangerous dose of iron can be as small as 30 mg/kg. Ferrous sulfate (hydrous) is 20% iron and ferrous fumarate is 33% iron. At least 30 children have died from ingestion of iron compounds. No significant toxic reactions have occurred after overdoses of any children's-size multiple vitamins with iron.

The toxic effect of iron is due to unbound iron in the serum. Soluble ferric or ferrous iron salts also cause corrosive damage to the stomach and small intestine.

The pathologic findings in fatal cases include pulmonary edema and hemorrhages, dilatation of the heart, and hemorrhagic and necrotic gastroenteritis. Iron pigment may be found in the stomach, liver, lungs, and kidneys. Degenerative changes may be found in the lymph nodes, liver, and kidneys. Venous thromboses are found in the mucosa of the small intestine.

Clinical Findings

The principal manifestations of poisoning with the iron compounds are vomiting, diarrhea, and circulatory collapse.

A. Acute Poisoning: (From ingestion.) Lethargy, nausea and vomiting, upper abdominal pain, tarry stools, diarrhea, fast and weak pulse, hypotension, dehydration, acidosis, and coma occur within one-half to one hour following ingestion of iron salts. All symptoms may clear in a few hours and the patient may be asymptomatic for 24 hours, after which symptoms return, with cyanosis, pulmonary edema, shock, convulsions, acidosis, anuria, hyperthermia, and death in coma within 24–48 hours. Liver necrosis may occur 2 days after ingestion.

Injection of iron-dextran has caused fever, tachycardia, enlargement of lymph nodes, skin rash, back pain, and, in some cases, anaphylactoid reactions.

B. Chronic Poisoning: Administration of parenteral iron preparations in excess dosage causes exogenous hemosiderosis with damage to the liver and pancreas. Injection of large amounts of iron-dextran complex (Imferon) intramuscularly in experimental animals has caused sarcoma. However, injection of 953 mL of iron-dextran in one patient did not result in sarcoma.

C. Laboratory Findings:

1. Increased red blood cell count and hemoglobin indicate hemoconcentration.

2. Stools may contain gross or occult blood.

3. Serum iron levels above 400–500 $\mu g/dL$ are a cause for concern; iron levels over 500 $\mu g/dL$ in a symptomatic patient are an indication for chelation therapy with deferoxamine (see below).

4. Measurements of iron-binding capacity are not usually helpful.

5. Iron medications are opaque in x-rays of the abdomen, but an absence of opaque material on x-ray does not exclude the possibility of iron ingestion.

Prevention

Iron medications must be stored safely. Parenteral iron preparations are contraindicated in hemochromatosis and in the presence of renal or hepatic damage. Slow-release iron tablets are especially hazardous.

Treatment

A. Emergency Measures:

1. Establish airway and maintain respiration.

2. If the serum iron determination will be delayed and the patient has a history of excessive iron ingestion and symptoms more serious than nausea and vomiting, consider giving deferoxamine, 40 mg/kg intravenously (see below).

3. Draw blood for determination of hemoglobin level, white blood cell count, serum iron level, electrolyte concentrations, and blood typing.

4. In patients not in shock or coma, induce emesis with syrup of ipecac if the patient has not vomited. If gastric lavage is performed as well, add sodium bicarbonate, 20 g/L, and leave sodium bicarbonate solution in the stomach.

5. Start an infusion of isotonic saline or dextrose solution to correct electrolyte disturbances and dehydration. Maintain blood pressure by blood or plasma transfusion.

6. Order an abdominal x-ray only if large numbers of ferrous sulfate tablets were ingested.

B. Antidote:
If there are iron tablets visible on x-ray, symptoms or signs of iron poisoning, or pink ("vin rosé") urine with good urine output, give chelation therapy with deferoxamine, 15 mg/kg/h by continuous intravenous infusion to a maximum of 80 mg/kg in each 12-hour period. Monitor blood pressure during administration of deferoxamine, and reduce the rate of administration if the blood pressure falls. Single doses should not exceed 1 g and the maximum in 24 hours should not exceed 6 g. Deferoxamine is hazardous in patients with severe renal disease or anuria, and dialysis is necessary in such cases. Injected deferoxamine is associated with a high risk and should be reserved for serious poisoning. Continue deferoxamine therapy until the patient is free of symptoms and signs for 24 hours.

C. General Measures:
Treat shock (see p 66) and acidosis (see p 49). Maintain adequate intravascular volume and tissue perfusion by blood transfusion or other intravenous therapy. Exchange transfusion has also been used in small infants. Maintain urine output at 1 mL/kg/h. Gastrotomy may be necessary to remove a bolus of iron tablets.

Prognosis

If the patient is asymptomatic at the end of 48 hours, recovery is likely.

Table 32—2. Miscellaneous drugs and chemicals.*

Agent	Clinical Findings
Acetohydroxamic acid (Lithostat)	Headache, depression, nausea and vomiting, diarrhea, hemolytic anemia, alopecia, rash, phlebitis, palpitation.
Adenosine phosphate	Local erythema, rash, flushing, palpitation, anaphylaxis.
Allopurinol (Zyloprim)	Rash, fever, nausea, vomiting, diarrhea, leukopenia, eosinophilia, reversible liver impairment. The possibility of cataract formation has been suggested.
Aluminum hydroxide	Delays absorption of drugs.
p-Aminobenzoic acid (10 g or more daily), octyl dimethyl p-aminobenzoic acid	Nausea, vomiting, acidosis, methemoglobinemia, and sensitivity reactions, including fever and rash, to any quantity.
Aminocaproic acid (Amicar)	Rash, hypotension, nausea, diarrhea, delirium, thrombotic episodes or cardiac and hepatic necrosis.
Angiotensin amide (Hypertensin)	Hypertensive and sensitivity reactions.
Arginine (R-Gen)	Flushing, nausea and vomiting, headache, abdominal pain, decreased platelet count, thrombocytopenia, acrocyanosis, elevated BUN, sensitization.
Arginine glutamate (Modumate)	Vomiting.
Aspartic acid (Spartase)	Nausea, abdominal discomfort, diarrhea.
Azuresin (Diagnex-Blue)	Rarely, allergic urticaria and itching.
Bentiromide (Chymex)	Diarrhea, headache, nausea and vomiting.
Benzophenones	Irritation, sensitization.
Betaine hydrochloride	Nausea, vomiting, diarrhea.
Bromelains (Ananase)	Sensitivity reactions, menstrual irregularities, gastrointestinal disturbances.
Calcium carbonate	Increased gastric acid secretion.
β-Carotene (Solatene)	Diarrhea.
Cellulose sodium phosphate	Diarrhea, hyperoxaluria, hypomagnesemia.
Chenodiol (Chenix)	Elevated serum liver enzyme levels, hepatitis, diarrhea, leukopenia, increased serum cholesterol.
Cholanic acid	Diarrhea.
Cholestyramine (Questran)	Constipation, vitamin K deficiency, rash, mucous membrane irritation, osteoporosis, eosinophilia.
Chymopapain (Chymodiactin, Diskase)	Hypersensitivity, anaphylaxis, transverse myelitis, rash, back pain.
Chymotrypsin (Chymar, Cytolav, Enzeon)	Anaphylactic reactions; ulceration, pain, and swelling at injection site.
Colestipol (Colestid)	Constipation, headache, fatigue, elevation of liver enzymes, sensitivity reactions.
Collagenase (Biozyme-C)	Burning, pain, erythema, hypersensitivity.
Congo red	Severe substernal pain, cold sweats, impairment of vision, vomiting, sudden death after IV administration.
Copper oleate (Cuprex)	Edema, itching, burning.

*Treatment: Withdraw drug.

Table 32–2 (cont'd). Miscellaneous drugs and chemicals.*

Agent	Clinical Findings
Cromolyn (Intal)	Bronchospasm, laryngeal edema, irritation, rash, dysuria.
Cyclamate	Diarrhea. A breakdown product found in human urine, cyclohexylamine, has caused chromosome breaks in experimental animals.
Cyclosporin A	Kidney and liver damage.
Deoxyribonuclease (Dornase)	Sensitivity reactions.
Dexpanthenol (Ilopan)	Hypersensitivity reactions, potentiation of parasympathomimetic agents.
Dextranomer (Debrisan)	Pain, bleeding, blistering, erythema.
Digalloyl trioleate	Sensitivity reactions.
Dimethyl sulfoxide	Irritant, narcotic, convulsant. Visual disturbances. Large IV doses cause kidney and liver damage and hemolysis.
Etidronate (Didronel)	Nausea, vomiting, diarrhea, hypocalcemia.
Fibrinolysin-desoxyribonuclease (Elase)	Skin irritation.
Florantyrone (Zanchol)	Diarrhea.
Folic acid (Folvite)	Sensitivity reactions, rash, bronchospasm, anaphylaxis.
Fructose	Metabolic acidosis after IV injection.
γ-Globulin	Cardiac arrhythmias, hypotension, fever, renal impairment; sensitivity reactions, including anaphylaxis.
Guaifenesin	Emesis.
Hyaluronidase (Wydase)	Sensitivity reactions.
Isotretinoin (Accutane)	Cheilitis, desquamation, hair loss, hypertriglyceridemia, joint and muscle pain, fatigue.
Lactulose	Potassium depletion.
Lithium salts (Eskalith, Lithane, Lithonate)	Diarrhea, vomiting, drowsiness, skin eruptions, muscular weakness, lack of coordination, slurred speech, athetotic movements, convulsions, coma, blood pressure fall. Serum level should not exceed 1.5 meq/L. Long administration has caused thyroid enlargement, nephrosis, and bone marrow depression.
Magnesium trisilicate	Silicate urinary stones.
Methylene blue	Quadriplegia after intrathecal injection.
MSG (monosodium glutamate)	Feeling of pressure in head, tightness of face; seizures.
Nicotinic acid	Depressed liver function, activation of peptic ulcer. After IV administration, fall of blood pressure may be severe, and anaphylactic reactions occur rarely.
Pancreatin	Gastrointestinal distress, hypersensitivity, hyperuricemia, oral ulceration.
Pancrelipase	Gastrointestinal distress, hyperuricemia.
Poison ivy extract, alum-precipitated	Gastrointestinal upset, joint swelling, purpura.
Protamine sulfate	Hypertension, sensitivity.

*Treatment: Withdraw drug.

Table 32–2 (cont'd). Miscellaneous drugs and chemicals.*

Agent	Clinical Findings
Protein hydrolysates	Brain damage in animals. Sudden death has occurred in those on restricted protein hydrolysate diets, possibly from potassium or magnesium deficiency.
Renacidin	Injurious to kidney and other organs. Not to be used above the ureterovesical junction.
Saccharin	5 g has caused nausea, vomiting, diarrhea.
Sodium chloride	In infants, excessive amounts cause coma and convulsions that may be persistent owing to vascular injury. Dialysis is lifesaving.
Sodium polystyrene sulfonate (Kayexalate)	Gastrointestinal upset, fecal impaction, hypokalemia.
Succus cineraria maritima (*Senecio maritima*)	Sensitivity reactions, irritation.
Sucralfate (Carafate)	Gastrointestinal distress, rash, itching.
Sutilains (Travase)	Pain, rash, bleeding.
Tartrazine (FD&C yellow No. 5)	Life-threatening allergic reactions, cross-reaction to aspirin.
Terpin hydrate	Liver injury from excessive use.
Tretinoin (Retin-A)	Skin or mucous membrane irritation.
Trioxsalen (Trisoralen) Methoxsalen	Nausea and epigastric discomfort; possible increased sensitivity to sun or ultraviolet light after overdosage.
Tromethamine (THAM)	Sloughs from perivascular injection. May depress respiration.
Vitamin A (20–100 times daily requirement)	Painful nodular periosteal swelling, osteoporosis, itching, skin eruptions and ulcerations, anorexia, increased intracranial pressure, irritability, drowsiness, alopecia, liver enlargement (occasionally); and diplopia, papilledema, and other symptoms suggesting brain tumor.
Vitamin B_1 (thiamine)	Drug fever and anaphylaxis after IV administration.
Vitamin B_{12} (cyanocobalamin)	Sensitivity reactions, gastrointestinal distress, thrombosis, itching, rash.
Vitamin C	Amounts up to 10 g or more daily may cause diarrhea.
Vitamin D, calcitriol, calciferol, calcifidiol, ergocalciferol (150,000 units or more daily)	Weakness, nausea, vomiting, diarrhea, anemia, and decrease in renal function with polyuria, increase in potassium loss, acidosis, proteinuria, and moderate elevation of blood pressure. Serum calcium and NPN are raised. Calcium deposits are seen in the cornea and conjunctiva; less commonly, strabismus, epicanthal folds, papilledema, slow pupillary reaction to light, iritis, and cataract occur. X-rays show metastatic calcification in the kidney, heart, aorta, blood vessels, and skin. Excessive doses during pregnancy are suspected of causing retardation and congenital heart defects in children. Give calcium disodium edetate orally to increase fecal loss of calcium.

*Treatment: Withdraw drug.

Table 32–2 (cont'd). Miscellaneous drugs and chemicals.*

Agent	Clinical Findings
Vitamin E (α-tocopherol)	Gastrointestinal distress, fatigue, rash, increased serum cholesterol. IV injection in premature infants can cause pulmonary deterioration, thrombocytopenia, liver failure, ascites, kidney damage, sepsis, and necrotizing enterocolitis; these effects may be due to the polysorbate contained in the preparation.
Vitamin K	Hemolytic anemia, hyperbilirubinemia, icterus, impairment of function and enlargement of liver; deaths in newborn infants from excessive doses. Total dose should not exceed 3 mg of menadiol or 1 mg of menadione. Excessive doses have caused decreased liver function and hypoprothrombinemia in adults.
Vitamin K₁ (phytonadione)	IV administration is hazardous. Deaths have occurred at injection rates greater than 1 mg/min.

*Treatment: Withdraw drug.

OXYGEN

O_2 therapy is used in the treatment of many medical conditions in which inadequate circulation, O_2 transport, or respiration is present or suspected.

O_2 concentrations above 40% in the newborn increase the incidence of retrolental fibroplasia. A suggested mechanism is the induction of retinal vasoconstriction. Oxygen therapy is also believed to play a role in infant respiratory distress syndrome.

In adult humans, concentrations over 21% cause damage related to the duration of exposure; 100% O_2 causes pulmonary irritation and reduced vital capacity in about 50% of those exposed for 8–24 hours.

Pure O_2 at pressures of 2–3 atmospheres causes almost immediate adverse effects by means of direct central nervous system injury.

Pathologic Findings

A. Retrolental Fibroplasia: The earliest change is the appearance of new blood vessels in the nerve fiber layer of the retina. Later changes include the spreading of these vessels through the retina into the vitreous humor. Evidence of hemorrhage from these new blood vessels is found, and this is organized by fibrosis. As this fibrosed tissue contracts, it becomes detached and folded and forms the membrane behind the lens that is called "retrolental fibroplasia."

B. Pulmonary Damage in Adults: Administration of O_2 in concentrations above 20% at or above atmospheric pressure causes pulmonary damage characterized by capillary congestion, alveolar proteinaceous exudate, intra-alveolar hemorrhage, hyaline membrane,

Table 32–3. Diagnostic agents.

Agent	Clinical Findings
Acetrizoate* (Urokon) Diatrizoate* (Hypaque) Diprotrizoate* (Miokon) Iocetamic acid (Cholebrine) Iodamine (Renovue) Iodipamide* (Cholografin) Iodohippurate* (Hippuran) Iodomethamate* Iodopyracet* (Diodrast) Iopanoic acid* Iothalamate* (Conray) Metrizamide (Amipaque)	Reactions include a feeling of generalized warmth, nausea, and vomiting. Other side effects include flushing of the face and neck, urticaria, fall of blood pressure, hyperpnea, generalized itching and weakness, lacrimation, salivation, edema of the glottis, bouts of coughing, choking sensations, and cyanosis. Although these symptoms usually disappear in 15–30 minutes, they may progress rapidly and result in death from bronchial constriction or cardiovascular collapse. Prior to injection of a water-soluble organic iodine compound, epinephrine, 1:1000, should be prepared in a syringe for injection in case of a reaction. After injecting the first 1 mL of iodine compound, wait 30–60 seconds to observe any immediate reactions. The rest of the injection should then be given slowly. Doses of contrast media exceeding 3 mL/kg have sometimes caused renal medullary necrosis.
p-Aminohippurate	Nausea, vomiting, sudden warmth.
Betazole (Histalog)	Flushing, headache, syncope, respiratory difficulty.
Chloriodized oil* Ethiodized oil* Propyliodone*	Irritation or sensitivity reactions of skin or mucous membranes.
Evans blue	Hypersensitivity reactions, staining.
Histoplasmin	Hypersensitivity reactions, induration, local reaction.
Indigotindisulfonate (Indigo carmine)	Sensitivity reactions, rash, bronchospasm, hypertension, bradycardia.
Indocyanine green (Cardio-Green)	Sweating, itching, headache.
Iodoalphionic acid* Ipodate*	Nausea, vomiting, diarrhea. Ipodate also causes dysuria, urticaria, headache, increase in serum bilirubin, and, rarely, hypotension.
Iophendylate* Iophenoxic acid*	Reactions after intraspinal injection include backache and transient fever. The bulk of the injected material should be removed if possible.
Pentagastrin	Gastrointestinal distress, tachycardia, hypotension.
Phenolsulfonphthalein (phenol red)	Hypersensitivity reactions.
Saralasin (Sarenin)	Nausea, dizziness, headache, hypotension, hypertension, extrasystoles.
Sincalide (Kinevac)	Nausea, dizziness, flushing, possible extrusion of gallstones.
Sodium tyropanoate (Bilopaque)	Gastrointestinal upset, allergic skin reactions, laryngotracheal edema.
Sulfobromophthalein	Anaphylactoid reaction from IV injection.
Thorium dioxide	Renal damage, local inflammatory reactions, multiple granulomas, malignant tumors.

*For treatment, see p 364.

edema, fibroblastic proliferation, and hyperplasia of alveolar cells. Damage is proportionate to the concentration and duration of exposure.

Clinical Findings

The principal manifestations of exposure to elevated O_2 concentrations are blindness and pulmonary changes.

A. Retrolental Fibroplasia: Concentrations of O_2 over 40% may cause visible vasoconstriction and even obliteration of retinal vessels in premature infants. Two to 6 weeks after birth, dilatation and tortuosity of the retinal vessels begin to appear. The lesions may progress rapidly to hemorrhages and edema followed by membrane formation through retinal detachment, or they may regress without impairment of vision.

B. Pulmonary Irritation: O_2 concentrations above 60% cause irritation of the respiratory tract, cough, decrease in vital capacity, and substernal distress in a high percentage of subjects when exposure is continued for 24 hours. As the concentration of O_2 is increased above 60%, the incidence of symptoms increases rapidly. One patient developed irreversible pulmonary damage after about 16 hours of exposure to hyperbaric O_2.

C. Oxygen Poisoning: Inhalation of pure O_2 at elevated pressures, such as those that occur during marine diving, causes the rapid development of nervousness, hilarity, impaired judgment, paresthesias, muscular twitching or spasms, unconsciousness, and even convulsions. The latent period prior to the onset of symptoms depends on the pressure: at 3 atmospheres (66 feet of sea water), the latent period is about 2 hours; at 4 atmospheres (88 feet of sea water), it is 30 minutes. The interval is shortened by exercise.

Prevention

A. Retrolental Fibroplasia: Prolonged O_2 therapy at concentrations above 40% should be avoided by the use of equipment that allows adequate dilution of O_2 with air. Reliable methods include the use of tanks containing 60% nitrogen and 40% oxygen and the use of devices that mix O_2 from a high-pressure tank with sufficient air so that the final concentration of O_2 is 40%. O_2 should be given to premature infants only when it is definitely indicated by cyanosis and respiratory distress. Irregular respiration is not an indication for O_2 therapy. When O_2 therapy is necessary, use should be based on frequent arterial O_2 measurements. The O_2 concentration under operating conditions should be tested at least every 30 minutes by a reliable O_2 analyzer.

If proper control of O_2 therapy cannot be maintained, the use of O_2 for premature infants must be discontinued until reliable control can be instituted.

B. Oxygen Poisoning: Pure O_2 should not be breathed at pressures higher than atmospheric pressure. O_2 should not be used for div-

Table 32—4. Anticancer agents.

Name	Clinical Findings (In Addition to Those on p 459)
Aminopterin	Lymphopenia, fetal death or abnormalities, stomatitis.
Asparaginase (Elspar)	Sensitization, depressed liver function, reductions in clotting factors, elevated BUN, pancreatitis, depression, fever.
Azaribine (Triazure)	Renal damage, CNS depression, thromboembolic episodes.
Azaserine	Liver damage, stomatitis.
Azathioprine (Imuran)	Mouth lesions, skin rash, fever, alopecia, arthralgia, steatorrhea, jaundice, shock, plasmacytosis, anemia.
Bleomycin (Blenoxane)	Pulmonary fibrosis with 1% mortality. Fever, chills, vesiculation, hyperpigmentation.
Busulfan (Myleran)	Depression of erythropoiesis leading to aplastic anemia, diffuse pulmonary fibrosis, precipitation of uric acid in kidney tubules, hemorrhages.
Carmustine (BCNU, Bicnu), Lomustine (CCNU, CeeNU), Semustine (methyl-CCNU)	Liver function alteration, ataxia, dysarthria, CNS depression, renal damage, pulmonary damage.
Chlorambucil (Leukeran)	Interstitial pneumonia. Convulsions and coma after administration of 5 mg/kg orally, followed by recovery.
6-Chloropurine	Liver damage.
Cisplatin (Platinol)	Renal damage, hemolysis, tetany.
Cyclophosphamide (Cytoxan)	Alopecia, myocardial damage, interstitial pneumonitis.
Cytarabine (Cytosar)	Nausea, vomiting, megaloblastosis.
Dacarbazine (DTIC-Dome)	Diarrhea.
Dactinomycin (actinomycin D, Cosmegen)	Cheilosis, glossitis, oral ulceration.
Daunorubicin (6-diazo-5-oxonorleucine, DON)	Stomatitis, myocardial damage.
Doxorubicin (Adriamycin)	Irreversible myocardial toxicity.
Etoposide (VePesid)	Diarrhea, hypotension, sensitivity reactions, alopecia, fever.
Floxuridine 5-Fluorouracil	Diarrhea, alopecia, dermatitis, hyperpigmentation.
Guanazolo	Diarrhea, erythematous skin excoriations.
Hydroxyurea	Maculopapular rash, facial erythema, dysuria, alopecia, fever, drowsiness, disorientation, hallucinations, convulsions, impairment of renal tubular function.
Leucovorin	Hypersensitivity.
Mechlorethamine (nitrogen mustard, Mustargen)	Lymphopenia, thrombosis at site of injection, necrosis following extravascular injections, precipitation of uric acid in kidney tubules.
Melphalan (Alkeran)	Hypocalcemia, reversible lung damage.
6-Mercaptopurine (Purinethol)	Hepatic necrosis.
Methotrexate (amethopterin)	Anemia, diarrhea, ulcerative stomatitis, melena, dermatitis, alopecia, liver injury. Neurotoxocity after intrathecal injection.

Table 32–4 (cont'd). Anticancer agents.

Name	Clinical Findings (In Addition to Those in Text [below])
Mitomycin (Mutamycin)	Alopecia, pulmonary damage.
Pipobroman (Vercyte)	Vomiting, abdominal cramping, diarrhea, skin rash.
Plicamycin (Mithracin)	Bleeding, fever, abnormal liver function.
Procarbazine (Matulane)	Myalgia, arthralgia, fever, weakness, dermatitis, alopecia, paresthesias, hallucinations, tremors, convulsions, coma.
Streptozocin (Zanosar)	Possible liver and kidney damage.
Thioguanine	Jaundice.
Thiotepa (triethylenethio-phosphoramide)	Lymphopenia, precipitation of uric acid in kidney tubules.
Triethylenemelamine (TEM)	Lymphopenia.
Uracil mustard	Rash, alopecia.
Urethan	Vomiting, coma, hemorrhages; kidney and liver injury.
Vinblastine (Velban)	Stomatitis, ileus, mental depression, paresthesias, loss of deep reflexes, and even permanent CNS damage.
Vincristine (Oncovin)	Alopecia, paresthesias, neuritic pain, motor difficulties, loss of tendon reflexes.

ing equipment or submarine escape equipment unless the partial pressure of O_2 can be kept below 200 mm Hg.

Treatment

A. Retrolental Fibroplasia: No specific treatment is effective.

B. Pulmonary Irritation: Reduce the concentration of O_2 to 60% or less. Interrupt O_2 therapy frequently.

C. Oxygen Poisoning: Reduce the O_2 concentration below a partial pressure of 200 mm Hg.

Prognosis

Complete blindness may result in as many as 10% of premature infants who show evidence of retrolental fibroplasia.

ANTICANCER AGENTS

Overdosage with many of the agents listed in Table 32–4 causes leukopenia, granulocytopenia, thrombocytopenia, hypoplasia of all elements of bone marrow, nausea and vomiting, and anorexia.

Treatment of poisoning with these agents consists of discontinuing the drug, giving blood transfusions, and treating bone marrow depression. Treat overdoses of methotrexate by giving leucovorin calcium (folinic acid), 3–6 mg intramuscularly daily. Sodium thiosulfate can be used to antagonize immediately the effects of mechlorethamine.

COLCHICINE & COLCHICUM

Colchicine and colchicum are used in the treatment of gout. An alkaloid, colchicine, is present in all parts of the meadow saffron *(Colchicum autumnale)*. Another alkaloid, demecolcine, has also been isolated from the plant. The tincture of colchicum is made from the seeds.

The fatal dose of colchicine for adults is 20 mg. The fatal dose of tincture of colchicum may be as small as 15 mL. Fatalities occur in about 50% of those seriously poisoned. Colchicine has also caused thrombocytopenia with hemorrhages, leukopenia, or liver damage.

Colchicine is apparently converted in the body to oxydicolchicine, which, in excessive doses, is extremely irritating to all cells. The pathologic findings in fatal cases are congestion and degenerative changes in the gastrointestinal tract and kidneys.

Clinical Findings

The principal manifestations of poisoning with these compounds are vomiting, diarrhea, and collapse.

A. Acute Poisoning: After 3–6 hours, overdose causes burning in the throat, vomiting, watery to bloody diarrhea, abdominal pain, oliguria, fall of blood pressure, anuria, cardiovascular collapse, delirium, convulsions, and muscular weakness with respiratory failure. Sudden death may occur after rapid intravenous administration of 2 mg of colchicine.

B. Chronic Poisoning: Repeated administration of demecolcine and colchicine sometimes causes pancytopenia, thrombocytopenia with hemorrhages, leukopenia, malabsorption, oliguria, and hepatitis.

C. Laboratory Findings: Urinalysis may show hematuria, proteinuria, or hemoglobin casts. In demecolcine poisoning, all formed elements of the blood are decreased.

Prevention

Begin gout therapy with doses of colchicine no larger than 0.5 mg, and do not repeat doses oftener than every hour. Discontinue at onset of diarrhea or other toxic manifestations. Keep colchicine away from children. Since effective doses are approximately 80% of toxic doses, cautious use is imperative.

Treatment

A. Emergency Measures:

1. Discontinue medication if any symptoms of poisoning occur.

2. Delay absorption of ingested poison by giving tap water, milk, or activated charcoal and then remove by gastric lavage or emesis (see pp 21–28).

3. Treat shock by intravenous administration of saline, glucose, or blood (see p 66).

4. Give artificial respiration if muscular weakness is present. Give O_2 for cyanosis.

B. General Measures:

1. Keep the patient warm and quiet.

2. Give morphine sulfate, 2–10 mg, as necessary to relieve abdominal cramps.

3. For pancytopenia, give repeated blood transfusions.

C. Special Problems: Treat anuria or oliguria (see p 72).

Prognosis

If the administration of fractional doses of colchicine is discontinued at the onset of nausea and vomiting, recovery ordinarily occurs. Single doses of 4–8 mg orally or 2 mg intravenously may lead to fatalities in spite of therapy.

INTERACTIONS
(See p 17.)

Vitamin K displaces bilirubin from plasma protein binding and drives bilirubin into tissues, with increased brain injury in newborn infants (kernicterus).

Lithium increases the toxicity of haloperidol.

Combination of vinblastine and bleomycin causes Raynaud's disease.

Allopurinol enhances the effects of azathioprine and 6-mercaptopurine.

Sodium restriction and diuretics that induce sodium loss increase the toxicity of lithium.

PHARMACOKINETICS & TOXIC CONCENTRATIONS
(See p 89.)

	pK$_a$	t$_{1/2}$	V$_d$	% Binding
Allopurinol	9.4	2–30		0–4.5
Azathioprine		3		30
Colchicine	1.7, 12.4	0.32	2.19	
Cyclophosphamide		3–11		0–10
Cytarabine	4.3	1.9–2.6		
Daunorubicin		6–63		
5-Fluorouracil	8.1	0.17–0.33		
Lithium*		7–35	0.4–1.4	14
6-Mercaptopurine	7.6	1.5		
Methotrexate	4.3, 5.5	3.5, 27		50
Vinblastine	5.4, 7.4	3	1.4–1.7	
Vincristine	5.0, 7.4	1.5		

*Toxic concentration, 1 mmol/L.

References

Disulfiram & Thiocarbamates

Benitz WE: Disulfiram intoxication in a child. *J Pediatr* 1984;**105**:487.

Garnier R et al: Acute thioproline poisoning. *J Toxicol Clin Toxicol* 1982;**19**:289.

Kirubakaran V et al: Acute disulfiram overdose. *Am J Psychiatry* 1983; **140**:1513.

Lacoursiere RB, Smatek R: Adverse interaction between disulfiram and marihuana. *Am J Psychiatry* 1983;**140**:243.

Iron Salts

Lovejoy FH Jr: Chelation therapy in iron poisoning. *J Toxicol Clin Toxicol* 1982;**19**:871.

Anticancer Agents

Blank DW et al: Acute renal failure and seizures associated with chlorambucil overdose. *J Toxicol Clin Toxicol* 1983;**20**:361.

Bressler RB et al: Water intoxication following moderate-dose intravenous cyclophosphamide. *Arch Intern Med* 1985;**145**:548.

Chapman JR et al: Reversibility of cyclosporin nephrotoxicity after three months' treatment. *Lancet* 1985;**1**:128.

Collins JA: Hypersensitivity reaction to doxorubicin. *Drug Intell Clin Pharm* 1984;**18**:402.

Hirsh JD, Conlon PF: Implementing guidelines for managing extravasation of antineoplastics. *Am J Hosp Pharm* 1983;**40**:1516.

Hirst M et al: Occupational exposure to cyclophosphamide. *Lancet* 1984;**1**:186.

Hrushesky WJM et al: Twenty-four hour mean pulse: Simple predictor of dox-orubicin-induced cardiac damage. *Am J Med* 1984;**77**:399.

Kolmodin-Hedman B et al: Occupational handling of cytostatic drugs. *Arch Toxicol* 1983;**54**:25.

Saltiel E, McGuire W: Doxorubicin cardiomyopathy. *West J Med* 1983;**139**:332.

Smith FP, McCabe MS: Preventing chemotherapy-induced alopecia. *Am Fam Physician* (July) 1983;**28**:182.

Venitt S et al: Monitoring exposure of nursing and pharmacy personnel to cytotoxic drugs: Urinary mutation assays and urinary platinum as markers of absorption. *Lancet* 1984;**1**:74.

Diagnostic Agents

Berkseth RO, Kjellstrand CM: Radiologic contrast-induced nephropathy. *Med Clin North Am* 1984;**68**:351.

Elliott RL et al: Prolonged delirium after metrizamide myelography. *JAMA* 1984;**252**:2057.

Nicot GS et al: Transient glomerular proteinuria, enzymuria, and nephrotoxic reaction induced by radiocontrast media. *JAMA* 1984;**252**:2432.

Lithium & Sodium

Addleman M et al: Survival after severe hypernatremia due to salt ingestion by an adult. *Am J Med* 1984;**78**:176.

Amdisen A: Lithium and drug interactions. *Drugs* 1982;**24**:133.

Cairns SR et al: Persistent nephrogenic diabetes insipidus, hyperparathy-roidism, and hypoparathyroidism after lithium treatment. *Br Med J* 1985;**290**:516.

Clendenin NJ et al: Potential pitfalls in the evaluation of the usefulness of hemodialysis for the removal of lithium. *J Toxicol Clin Toxicol* 1982;**19**:341.

El-Mallakh RS: Treatment of acute lithium toxicity. *Vet Hum Toxicol* 1984;**26**:31.

Fenvez AZ et al: Lithium intoxication associated with acute renal failure. *South Med J* 1984;**77**:1472.

Hansen HE: Renal toxicity of lithium. *Drugs* 1981;**22**:461.

Lewis DA: Unrecognized chronic lithium neurotoxic reactions. *JAMA* 1983;**250**:2029.

Mastrangelo MR et al: Spontaneous rupture of the stomach in a healthy adult man after sodium bicarbonate ingestion. *Ann Intern Med* 1985;**101**:649.

Parfrey PS et al: Severe lithium intoxication treated by forced diuresis. *Can Med Assoc J* 1983;**129**:979.

Puczynski MS et al: Sodium intoxication caused by use of baking soda as a home remedy. *Can Med Assoc J* 1983;**128**:821.

Dietary Additives, Vitamins, & Oxygen

Baxi SC, Dailey GE III: Hypervitaminosis A: A cause of hypercalcemia. *West J Med* 1982;**137**:429.

Benke PJ: The isotretinoin teratogen syndrome. *JAMA* 1984;**251**:3267.

Coates AL et al: Oxygen therapy and long-term pulmonary outcome of respira-tory distress syndrome in newborns. *Am J Dis Child* 1982;**136**:892.

Cordle F, Miller SA: Using epidemiology to regulate food additives: Saccharin case control studies. *Public Health Rep* 1984;**99**:365.

Jibani M et al: Prolonged hypercalcaemia after industrial exposure to vitamin D₃. *Br Med J* 1985;**290**:748.

Kemmann E et al: Amenorrhea associated with carotenemia. *JAMA* 1983;**249**:926.

Lawton JM et al: Acute oxalate nephropathy after massive ascorbic acid administration. *Arch Intern Med* 1985;**145**:950.

MacCara ME: Tartrazine: A potentially hazardous dye in Canadian drugs. *Can Med Assoc J* 1982;**126**:910.

Masked hypervitaminosis A and liver injury. *Nutr Rev* (Oct) 1982;**40**:303.

Podell RN: Vitamin A overdose. *Postgrad Med* (Sept) 1983;**74**:297.

Vitamin A and teratogenesis. (Editorial.) *Lancet* 1985;**1**:319.

Warin RP, Smith RJ: Role of tartrazine in chronic urticaria. *Br Med J* 1982;**284**:1443.

Miscellaneous

McGrath KG et al: Anaphylactic reactivity to streptokinase. *JAMA* 1984;**252**:1314.

Shah D et al: Generalized epileptic fits in renal transplant recipients given cyclosporin A. *Br Med J* 1984;**289**:1347.

VI. Animal & Plant Hazards

Reptiles | 33

SNAKES
(Tables 33–1, 33–2, 33–3, and 33–4)

Poisonous snakes occur throughout most parts of the tropical and temperate zones of the world. They are more numerous in tropical or semitropical areas.

The degree of toxicity resulting from snakebite depends on the potency of the venom, the amount of venom injected, and the size of the person bitten. Table 33–1 shows the smallest dose by intraperitoneal or intravenous injection that kills 50% of a group of experimental mice (LD50) and the amount of dried venom in the venom glands of an adult specimen. The amount of venom injected by the snake may vary from 0 to 75% of the total stored in the gland.

In 1979, there were 5 deaths from venomous reptile bites in the USA; each year, several thousand patients receive antiserum. Worldwide, deaths have been estimated at 30,000–40,000.

Pathologic Physiology

Poisoning may occur from injection or absorption of venom through cuts or scratches.

Snake venoms are complex and include proteins, some of which have enzymatic activity. The effects produced by venoms include neurotoxic effects with sensory, motor, cardiac, and respiratory difficulties; cytotoxic effects on red blood cells, blood vessels, heart muscle, kidneys, and lungs; defects in coagulation; and effects from local release of substances by enzymatic action.

Pathology

The pathologic findings in nervous tissue include changes in Nissl's granules, fragmentation of the reticulum of the nerve cells, opacity of the nuclei, and fragmentation and swelling of the nucleoli. Acute granular degeneration may be seen in the cells of the anterior medulla. Loss of staining characteristics is also present. Other findings are widespread gross and petechial hemorrhages, necrosis and desquamation of the renal tubules, cloudy swelling and granular changes in the cells of other organs, and extensive local hemorrhages at the site of the wound.

Table 33–1. Venoms of important poisonous snakes.*

Snake	Average Length of Adult (inches)	Approximate Yield, Dry Venom (mg)	LD50 (mg/kg)
North America:			
Rattlesnakes (Crotalus)			
Eastern diamondback (Crotalus adamanteus)	33–65	370–720	1.68
Western diamondback (Crotalus atrox)	30–65	175–325	3.71
Timber (Crotalus horridus horridus)	32–54	95–150	2.63
Prairie (Crotalus viridis viridis)	32–46	25–100	1.61
Great Basin (Crotalus viridis lutosus)	32–46	75–150	2.20
Southern Pacific (Crotalus viridis helleri)	30–48	75–160	1.29
Red diamond (Crotalus ruber ruber)	30–52	125–400	3.70
Mojave (Crotalus scutulatus)	22–40	50–90	0.21
Sidewinder (Crotalus cerastes)	18–30	18–40	4.00
Moccasins (Agkistrodon)			
Cottonmouth (Agkistrodon piscivorus)	30–50	90–148	4.00
Copperhead (Agkistrodon contortrix)	24–36	40–72	10.50
Cantil (Agkistrodon bilineatus)	30–42	50–95	2.40
Coral snakes (Micrurus)			
Eastern coral snake (Micrurus fulvius)	16–28	2–6	0.97
Central and South America:			
Rattlesnakes (Crotalus)			
Cascabel (Crotalus durissus terrificus)	20–48	20–40	0.30
American lance-headed vipers (Bothrops)			
Barba amarilla (Bothrops atrox)	46–80	70–160	3.80
Bushmaster (Lachesis mutus)	70–110	280–450	5.93
Asia:			
Cobras (Naja)			
Asian cobra (Naja naja)	45–65	170–325	0.40
Kraits (Bungarus)			
Indian krait (Bungarus caeruleus)	36–48	8–20	0.09
Vipers (Vipera)			
Russell's viper (Vipera russellii)	40–50	130–250	0.08
Pit vipers (Agkistrodon)			
Malayan pit viper (Agkistrodon rhodostoma)	25–35	40–60	6.20
Africa:			
Vipers			
Puff adder (Bitis arietans)	30–48	130–200	3.68
Saw-scaled viper (Echis carinatus)	16–22	20–35	2.30
Mambas (Dendroaspis)			
Eastern green mamba (Dendroaspis angusticeps)	50–72	60–95	0.45
Australia:			
Tiger snake (Notechis scutatus)	30–56	30–70	0.04
Europe:			
European viper (Vipera berus)	18–24	6–18	0.55
Indo-Pacific:			
Beaked sea snake (Enhydrina schistosa)	30–48	7–20	0.01

*All tables in this chapter are modified from *Poisonous Snakes of the World.* Navmed P-5099. US Department of the Navy, Bureau of Medicine and Surgery, 1968. US Government Printing Office, Washington, DC 20402.

Table 33–2. Symptoms and signs of crotalid bites.

	North American Rattlesnakes (Crotalus)	Central and South American Rattlesnakes (Crotalus)	North American Moccasins (Agkistrodon)	American Lance-headed Vipers (Bothrops)	Asian Lance-headed Vipers (Trimeresurus)	Malayan Pit Viper (Agkistrodon)
Swelling and edema	+++	++	++	+++	+++	++
Pain at site of bite	++	++	+	+++	++	++
Discoloration of skin	+++	+	+	+++	+++	++
Vesicles	+++		+	+++	+++	++
Ecchymosis	+++	+	++	+++	+++	+++
Superficial thrombosis	++			++		
Necrosis	++		+	+++	+	+
Sloughing of tissue	++			+++	+	+
Lassitude	++	+++	+	++	++	++
Thirst	++	++	+	+++	+	++
Nausea or vomiting (or both)	++	++	+	++		
Weak pulse and changes in rate	+++	+++	+	+++	++	++
Hypotension or shock	+++	+	+	+++	++	++
Sphering or destruction of red cells	+++			+++		
Increased bleeding time	++	+		++	+	+
Increased clotting time	+++	+		+++	++	+++
Hemorrhage	+++		+	++	++	++
Anemia	++			++	+	+
Glycosuria	++		+	++		
Proteinuria	++		+	++	+	+
Tingling or numbness	++	+++	+	+	+	
Fasciculations	+	+++	+	+	+	
Muscular weakness or paralysis	+	++		+		
Ptosis of lids	+	++		+		
Blurring of vision	+	+++		++		
Respiratory distress	++	+++	+	++		
Swelling of regional lymph nodes	++	+	+	++	+	

Table 33–3. Symptoms and signs of elapid bites.

Symptoms and Signs	Cobras (Naja)	Kraits (Bungarus)	Mambas (Dendroaspis)	Taipan (Oxyuranus)	Coral Snakes (Micrurus)
Pain at site of bite	++	+	+	+	++
Localized edema	+				+
Drowsiness, lassitude	+++	+++	++	+++	+++
Feeling of thickened tongue and throat, slurring of speech, difficulty in swallowing	+++	+++	+++	+++	++
Ptosis of lids	+++	+++	++	+++	++
Changes in respiration	++	+++	++	+++	++
Headache	++	++	++	+++	++
Blurring of vision	++	++	+++	+++	+
Weak pulse and changes in rate	++	++	++	+	++
Hypotension or shock	++	+++	++	+	+
Excessive salivation	+++	+++	+++	+	+++
Nausea and vomiting	+	++	+++	+++	+
Abdominal pain	+	+++	+++	+++	+
Pain in regional lymph nodes	+	++			+
Localized discoloration of skin	++				+
Localized vesicles	+				
Localized necrosis	+				
Muscle weakness, paresis, or paralysis	++	+++	++	++	+
Muscle fasciculations	+	+	+	+	+
Numbness of affected area	++	+++	+	+	+++
Convulsions	+	+			+++

Table 33–4. Symptoms and signs of viperid bites.

Symptoms and Signs	Russell's Viper (Vipera russellii)	Saw-Scaled Viper (Echis carinatus)	Levantine Viper (Vipera lebetina) and Related Species	European Viper (Vipera berus)	Puff Adder (Bitis arietans)
Swelling and edema	++	+++	++	++	++
Pain at site of bite	+++	+++	++	++	+++
Discoloration of skin	+++	++	++	++	+++
Weakness	++	++	+	++	++
Nausea or vomiting (or both)	++	+	+++	++	++
Abdominal pain	++	+	+++	+	++
Diarrhea	++	+++	+++		++
Thirst	++		+	++	+
Chills or fever	++	++	++		+
Swelling of regional lymph nodes	+	+	++	++	++
Facial edema	+		++	+	+
Dilatation of pupils	++	+	+	+	+
Weak pulse and changes in rate	++	+	++	+	
Proteinuria	++	++	++		+
Hypotension	++	++	++	+	++
Shock	++	++	++	+	++
Hemorrhage*	++	+++	+	+	++
Anemia	++	++	+		
Vesicles	++	++	++	+	++
Ecchymosis	++	+	++	+	++
Necrosis	++	+	+		+
Decreased platelets	+	+	+		+
Prolonged clotting time	+++	+++	++		+

*Usually limited to area of wound in puff adder and European viper bites. However, bleeding from the gums, intestine, and urinary tract may occur, particularly in saw-scaled viper and Russell's viper envenomizations.

Clinical Findings

The diagnosis of a poisonous snakebite depends on finding one or more puncture wounds or tooth marks and any one of the following signs of envenomization: local swelling, local pain, ecchymosis, blurring of vision, any evidence of muscular weakness, drowsiness, nausea, vomiting, salivation, or sweating. (See Tables 33–1, 33–2, 33–3, and 33–4.)

A. Crotalid Envenomization: Swelling, edema, and local pain beginning within 10 minutes. Discoloration of skin and ecchymosis develop over several hours and progress to petechiae and hemorrhagic vesiculations. Weakness, sweating, faintness, nausea, tender lymph nodes, and tingling or numbness of tongue, mouth, or scalp are common. Hemoglobin, blood volume, and platelets decrease.

B. Viperid Envenomization: Local pain, swelling, edema, skin discoloration, and ecchymosis occur. Bleeding from the wound and from the gums is common in severe Russell's and saw-scaled viper bites. The blood may fail to clot. Severe poisoning is indicated by swelling extending above the elbows or knees within 2 hours or by hemorrhages.

C. Elapid Envenomization: Cobra bites are characterized by pain within 10 minutes, but onset of swelling is slow. General symptoms include drowsiness, weakness, excessive salivation, and paralysis of the facial muscles, lips, tongue, and larynx. Blood pressure falls and respiration becomes difficult. Ptosis, blurring of vision, convulsions, and headache also occur. The kraits, mambas, and taipan and coral snakes cause less local reaction, but abdominal pain is more intense. Severe poisoning is indicated by neurotoxic signs occurring within 1 hour.

D. Envenomization by Sea Snakes: Bites cause little local pain, but there is pain in skeletal muscles, especially during motion. Paresthesias of the tongue and mouth, difficulty with swallowing, trismus, weakness of extraocular muscles, pupillary dilation, and ptosis also occur. Myoglobinuria is diagnostic.

Laboratory Findings

The levels of prothrombin, fibrinogen, fibrin products, hematocrit, hemoglobin, and platelets should be determined.

Prevention

People in snake-infested areas should wear shoes and heavy canvas leggings because more than half of all bites are on the lower parts of the legs.

Snake venom antiserum for snakes of the region should be readily available in areas where snakebites are frequent.

Avoid walking at night or in grass and underbrush. Do not climb rocky ledges without visual inspection. Do not kill snakes unnecessarily; many people are bitten in such attempts.

Treatment

Treatment of snakebite requires immediate identification and administration of appropriate antiserum. Bring the dead snake in with the patient, if possible.

A. Emergency Measures:

1. Immobilize the patient and the bitten part in a horizontal position. Wash the bitten area with water to remove surface venom. Avoid any manipulation of the bitten area. Do not allow the patient to walk, run, or take alcoholic beverages or stimulants. Transport the patient without delay to a medical facility for definitive treatment.

2. If symptoms develop rapidly and antiserum cannot be given, apply constricting bands just proximal and distal to the bite. A $\frac{1}{2} \times 24$ inch thin rubber band or $\frac{1}{8}$-inch-diameter thin-walled gum rubber tubing is satisfactory. (Bands are not helpful if they are applied more than 30 minutes after the bite or after giving antiserum.) The bands should occlude lymph drainage but not veins or arteries. Move the bands as swelling progresses. The bands should be left in place until antiserum can be given. Be prepared to cope with severe fall of blood pressure when the bands are released. Remove constricting bands completely 4–8 hours after antiserum is given.

3. Incision through the fang marks by untrained persons as an emergency measure is not advisable; it is too hazardous to underlying structures and at best removes only 20% of the venom.

B. Antidote:

1. Give specific antiserum intravenously (see pp 476–481) after testing for serum sensitivity (see below). Since antiserum can be dangerous to life, wait for clear evidence of systemic venom toxicity beyond nausea and vomiting before beginning administration. In coral snake bite, 1–5 vials of antivenom should be given as soon as possible, since the venom is fixed in neural tissues before symptoms occur. If there are any signs of envenomization, give 3–5 vials. The size of the initial dose of *Micrurus fulvius* antiserum depends on the extent of initial pain and the certainty that the bite actually injected venom. Overtreatment is common but preferable. In crotalid envenomization with minimal systemic symptoms and signs, give 3–5 vials of antivenom. If there is progressive swelling, paresthesia around the mouth, or any other systemic symptoms, an initial dose of up to 10 vials may be needed depending on the severity of symptoms. Dilute the initial dose of antiserum with 500 mL of 5% dextrose in saline and start a slow intravenous drip if the patient is not sensitive or has been desensitized. Cardiorespiratory resuscitation measures, including epinephrine, must be available. If no sensitivity reaction occurs in the first 5 minutes, in-

crease the flow rate in order to inject the total dose in 1 hour. If swelling does not progress and paresthesias disappear, give a second 500 mL of saline with 3–5 vials of antiserum over the next 4 hours. If swelling progresses and systemic symptoms increase, a total dose of antiserum up to 300 mL in the first 4 hours may be necessary. Antiserum is less useful after a delay of 4 hours and probably useless after 24 hours. A dose of 30 mL or more will ordinarily produce serum reactions.

Serum sensitivity is determined by injecting into the skin (intradermally) 0.02 mL of antiserum diluted 1:100 in 0.9% saline solution with a control injection of 0.9% saline for comparison. Examine in 10 minutes. A positive reaction is indicated by a wheal or swelling surrounded by redness. The test can also be done by placing a drop of diluted antiserum in the conjunctival sac. Congestion, lacrimation, and itching indicate a positive reaction. Apply 1:1000 epinephrine locally to limit the reaction.

If the sensitivity test is positive, desensitize the patient by injecting 0.05 mL of 1:100 dilution subcutaneously. Double the amount injected every 5 minutes until 1 mL of 1:10 dilution is given; then, if no reaction occurs, begin a slow intravenous drip of 1:50 dilution as above. Reactions are controlled by the repeated injection of epinephrine, 1:1000 solution, and administration of diphenhydramine, 50 mg intravenously, as necessary.

2. Even in the absence of a skin sensitivity reaction to a test injection, serum sickness occurs in about 30% of patients given 3 vials of antiserum and in more than 90% of those given 6 vials or more.

C. General Measures:

1. Monitor blood pressure, pulse, respiration, central venous pressure, hematocrit, hemoglobin products in urine, and catheterized urine output. Repeat the blood coagulation profile every 4 hours as necessary. Measure the circumference of the affected extremity at several places every 15 minutes to monitor progression of swelling and to determine the need for additional antivenom.

2. In antiserum reactions, give prednisone, 45–60 mg daily in divided doses, but avoid giving corticosteroids for 24 hours after antivenom administration, if possible.

3. Maintain blood pressure (see p 66). Central venous pressure should exceed 5 cm of water. Intravenous fluid needs may reach 1 L/h. If the hemoglobin level falls below 10 g/dL, give packed red blood cells or whole blood to raise the hemoglobin level to 12 g/dL.

4. If the fibrinogen level is low, give human fibrinogen intravenously. Platelet transfusion may be necessary. Other coagulopathies require replacement with specific factors, fresh whole blood, or plasma.

5. For convulsions or respiratory paralysis, give artificial respiration. Respiratory paralysis for up to 10 days is compatible with recovery after elapid envenomization.

6. Treat renal failure by fluid and electrolyte restriction or hemodialysis.

7. Give tetanus antitoxin or, if the patient has already been immunized, tetanus toxoid.

8. For infection in the bitten area, give organism-specific chemotherapy.

9. Control pain by the use of aspirin or codeine. Avoid depressant narcotics.

Prognosis

Adequate, early, specific antiserum treatment will reduce the mortality rate from all snakebites below 10%.

GILA MONSTER

The Gila monster (*Heloderma* species), the only poisonous lizard, lives in desert areas of the southwestern USA and northern Mexico. This lizard does not have fangs like many poisonous snakes. Instead, grooves in the front teeth carry the poison.

The fatal dose of the venom is not known, but toxicity is presumably comparable to some snake venoms, since severe injury may follow a scratch from the teeth of the Gila monster. The venom causes enzymatic tissue destruction. The pathologic findings are similar to those from rattlesnake bite.

Fatal poisoning is rare, since the lizard is uncommon and is not likely to bite unless handled.

Clinical Findings

Symptoms and signs (from a bite or tooth-scratch from a Gila monster) include nausea and vomiting, local swelling and pain that spreads rapidly, cyanosis, respiratory depression, and weakness. The laboratory findings are not characteristic.

Treatment

A. Emergency Measures: If, in biting, the lizard is tenacious, cut the muscles at the angle of the lizard's jaw to loosen it. Enforce complete inactivity of the victim, as for snakebite (see p 473).

B. Antidote: No specific antiserum is available.

C. General Measures: See p 474 for the general measures used in the treatment of snakebite.

Prognosis

The mortality rate is about 1% in adults, about 5% in children.

SOURCES OF ANTISERA FOR
POISONOUS SNAKES

This section lists the sources of antisera, the venoms used in preparation of the antisera, and possible neutralizing potency against other venoms. When used against venoms of heterologous species, antivenin should be given in doses 2–4 times as large as those recommended for the homologous species.

NORTH AMERICA

United States. Wyeth Laboratories, Box 8299, Philadelphia, PA 19101. (Telephone: [215] 688–4400.)

> **Antivenin (Crotalidae) Polyvalent.** *Crotalus adamanteus, Crotalus atrox, Crotalus durissus terrificus, Bothrops atrox*. Neutralizes most crotalid venoms.

> **Antivenin *Micrurus fulvius* (coral snake).** *Micrurus fulvius fulvius*. Also neutralizes *Micrurus nigrocinctus* but not *Micrurus mipartitus* or *Micruroides euryxanthus*.

Mexico. Instituto Nacional de Higiene, Czda. M. Escobedo No. 20, Mexico 13, DF.

> **Suero Anticrotálico.** *Crotalus durissus* subspecies, *Crotalus basiliscus*. Reported to neutralize venoms of all Mexican crotalids.

> **Suero Antibotrópico.** *Bothrops atrox*.

> **Suero Antiviperino.** *Crotalus durissus* subspecies, *Crotalus basiliscus, Bothrops atrox*.

Mexico. Laboratorios MYN, S.A., Av. Coyoacan 1707, Mexico 12, DF.

> **Suero Anticrotálico MYN Liofilizado.** Different Mexican crotalids. Neutralizes *Crotalus durissus* venom and others.

> **Suero Antibotrópico MYN Liofilizado.** *Bothrops atrox*.

> **Suero Antiviperino MYN Liofilizado.** Different Mexican crotalids and *Bothrops atrox*.

> **Suero Antiofidico MYN Polivalente (Liquido).** Mexican crotalids and *Bothrops atrox*.

Costa Rica. Instituto Clodomiro Picado, Universidad de Costa Rica, Cuidad Universitaria "Rodrigo Facio."

> **Suero Polivalente.** *Bothrops atrox, Crotalus durissus, Lachesis muta*.

Suero Anti-Coral. *Micrurus nigrocinctus, Micrurus alleni.*
Suero Anti-*Micrurus*. *Micrurus mipartitus.*
Suero Anti-Laquético. *Lachesis mutus stenophyrs.*

SOUTH AMERICA*

Argentina. Instituto Nacional de Microbiologia, Velez Sarsfield 563, Buenos Aires.
    Bivalente Anti-Botrópico. *Bothrops alternatus, Bothrops neuweidi.*
    Polivalente Anti-Botrópico y Anti-Crotálico. *Crotalus durissus terrificus, Bothrops alternatus, Bothrops neuweidi.*
    Polivalente Misiones. *Crotalus durissus terrificus, Bothrops alternatus, Bothrops neuweidi, Bothrops jajaraca (jararaca), Bothrops jararacussu.*
    Monovalente Anti-Elapidico (Liofilizado).

Brazil. Instituto Pinheiros Productos Therapeuticos, Caixa Postal 951, São Paulo.
    Sôro Anti-Botrópico. *Bothrops alternatus, Bothrops atrox, Bothrops jajaraca (jararaca), Bothrops jararacussu, Bothrops cotiara.* Reported to neutralize the venom of *Lachesis mutus* in large doses.
    Sôro Anti-Ophidico. Same as Anti-Botrópico plus *Crotalus durissus terrificus.* Reported to neutralize the venom of *Lachesis mutus* in large doses.
    Sôro Anti-Crotálico. *Crotalus durissus terrificus.*

Brazil. Instituto Butantan, Caixa Postal 65, São Paulo.
    Sôro Anti-Crotálico. *Crotalus* species.
    Sôro Anti-Laquético. *Lachesis mutus.*
    Sôro Anti-Elapidico. *Micrurus* species.
    Sôro Anti-Botrópico. *Bothrops* species. Reported to neutralize the venom of *Lachesis mutus* in large doses.
    Sôro Anti-Ophidico. *Bothrops* species and *Crotalus* species. Reported to neutralize the venom of *Lachesis mutus* in large doses.
    Sôro Anti-Botrópico-Laquético. *Bothrops jararaco* and *Lachesis mutus.*

Colombia. Instituto Nacional de Salud. Avenida El Dorado Con Carrera 50, Zonas 6, Apartados Aereus 80080 Y, 80334 Bogotá DE, Colombia.

*See also Europe, Germany: Behringwerke AG.

Polyvalente. *Bothrops atrox, Crotalus durissus terrificus.*

Venezuela. Laboratorio Behrens, Calle Real do Capellin, Apartado 62, Caracas, DF.

    Suero Antibotrópico. *Bothrops atrox,* "tigra mariposa" *(Bothrops).* The name "tigra mariposa" is applied to at least 2 species of *Bothrops* in Venezuela; it is not clear which species' venom is used in preparation of the antivenin.

    Suero Anticrotálico. *Crotalus durissus* subspecies.

    Suero Antiofidico Polivalente. *Bothrops atrox,* "tigra mariposa" *(Bothrops).* (See above.)

PACIFIC

Australia. Commonwealth Serum Laboratories, Poplar Road, Parkville, Melbourne, Victoria.

    Brown Snake Antivenene. *Demansia textilis.* Neutralizes venoms of other species of *Demansia* such as *Demansia olivacea.*

    Death Adder Antivenene. *Acanthophis antarcticus.*

    Malayan Cobra Antivenene. *Naja naja sputatrix.*

    Black Snake Antivenene. *Pseudechis papuanus.* Neutralizes *Pseudechis porphyriacus* and *Pseudechis australis* venoms.

    Sea Snake Antivenene. *Enhydrina schistosa* and other sea snakes.

    Taipan Antivenene. *Oxyuranus scutellatus.* Neutralizes *Pseudechis australis* and *Demansia textilis* venoms.

    Tiger Snake Antivenene. *Notechis scutatus.* Neutralizes the venoms of all important venomous snakes of the Australian and New Guinea region to some extent.

    Polyvalent (Aust/NG) Antivenene. (For unidentified snakes of Australia and New Guinea.)

Japan. The Chemo-Sero-Therapeutic Research Institute, Kumamoto City.

    Antivenin Habu. *Trimeresurus flavoviridis.*

Japan. Takeda Chemical Industries, Osaka.

    Antivenin Mamushi. *Agkistrodon halys blomhoffii.*

Philippine Republic. Serum and Vaccine Laboratories, Alabang, Muntinlupa, Rizal, Republic of the Philippines.

    Philippine Cobra Antivenene. *Naja naja philippinensis.*

EUROPE

Austria. Serotherapeutisches Institute Wien, Triesterstrasse 50, 1100
X Wien. Distributor of antisera for European vipers.

France. Institut Pasteur, 36 Rue du Docteur Roux, Paris 15.
    Ipser V. *Vipera aspis, Vipera berus.*
    Ipser Europe. *Vipera aspis, Vipera berus, Vipera ammodytes.*
    Anti *Bungarus*. *Bungarus fasciatus.*
    Anti *Cerastes*. *Cerastes cerastes, Cerastes vipera.*
    Anti *Bothrops*. *Bothrops atrox.*
    Anti Cobra. *Naja naja.*
    Polyvalent. *Cerastes, Echis, Naja,* and *Vipera* of Middle East.
    Anti Viper. (Middle East). *Vipera lebetina, Vipera xanthina
        palaestinae.*
    Anti *Bitis Echis Naja*. *Bitis gabonica, Bitis lachesis, Bitis nasi-
        cornis, Echis carinatus, Naja haje, Naja melanoleuca,
        Naja nigricollis, Naja nivea, Haemachatus haemacha-
        tus.*
    Anti *Dendroaspis*. *Dendroaspis angusticeps, Dendroaspis
        jamesoni, Dendroaspis polylepis, Dendroaspis viridis.*

Germany. Behringwerke AG, Postschliessfach 167, 355 Marburg-
Lahn.
    Serum Nordafrika. *Bitis gabonica, Bitis arietans, Cerastes
        cerastes, Cerastes vipera, Vipera lebetina, Echis carina-
        tus, Naja nigricollis, Naja haje.*
    Serum Zentralafrika. *Bitis gabonica, Bitis arietans, Bitis nasi-
        cornis, Haemachatus haemachatus, Naja nigricollis,
        Naja haje.*
    Serum Naher- und Mittlerer Orient. *Cerastes cerastes, Echis
        carinatus, Vipera ammodytes, Vipera lebetina, Naja
        haje.*
    Serum Europa. *Vipera ammodytes, Vipera lebetina.*
    Serum Mittel- und Sudamerika. *Crotalus durissus terrificus,
        Bothrops atrox, Bothrops jajaraca (jararaca).*
    Serum Kobra. *Haemachatus haemachatus, Naja haje, Naja
        nivea, Naja nigricollis.*

Italy. Instituto Sieroterapico e Vaccinogeno "SCLAVO," Via
Fiorentina, 53100 Siena.
    Antiophidio Serum. *Vipera ammodytes, Vipera aspis, Vipera
        berus.* Reported to be effective against venoms of all Eu-
        ropean vipers.

USSR. Tashkent Institute, Ministry of Health, Moscow. The product names are only approximations of the Russian.

Cobra Antivenin. *Naja naja oxiana.*

Echis **Antivenin.** *Echis carinatus.*

Gyurza Antivenin. *Vipera lebetina.*

Gyurza Polyvalent Antivenin. *Vipera lebetina, Naja naja oxiana.*

Echis **Polyvalent Antivenin.** *Echis carinatus, Naja naja oxiana.*

Yugoslavia. Institute for Immunology, Rockefellerova 2, Zagreb.

Serum Antiviperinum. *Vipera ammodytes, Vipera aspis, Vipera berus.*

AFRICA*

Algeria. Institut Pasteur d'Algerie, Rue Docteur Laveran, Alger.

Serum Antiviperin. *Cerastes cerastes, Vipera lebetina.*

Republic of South Africa. South African Institute for Medical Research, PO Box 1038, Johannesburg.

Echis carinatus **Antivenom.** *Echis carinatus* and *Cerastes* species.

Mamba Antivenom. *Dendroaspis* species.

Boomslang Antivenom. *Dispholidus typus.*

Polyvalent Antivenin *(Haemachatus, Naja, Bitis, Dendroaspis).* Vipers, mambas, ringhals, and cobras.

ASIA*

India. Central Research Institute, Kasauli, RI, Punjab.

Polyvalent Antivenin. *Bungarus caeruleus, Naja naja, Echis carinatus, Vipera russellii.*

India. Haffkine Bio-Pharmaceutical Corporation, Parel, Bombay 400 012.

Polyvalent Anti-Snake Venom Serum.

Bungarus **Anti-Snake Venom Serum.** *Bungarus caeruleus, Echis carinatus, Naja naja.*

Agkistrodon **Antivenin.** *Agkistrodon rhodostoma.*

Bungarus **Antivenin.** *Bungarus fasciatus.*

Cobra Antivenin. *Naja naja sputatrix.*

*See also Europe, Germany: Behringwerke AG.

Indonesia. Perusahaan Negara Bio Farma (Pasteur's Institute), 9 Djalan Pasteur, Postbox 47, Bandung.

    ABM Antivenin. *Bungarus fasciatus, Naja naja sputatrix, Agkistrodon rhodostoma.*

Iran. Institut d'Etat des Serum et Vaccins Razi, Boite postale 656, Teheran (Hessarak-Karadj).

    Monovalent antivenins against venoms of *Vipera lebetina, Vipera latifii, Naja naja oxiana, Echis carinatus, Pseudocerastes persicus,* and *Agkistrodon halys.*

    Polyvalent Antivenin for Iran. *Naja naja oxiana, Echis carinatus, Vipera lebetina, Pseudocerastes persicus, Vipera xanthina, Agkistrodon halys.*

Israel. Rogoff Wellcome Research Laboratories, Beilinson Hospital, POB 85, Petah Tikva.

    Echis coloratus **Antiserum.** *Echis coloratus.*

    Vipera palaestinae **Antiserum.** *Vipera palaestinae.*

Taiwan. Taiwan Serum and Vaccine Laboratory, 151 Tongshin Street, Nang Kang, Taipei. Supplied only to Taiwan addressees.

    Bungarus **Monovalent.** *Bungarus multicinctus.*

    Naja **Monovalent.** *Naja naja atra.*

    Agkistrodon **Monovalent.** *Agkistrodon acutus.* Reported to neutralize Chinese habu venom.

    Neurotoxic Polyvalent. *Bungarus multicinctus, Naja naja atra.*

    Hemorrhagic Polyvalent. *Trimeresurus mucrosquamatus, Trimeresurus stejnegeri.* Reported to neutralize *Agkistrodon* venom to a limited extent.

Thailand. Queen Saovabha Memorial Institute, Rama IV Street, Bangkok.

    Banded Krait Antivenin. *Bungarus fasciatus.*

    Cobra Antivenin. *Naja naja.*

    Green Pit Viper Antivenin. *Trimeresurus popeorum.*

    King Cobra Antivenin. *Naja hannah.*

    Russell's Viper Antivenin. *Vipera russellii.*

    Malayan Pit Viper Antivenin. *Agkistrodon rhodostoma.*

Viet Nam. Institut Pasteur, Nha Trang.

    Sea Snake Antivenin. *Lapemis hardwickii.*

References

Cable B et al: Prolonged defibrination after a bite from a "non-venomous" snake *(Rhabdophis subminatus)*. *JAMA* 1984;**251**:925.

Curry SC et al: Death from a rattlesnake bite. *Am J Emerg Med* 1985;**3**:227.

Kunkel DB et al: Reptile envenomations. *J Toxicol Clin Toxicol* 1983;**21**:503.

Otten EJ: Antivenin therapy in the emergency department. *Am J Emerg Med* 1983;**1**:82.

Otten EJ, McKimm D: Venomous snakebite in patient allergic to horse serum. *Ann Emerg Med* 1983;**12**:624.

Warrell DA et al: Severe neurotoxic envenoming by the Malayan krait *Bungarus candidus*. *Br Med J* 1983;**286**:678.

BLACK WIDOW SPIDER

The black widow spider *(Latrodectus mactans)*, also called "hourglass" spider, may be found throughout the USA and even in Canada but is most numerous in the warmer areas. Other members of the *Latrodectus* genus are common throughout the temperate and tropical zones. These spiders inhabit woodpiles, outhouses, brush piles, and dark corners of barns, garages, and houses. Only the female is dangerous. It is jet black with a globular abdomen that is ordinarily marked with orange or red spots in the shape of an hourglass.

The toxicity of the venom is probably greater than that of the snake venoms, but the spider injects only a minute amount of poison. The bite is ordinarily only dangerous to life in children weighing less than 15 kg. The venom of the black widow spider causes various neurologic effects that have not been completely elucidated. The pathologic findings are not characteristic.

The number of bites is about 500 per year, but the fatality rate is below 1% of those bitten.

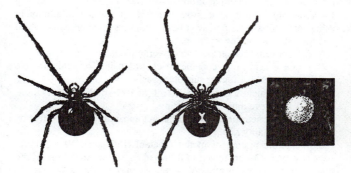

Figure 34–1. Black widow spider *(Latrodectus mactans)*. (Life size.) *Left:* Dorsal view. *Center:* Ventral view. *Right:* Egg sac.

Clinical Findings

The principal manifestation of black widow spider bite is immediate muscle spasm. Symptoms and signs consist of slight pain, blanching, and swelling at the site of the bite, progressing rapidly to pain in the chest, abdomen, and joints and to nausea, salivation, and sweating. Breathing later becomes labored, and muscular pain, tightness, and cramping extend throughout the body. The abdominal, chest, or back muscles are rigid, and the patient, in contrast to patients with acute abdominal emergencies, is extremely restless. Recovery begins after 12–24 hours and is complete within a week.

Prevention

Prevention depends on the destruction of black widow spiders wherever found. The bottoms of outdoor privy seats should be sprayed with creosote every 3 months to repel the spiders. Rubbish and wood-piles should not be moved without the wearing of gloves and a heavy shirt buttoned at the wrists.

Shoes, wearing apparel, and sleeping accommodations should be inspected for black widow spiders prior to use.

Treatment

A. Emergency Treatment:

1. Enforce complete rest. Establish airway and maintain respiration.

2. Apply cold packs to the bite for several hours.

3. For funnel-web spider bite, apply an arterial tourniquet until a medical facility can be reached.

B. Antidote: Give antiserum (see p 488), 1–2.5 mL diluted in 50 mL of 5% dextrose in saline intravenously over 15 minutes after testing for sensitivity. To test for sensitivity, inject 0.1 mL of 1:10 dilution in saline intradermally. A positive reaction consists of an urticarial wheal surrounded by a zone of erythema.

C. General Measures: Avoid overtreatment.

1. Give aspirin or codeine to control pain. In children, give codeine phosphate, 1 mg/kg subcutaneously.

2. Give calcium gluconate, 10 mL of 10% solution slowly intravenously to relieve muscular cramping.

3. Cortisone relieves symptoms but apparently has no effect on the overall mortality rate.

4. Administration of methocarbamol (Robaxin), 10 mL intravenously over a 5-minute period followed by 10 mL in 250 mL of 5% glucose over 2 hours, is reported to relieve muscle spasms.

5. For funnel-web spider bite, atropine and diazepam are effective.

Prognosis

Death from spider bite in previously well individuals is unlikely. Recovery is usually complete within a week.

BROWN RECLUSE SPIDER
(Violin Spider)

The brown recluse spider *(Loxosceles reclusa),* found in 25 states ranging from Hawaii to New Jersey and Texas to Illinois, has caused more than 10 deaths. It is light yellow to medium dark brown with a darker brown violin-shaped patch on the back. The body is $\frac{3}{8}$–$\frac{1}{2}$ inch long, $\frac{1}{4}$ inch wide, and $\frac{3}{4}$–1 inch toe-to-toe. It is found in dark, undisturbed places. The female is more dangerous than the male.

The venom causes necrosis by activating the clotting mechanism to form microthrombotic aggregates that plug arterioles and venules.

Clinical Findings

The principal manifestation of recluse spider bite is cutaneous necrosis.

The bite is initially painless, with pain developing in 2–8 hours, followed by blisters, redness, swelling, bleeding, or ulceration. The untreated lesion increases in size for up to a week. Systemic symptoms and signs include cyanosis, hemoglobinuria, fever, chills, malaise, weakness, nausea and vomiting, joint pain, skin rash, and delirium. The onset of intravascular hemolysis can be detected early by determining hemoglobin and hematocrit every 6 hours for the first 48 hours.

Prevention

Wear gloves when investigating secluded areas, and carefully examine clothing that has been stored before use.

Treatment

The treatment is controversial. The use of maximum doses of systemic or local adrenocortical steroids, local phentolamine, excision, and exchange transfusion have all been recommended. Most bites resolve without treatment. Skin grafts are rarely necessary. Treat hemolytic reaction (see p 80).

Prognosis

Healing of necrotic areas may require 6–8 weeks. Death ordinarily occurs in the first 48 hours.

Table 34—1. Diagnosis and treatment of poisoning from other spiders.

Scientific and Common Name	Range	Clinical Findings	Treatment
Loxosceles laeta (brown spider)	South America	Cutaneous necrosis, jaundice, hemoglobinuria.	Specific antiserum.
Glyptocranium gasteracanthoides (pruning spider)	Peru	See *Latrodectus mactans*, p 484.	See p 484.
Atrax robustus (funnel-web spider)	Australia	Erythema, chills, collapse, cholinergic crisis.	See p 484.
Phoneutria fera (tarantula spider)	Brazil	See *L mactans*, p 484.	Give antiserum.
Lycosa erythrognata (tarantula spider), *Lycosa raptoria*	Brazil	See *L mactans*, p 484.	Give antiserum.
Ctenus nigriventer	Brazil	Necrosis, muscular cramps, respiratory failure.	Give antiserum.

SCORPIONS

Poisonous scorpions of the USA (*Centruroides gertschii* and *Centruroides sculpturatus*) live mainly in the arid Southwest. In Brazil, the poisonous species are *Tityus bahiensis* and *Tityus serrulatus*. In North Africa the poisonous scorpions are *Androctonus australis* and related species, *Buthus occitonus*, and *Buthacus arenicola*.

In areas inhabited by both poisonous scorpions and poisonous snakes, the mortality rate from scorpions may be higher because they live around homes and bites are more common. Scorpion venoms cause local, central nervous system, and cardiac effects.

Approximately 1000 stings in adults and children occur yearly in the southwestern USA, with about one fatality per year. Most of the deaths occur in children under 6 years of age. Reliable data on the incidence of stings are not available for other areas.

Clinical Findings

Local evidence of a sting is sometimes minimal or absent. The usual symptoms are a mild tingling or burning at the site of the sting, which may progress up the extremity. In severe cases, spasm in the throat, a feeling of thick tongue, restlessness, muscular fibrillation, abdominal cramps, convulsions, incontinence, hypertension, hypotension, oliguria, cardiac arrhythmias, pulmonary edema, and respiratory failure occur. Although the duration of symptoms is ordinarily 24—48 hours, neurologic manifestations may persist for up to 1 week. Laboratory tests are noncontributory.

Prevention

Specific antiserum should be available for immediate use in in-

Table 34–2. Diagnosis and treatment of poisoning
due to other insects and arachnids.

Name	Range	Clinical Findings	Treatment
Ticks: *Amblyomma americanum* *Dermacentor* species *Ixodidae* species	Southern and western USA, British Columbia, South Africa, Australia, Europe	Ataxia, weakness, paralysis coming on 12–24 hours after attachment of the tick. Respiratory failure may occur.	Remove the tick by applying kerosene or ether, by gentle traction with forceps, or by surgical excision. Apply moist heat.
Ticks: *Ornithodoros* species	Western USA	Severe pain and swelling, persisting for 1–2 weeks.	
Bee, wasp, yellow jacket	Worldwide	Single or multiple stings may cause severe fall of blood pressure, difficult breathing, collapse, peripheral neuritis, and hemoglobinuria. A sensitivity reaction may cause severe collapse, bronchial constriction, edema of the face and lips, and itching. Death may occur within 1 hour.	Epinephrine, 0.2–0.5 mL of 1:1000 subcut or IV. Give diphenhydramine, 50 mg subcut or IV, cautiously. Give hydrocortisone IV for severe collapse. Sensitive persons should carry treatment kits. Venom desensitization is possible.
Epyris californicus (wasp)	California	Numbness, itching, diarrhea, wheezing, prostration, sweating, drowsiness, with recovery in 30 minutes. See above under bee, wasp, and yellow jacket.	
Caterpillars	Worldwide	Redness, swelling, intense local pain, vomiting, shock, and sometimes convulsions from skin contact.	Give meperidine or diphenhydramine IM or calcium gluconate IV. Hydrocortisone may be useful.
Millipedes	Worldwide	Vesicular dermatitis with intense itching and burning lasting for 1–24 hours from skin contact.	Relieve itching by cold applications.
Scolopendra subspinipes (centipede)	Worldwide	Pain, redness, swelling.	Cold applications.
Solenopsis saevissima (fireant)	North and South America	Pain, swelling, edema, bullae.	Steroids may be useful.

fested areas. Spaces under houses and boardwalks should be tightly enclosed and sprayed regularly with creosote or other insecticides. Rubbish should not be left scattered where children play. Area treatment with insecticides is apparently ineffective in reducing the number of scorpions for more than a short time.

Treatment
A. Emergency Measures:
1. Immobilize the patient and the bitten part immediately. Apply a constriction band, as after snakebite (see p 473), to limit absorption of venom.

2. Give artificial respiration with O_2 if respiration is depressed.

3. Apply cold packs (10–15 °C) for the first few hours to help slow absorption.

B. Antidote: Inject specific scorpion antiserum (see below).

C. General Measures:
1. Control convulsions (see p 52). Diazepam may be useful.

2. Inject calcium gluconate, 10 mL of 10% solution slowly intravenously, to help relieve muscular cramps.

3. Inject a local anesthetic into the area of the bite to relieve pain unless the bite is on a digit.

4. Opiate analgesics may cause respiratory depression or potentiate postictal depression.

Prognosis
Fatalities are rare except in children under 6 years of age.

Rapid progression of symptoms in the first 2–4 hours after a sting indicates a poor outcome. Survival for 48 hours is ordinarily followed by recovery, although deaths have occurred 4 days after stinging.

ANTISERA AVAILABLE FOR SPIDERS & SCORPIONS

Algeria. Institut Pasteur d'Algerie, Alger.
    Serum Antiscorpionique. *Androctonus australis.*

Australia. Department of Health, Commonwealth Serum Laboratories, Melbourne, Victoria.
    Red-back Spider Antivenene. *Latrodectus hasseltii.*
    Sea Wasp Antivenene.
    Tick Antivenene. *Ixodes halocyclus.*

Brazil. Instituto Butantan, Caixa Postal 65, São Paulo.
    Serum Anti-aracnidico Polivalente. *Ctenus nigriventer, Lycosa raptoria, Tityus bahiensis, Tityus serrulatus.*

Serum Anti-escorpionico. *Tityus bahiensis, Tityus serrulatus.*
Serum Anti-loxoscelico. *Loxosceles* species.

Egypt. Serum and Vaccine Institute, Agouzam, Cairo.
   Anti-Scorpion Serum. Scorpions of North Africa.

Mexico. Laboratorios MYN, S.A., Av. Coyoacan 1707, Mexico 12,
      DF.
   Los Sueros Anti-alacran. *Centruroides suffusus suffusus, Centruroides noxius, Centruroides limpidus limpidus, Centruroides limpidus tecumanus, Centruroides limpidus infamatus, Centruroides sculpturatus.*

South Africa. The South African Institute for Medical Research, Hospital Street, Johannesburg.
   Scorpion Antivenom. *Parabuthus* species.
   Spider Antivenom. *Latrodectus* species.

Turkey. "Refik Saydam," Central Institute of Hygiene, Ankara.
   Scorpion Antiserum. *Prionurus crassicauda ol.*

USA. Antivenin Production Laboratory, Arizona State University,
      Tempe, AZ 85281.
   Scorpion Antivenin. *Centruroides sculpturatus.*

USA. Merck Sharp & Dohme, West Point, PA 19486.
   Antivenin *Latrodectus mactans.* Black widow spiders of North America.

Yugoslavia. Serum and Vaccine Institute, Rockefellerova 2, Zagreb.
   Serum Antilatrodectus Tredecimguttatus. *Latrodectus tredecimguttatus.*

References

Arthropods

Amitai Y et al: Scorpion sting in children: A review of 51 cases. *Clin Pediatr* 1985;**24**:136.

Curry SC et al: Envenomation by the scorpion *Centruroides sculpturatus*. *J Toxicol Clin Toxicol* 1983;**21**:417.

Ginsburg CM: Fire ant envenomation in children. *Pediatrics* 1984;**73**:689.

King LE Jr, Rees RS: Dapsone treatment of a brown recluse bite. *JAMA* 1983;**250**:648.

Rauber A: Black widow spider bites. *J Toxicol Clin Toxicol* 1983;**21**:473.

Ryan PJ: Preliminary report: Experience with the use of dantrolene sodium in the treatment of bites by the black widow spider, *Latrodectus hesperus*. *J Toxicol Clin Toxicol* 1983;**21**:487.

Wasserman GS, Anderson PC: Loxoscelism and necrotic arachnidism. *J Toxicol Clin Toxicol* 1983;**21**:451.

Hymenoptera

Green VA, Siegel CJ: Bites and stings of hymenoptera, caterpillar, and beetle. *J Toxicol Clin Toxicol* 1983;**21**:491.

SHELLFISH

Mussels, clams, oysters, and other shellfish growing in many marine locations become poisonous during the warm months (May to October) from feeding on certain dinoflagellates, including *Gonyaulax catenella*. One mussel, clam, or oyster may contain a fatal dose of poison. More than 10 deaths have been reported in the literature in the USA from this type of poisoning.

The poisonous principle contained in shellfish is a nitrogenous compound that produces a curarelike muscular paralysis. The pathologic findings in deaths from shellfish poisoning are not characteristic.

Clinical Findings

The principal manifestation of shellfish poisoning is respiratory paralysis.

After ingestion of poisonous shellfish, numbness and tingling of lips, tongue, face, and extremities occur and nausea and vomiting follow, progressing to respiratory paralysis. Convulsions may or may not occur.

Prevention

Do not eat fresh shellfish during the summer months (May to October). Check with local health department.

Treatment

Remove ingested shellfish by gastric lavage or emesis (see pp 21–28). Tracheal intubation and assisted ventilation with O_2 may be necessary if respiration is impaired.

Prognosis

The fatality rate is 1–10%. If the patient survives for 12 hours, recovery is likely.

FISH

The flesh of a number of fish found in tropical waters may be poisonous at certain times of the year. They apparently become poisonous by feeding on certain marine organisms. Some fish, such as puffers (family *Tetraodontidae*), triggerfish, and parrot fish, are poisonous during most of the year. Others, such as the moray eel, surgeon fish, moon fish, porcupine fish, filefish, and goatfish, are poisonous only a part of the year in some localities. The most common type of fish poisoning, known as ciguatera, occurs with fish that are ordinarily considered edible (grouper, surgeon fish, barracuda, pompano, mackerel, butterfly fish, snapper, sea bass, perch, wrasse, etc) but become sporadically poisonous in certain localities. Scombroid fish poisoning occurs after consumption of improperly prepared tuna and other scombroidei; it is due to growth of surface organisms in fish stored at ambient temperatures. Some of the toxic effects from scombroid fish poisoning may be the result of liberation of histaminelike amines during bacterial decomposition.

More than 300 species have been reported to cause outbreaks of fish poisoning. The puffer family seems to have the most potent toxin; the mortality rate may be as high as 50%. In other types of fish poisoning, the mortality rate ranges from less than 1% to as high as 10% depending on the physical condition of the individual, the amount of fish eaten, and the potency of the toxin. The incidence of poisoning may be as high as 5–50% of the population in tropical countries where fish forms a large part of the diet. In Hawaii, 50–100 cases are reported yearly, with a mortality rate of less than 1%.

The poison present in the flesh or viscera of the fish apparently exerts its primary effect on the peripheral nervous system, but the physiologic mechanism is as yet unknown. The pathologic findings are not characteristic.

Clinical Findings

The principal manifestations of ciguatera are vomiting and muscular paralysis. Scombroid poisoning causes vomiting.

A. Ciguatera: Symptoms of acute poisoning begin 30 minutes to 4 hours after ingestion and include numbness and tingling of the face and lips that spreads to fingers and toes. This is followed by nausea and vomiting, diarrhea, malaise, dizziness, abdominal pain, and muscular weakness. In severe poisoning, these symptoms progress to foaming at the mouth, muscular paralysis, dyspnea, or convulsions. Death may occur from convulsions or respiratory arrest within 1–24 hours. If the patient recovers from the immediate symptoms, muscular weakness and paresthesias of the face, lips, and mouth may persist for weeks. These paresthesias characteristically consist of reversed temperature sensations; thus, cold food or other cold objects cause a searing pain or an "electric shock" sensation, and hot things feel cold. Laboratory findings are not contributory.

B. Scombroid Poisoning: Symptoms include nausea and vomit-

Table 35–1. Venomous fish.

Name	Clinical Findings	Treatment
Sting-ray (*Urobatis halleri* and others)	Penetration of the skin by the barb in the tail of the sting-ray causes intense local pain, swelling, nausea and vomiting, abdominal pain, dizziness, weakness, generalized cramps, sweating, fall of blood pressure. Recovery occurs in 24–48 hours. Fatalities have occurred when the barb has penetrated the chest or abdomen.	1. Cleanse wound by irrigation and remove foreign material. 2. Soak wound in hot water (45–60 °C) for 30–60 minutes. 3. Surgically debride and close wound.
Scorpion fish (*Scorpaena guttata*)	Spines of the gill covers may penetrate skin and cause severe local pain and swelling, with extension of pain and swelling to involve the entire extremity.	1. Treat as for sting-ray. 2. For pain, give meperidine, 50–100 mg subcut.
Jellyfish or Portuguese Man-of-war (*Physalia* species)	Contact with these jellyfish causes urticarial wheals, numbness and pain of the extremities, severe chest and abdominal pain, abdominal rigidity, and dysphagia. Deaths are rare.	Inject 10 mL of 10% calcium gluconate IV to relieve muscular cramps. Apply aromatic spirits of ammonia in compress to remove the venom.
Jellyfish or sea wasp (*Chironex fleckeri*, *Chiropsalmus quadrigatus*)	Wheals, extreme pain, skin necrosis, respiratory and cardiac depression. Death occurs in minutes.	Apply occlusive tourniquet immediately. Give antiserum.*
Stonefish (*Synanceja trachynis*, *Synanceja horrida*)	Intense radiating pain with blanching, then cyanosis of the affected part, nausea and vomiting, fever, delirium, respiratory distress, and convulsions.	Treat as above for sting-ray and scorpion fish. Give specific antiserum.*

*Stonefish Antivenene *(Synanceja trachynis)*. Sea wasp Antivenene. Department of Health, Commonwealth Serum Laboratories, Melbourne, Victoria, Australia.

ing, cramps, diarrhea, facial flushing, headache, and burning in the mouth.

Prevention

Adequate prophylactic measures have not been developed, since some tropical fish that are considered edible may sometimes be poisonous. The following fish found in tropical waters should never be eaten: puffers, trunk or box fish, triggerfish, thorn fish, filefish, parrot fish, and porcupine fish. Scombroid fish should be refrigerated immediately after being caught.

Treatment

A. Emergency Measures: Remove the ingested fish by gastric lavage or emesis (see pp 21–28). Maintain adequate airway. Treat respiratory failure (see p 60).

B. General Measures: Treat convulsions (see p 52). Treat shock (see p 66). Administration of antihistamines is reported to relieve at least some of the symptoms from scombroid fish poisoning.

Prognosis

Mortality rates may vary from less than 1% to more than 50%. The lower rate may be expected when the fish is known to be a common type of edible fish.

References

Annual mussel quarantine—California, 1983. *MMWR* 1983;**32**:281.

Dickinson G: Scombroid fish poisoning syndrome. *Ann Emerg Med* 1982;**11**:487.

Engleberg NC et al: Ciguatera fish poisoning: A major common-source outbreak in the U.S. Virgin Islands. *Ann Intern Med* 1983;**98**:336.

Gonzaga RAF: Venomous fish stings on the European seashore. *Postgrad Med* (April) 1985;**77**:146.

Kizer KW: Marine envenomations. *J Toxicol Clin Toxicol* 1983;**21**:527.

Puffers, gourmands, and zombification. (Editorial.) *Lancet* 1984;**1**:1220.

AKEE

The unopened unripe fruit and the cotyledons of the tropical akee *(Blighia sapida)* are poisonous. In Cuba and Jamaica, up to 50 cases of poisoning (with some deaths) occur yearly. Approximately 85% of these cases of poisoning are in children. Poisoning has not been reported from Florida, where the akee is also grown. One unripe fruit contains a lethal dose of the poison, which is soluble in boiling water.

The toxic effects produced by akee are as yet poorly understood. The pathologic findings in the brain are congestion and hemorrhages in the subarachnoid space and parenchyma. The lungs show congestion and serous exudate. The liver and kidneys reveal marked fatty degeneration; less marked degenerative changes are seen in the heart and brain.

Clinical Findings

The principal manifestations of akee poisoning are vomiting, circulatory collapse, and hypoglycemia.

A. Symptoms and Signs: (From ingestion.) Nausea, vomiting, and abdominal discomfort usually begin within 2 hours after ingestion. The patient recovers from this attack and is free of symptoms for 2–6 hours. Vomiting or retching may then return, followed shortly by convulsions, coma, hypothermia, hypoglycemia, and fall of blood pressure. In fatal cases, death occurs within 24 hours after ingestion of the fruit.

B. Laboratory Findings:

1. The blood chloride is increased and the blood glucose low.

2. The red and white blood cell counts are decreased.

3. Hepatic cell function may be impaired as revealed by appropriate tests (see p 75).

Prevention

Only fully opened fruit should be picked. Fallen, unripe fruit should be burned to prevent children from eating it. The fruit capsule and seeds are both toxic.

If fruit is cooked, the water should be discarded and not used for further cooking.

Treatment

A. Emergency Measures: Remove the poison by gastric lavage or emesis (see pp 21–28).

B. Antidote: None is known. Alcohol was at one time thought to be a useful antidote, but experiments indicate that it is not effective.

C. General Measures: Control convulsions (see p 52). Give carbohydrates as 5% glucose intravenously or as sugar dissolved in fruit juice orally to protect the liver and maintain blood sugar. Treat uremia (see p 72).

Prognosis

Recovery is rare after the onset of convulsions or coma. Patients having only the primary attack of vomiting recovery completely in a few days.

CASTOR BEAN & JEQUIRITY BEAN

The castor bean plant *(Ricinus communis)* is grown for commercial and ornamental purposes. The residue or pomace after castor oil extraction of castor beans gives rise to dust that may cause sensitivity reactions or poisoning.

Jequirity (rosary bean, love beads, *Abrus precatorius*) is grown as an ornamental vine in tropical climates. The beans are 6 mm long and are bright orange with one black end. They are used as rosary beads and as decorations for costumes.

Ingestion of only one castor bean or jequirity bean has apparently caused fatal poisoning when the bean was thoroughly chewed. If the beans are swallowed whole, poisoning is unlikely because the hard seed coat prevents rapid absorption. In a recent report, no toxicity was found in 3 cases of castor bean ingestion.

Ricin, a toxic albumin found in castor beans, and abrin, a similar albumin found in jequirity beans, cause agglutination and hemolysis of red blood cells at extreme dilutions (1:1,000,000). They are also injurious to all other cells and are heat-labile.

The pathologic findings in fatal cases of castor bean or jequirity bean poisoning include hemorrhage and edema of the gastrointestinal tract, hemolysis, and degenerative changes in the kidneys.

Clinical Findings

The principal manifestations of poisoning with these beans are vomiting, diarrhea, and circulatory collapse.

A. Acute Poisoning: (From ingestion.) After 2 hours to several days, burning of the mouth, nausea and vomiting, diarrhea, abdominal pain, drowsiness, disorientation, cyanosis, stupor, circulatory collapse, retinal hemorrhage, hematuria, convulsions, and oliguria may begin and progress to death in uremia up to 12 days after poisoning. The vomitus and stools may contain blood.

B. Chronic Poisoning: (From inhalation of dust from castor bean pomace.) Dermatitis and inflammation of the nose, throat, and eyes. Instances of asthmatic attacks have also been reported from exposure to the dust.

C. Laboratory Findings: The urine may contain protein, casts, red blood cells, and hemoglobin. The blood may show an increase in blood urea nitrogen and nonprotein nitrogen.

Prevention

Children should not be allowed access to castor beans or jequirity beans. Dust from handling castor bean pomace should be controlled by proper air exhaust.

Treatment

A. Acute Poisoning:

1. Emergency measures–Remove ingested beans by gastric lavage or emesis (see pp 21–28). Catharsis is also useful. Maintain circulation by blood transfusions (see p 66).

2. General measures–Alkalinize the urine by giving 5–15 g of sodium bicarbonate daily to prevent precipitation of hemoglobin or hemoglobin products in the kidneys. Control convulsions with diazepam (see Table 4–3).

3. Special problems–Treat anuria (see p 72). For dehydration, maintain central venous pressure by giving fluids.

B. Chronic Poisoning: Remove from exposure.

Prognosis

The fatality rate is approximately 5%. Death may occur up to 14 days after poisoning.

Rauber A, Heard J: Castor bean toxicity: A new perspective. *Vet Hum Toxicol* 1985;**27**:498.

FAVA BEANS

Fava beans *(Vicia faba)*, or horse beans, are grown commercially for use as a food.

Severe reactions occur occasionally following ingestion of fava beans or inhalation of the pollen of growing plants.

At least 8 cases of favism have been reported in the USA. Deaths have not been reported in the USA but have occurred in Italy.

Table 36–1. Plants commonly involved in poisoning.*

Name	Poisonous Part of Plant, and Active Principle if Known	Clinical Findings	Treatment
Arum family: Calla lilly, elephant ear, jack-in-the-pulpit (*Dieffenbachia, Caladium, Alocasia, Colocasia, Philodendron, Arisaema triphyllum*)	All parts (oxalates and other toxins).	Severe irritation of mucous membranes, nausea and vomiting, diarrhea, salivation. Rare systemic effects.	Give demulcents: milk, oil, cooling drinks.
Oleander (*Nerium oleander*)	All parts (oleandrin).	Same as for digitalis, p 377.	As for digitalis (see p 378).
Pokeweed (*Phytolacca americana*)	All parts but especially root (saponins), glycoproteins.	Burning in the mouth and stomach, persistent vomiting and diarrhea, slowed respiration and weakness.	Remove ingested poison as outlined on pp 21–28.
Rhubarb (*Rheum* species)	Leafy part (oxalic acid).	Nausea, vomiting, diarrhea, abdominal pain, reduced urine formation, hemorrhages. See Oxalic acid, p 197.	Treat as for oxalic acid, p 198.
Solanaceae:			
Blue nightshade (*Solanum dulcamara*)	Leaves and fruit (solanine).	Abdominal pain, vomiting, diarrhea, mental and respiratory depression, hypothermia or fever, delirium, slow or fast pulse, shock.	Maintain respiration and circulation. Remove ingested poison as outlined on pp 21–28.
Black nightshade (*Solanum nigrum*)	Leaves and unripe berries (solanine).		
Jerusalem cherry (*Solanum pseudocapsicum*)	Leaves and unripe berries (solanine).		
Potato (*Solanum tuberosum*)	Green tubers, new sprouts (solanine).		
Yew (*Taxus*)	Wood, bark, leaves, seeds (taxine).	Nausea, vomiting, diarrhea, abdominal pain, dyspnea, dilated pupils, weakness, convulsions, shock, coma.	Remove ingested poison as outlined on pp 21–28.

*See also croton oil (*Croton tiglium*, p 437), deadly nightshade (*Atropa belladonna*, p 345), foxglove (*Digitalis purpurea, Digitalis lanata*, p 377). henbane (*Hyoscyamus niger*, p 345), jimsonweed (*Datura stramonium*, p 345), larkspur (*Delphinium* species, p 433), meadow saffron (*Colchicum autumnale*, p 460), monkshood (*Aconitum napellus, Aconitum columbianum*, p 433).

Fava beans induce agglutination and hemolysis in individuals who have a deficiency of the enzyme glucose-6-phosphate dehydrogenase. The pathologic findings are hemolysis and hemoglobin precipitation in the kidneys.

Clinical Findings

The principal manifestations of acute favism are jaundice and oliguria.

A. Symptoms and Signs: (From ingestion of beans or inhalation of pollen.) Fever, malaise, jaundice, dark urine, oliguria, pallor, enlargement of the spleen and liver beginning 1–2 days after ingesting the beans or 1–8 hours after inhaling the pollen from the plant.

B. Laboratory Findings: Anemia and increased serum bilirubin (see p 75). Nonprotein nitrogen may be increased if oliguria occurs. Hemoglobinuria may occur.

Prevention

In order to prevent development of sensitivity, fava beans should not be served as food to children under the age of 1 year.

Treatment

A. General Measures:

1. Give blood transfusions until anemia is corrected.

2. Alkalinize the urine with sodium bicarbonate, 2 g every 4 hours.

3. In the presence of normal renal function, maintain urine output by giving 2–4 L of fluid daily orally or intravenously.

4. Give hydrocortisone, 4–10 mg/h intravenously.

B. Special Problems: Treat anuria (see p 72).

Prognosis

Recovery is likely with adequate treatment.

HEMLOCK

The poisonous plants of the parsley family include poison hemlock *(Conium maculatum),* water hemlock *(Cicuta maculata* and other *Cicuta* species), and dog parsley *(Aethusa cynapium).*

Fatalities are reported at intervals of several years. A piece of *Cicuta maculata* 1 cm in diameter may produce fatal poisoning.

Cicuta species contain cicutoxin, a central nervous system stimulant like picrotoxin.

Conium maculatum and *Aethusa cynapium* contain a number of piperidine derivatives, including coniine, which cause peripheral mus-

Table 36-2. Additional poisonous plants.

Name	Poisonous Part of Plant, and Active Principle If Known	Clinical Findings	Treatment
Baneberry (*Actaea* species)	All parts.	Nausea, vomiting, diarrhea, shock.	*
Betelnut (*Areca catechu*)	Seed (arecoline).	Vomiting, diarrhea, difficult breathing, impaired vision, convulsions.	* . Give atropine, 2 mg subcut; repeat as necessary.
Bird of paradise (*Caesalpinia gilliesii, Poinciana* species)	Seed pod.	Nausea, vomiting, diarrhea.	* . Give milk, beaten eggs, liquid petrolatum; replace fluids.
Bleeding heart (*Dicentra* species)	All parts (alkaloids).	Ataxia, respiratory depression, convulsions.	*
Bloodroot (*Sanguinaria* species)	All parts (sanguinarine).	Vomiting, diarrhea, shock, coma.	*
Boxwood (*Buxus sempervirens*)	Leaves and twigs.	Nausea, vomiting, convulsions.	*
Buckeye, horse chestnut (*Aesculus* species)	Seed (a glycoside).	Nausea, vomiting, weakness, paralysis.	*
Burning bush (*Euonymus atropurpureus*), spindle tree (*Euonymus europaea*)	Fruit and leaves.	Nausea, vomiting, diarrhea, weakness, chills, coma, or convulsions.	*
Calabar bean (*Physostigma venenosum*)	Bean (physostigmine; see p 351).	Dizziness, faintness, vomiting, diarrhea, pinpoint pupils.	See p 352.
Celandine (*Chelidonium majus*)	All parts (chelidonine).	Nausea, vomiting, coma.	*
Cherry (*Prunus* species)	Seed, leaves (amygdalin).	Stupor, vocal cord paralysis, twitching, convulsions, and coma from chewing seeds. See cyanide poisoning (p 253).	* . Treat cyanide poisoning (see p 254).
Chinaberry (*Melia azedarach*)	Fruit and leaves.	Nausea, vomiting, diarrhea, paralysis.	*
Chrysanthemum	All parts (a resin).	Exudative dermatitis from sensitivity.	Wash skin.
Corn cockle (*Agrostemma githago*)	Seeds (githagin).	Nausea, vomiting, respiratory depression.	*

Crowfoot Family:		
Christmas rose (*Helleborus niger*)	All parts (helleborin and related alkaloids).	Severe gastrointestinal irritation with vomiting and diarrhea.	*
Crowfoot or buttercup (Ranunculaceae)	All parts.		
Marsh marigold (*Caltha palustris*)	All parts.		
Daffodil (*Narcissus pseudonarcissus*)	Bulb.	Nausea, vomiting, diarrhea.	*
Daphne	All parts.	Stomatitis, abdominal pain, vomiting, bloody diarrhea, weakness, convulsions, kidney damage.	
Elderberry (*Sambucus* species)	Leaves, shoots, bark, and roots (cyanogenic glycoside).	Dizziness, headache, nausea, vomiting, respiratory stimulation, tachycardia, convulsions.	*. Treat cyanide poisoning (see p 254).
Finger cherry (*Rhodomyrtus macrocarpa*)	Fruit.	Complete and permanent blindness within 24 hours.	*
Glory lily (*Gloriosa superba*)	All parts (gloriosine, colchicine).	Vomiting, diarrhea, fall of blood pressure, alopecia.	*. Maintain blood pressure, treat as for colchicine (see p 460).
Holly (*Ilex* species)	Berries.	Vomiting, diarrhea, narcosis.	*
Hyacinth	Bulb	Nausea, vomiting.	*
Hydrangea	All parts (possibly cyanogenic).	Gastroenteritis. Observe for cyanide symptoms.	*. Treat cyanide poisoning (see p 254).
Indian tobacco (*Lobelia inflata*)	All parts (α-lobeline).	Progressive vomiting, weakness, stupor, tremors, pinpoint pupils, unconsciousness (see Nicotine, p 131).	*. Give artificial respiration. Give atropine, 2 mg subcut.
Iris (Iridaceae)	Root.	Nausea, violent diarrhea, abdominal burning.	*
Jessamine (*Gelsemium sempervirens*)	All parts (gelsemine and related alkaloids).	Muscular weakness, convulsions, sweating, respiratory failure.	*. Give atropine, 2 mg subcut every 4 hours; artificial respiration.
Jetberry (*Rhodotypos scandens*)	Berries (cyanogenic glycoside).	Like cherry. See Cyanide, p 253.	See p 254.

*Remove ingested poison by activated charcoal, gastric lavage, or emesis (see pp 21–28). Treat symptoms.

Table 36–2 (cont'd). Additional poisonous plants.

Name	Poisonous Part of Plant, and Active Principle If Known	Clinical Findings	Treatment
Jute (*Corchorus olitorius, Corchorus capsularis*)	Fibrous stem.	Asthmatic attacks, rhinitis from sensitivity.	Avoid further exposure.
Laburnum, golden chain (*Laburnum anagyroides*), Kentucky coffee berry (*Gymnocladus dioica*)	Leaves, pod, and seeds (cytisine).	Burning in the mouth and abdomen, nausea, severe vomiting, diarrhea, prostration, irregular pulse and respiration, delirium, twitching, unconsciousness. Renal damage may occur.	*.
Lantana (*Lantana camara*)	All parts (lantanin).	Photosensitization with great increase in injury from sunlight.	Avoid sunlight.
	Green fruit.	Vomiting, lethargy, cyanosis, coma, dilated pupils, slowed respiration.	*. Administer O_2.
Laurel (*Kalmia* species)	All parts (andromedotoxin).	Salivation, increased tear formation, nasal discharge, vomiting, convulsions, slow pulse, low blood pressure, paralysis.	*. Treat as for veratrum (see p 509).
Lily-of-the-valley (*Convallaria* species)	All parts (digitalislike).	See Digitalis, p 377.	See p 378.
Locust (*Robinia pseudoacacia*)	Seed (robin).	Same as for castor bean, p 496.	Same as for castor bean, see p 497.
Lupin, lupine (*Lupinus* species)	All parts but especially in berries (lupinine and related alkaloids).	Paralysis, weak pulse, depressed breathing, convulsions.	*. Give artificial respiration, treat convulsions (see p 52).
Manchineel (*Hippomane mancinella*)	Sap.	Severe irritation, blistering, peeling of skin from contact with the sap.	Wash with soap and water or alcohol.
Mango (*Mangifera indica*)	Skin of fruit and sap of tree.	Dermatitis, nausea, vomiting, diarrhea.	Do not eat the peel, and avoid contact with the sap.
Mexican poppy (*Argemone mexicana*)	Leaves and seeds (alkaloids).	Vomiting, diarrhea, cardiac and visual effects.	*.

Plant	Toxic parts	Symptoms	Treatment
Mistletoe (*Phoradendron flavescens*)	All parts but especially in berries.	Vomiting, diarrhea, and slowed pulse similar to digitalis (see p 377).	Treat as for digitalis (see p 378).
Moonseed (*Menispermum canadense*)	Fruit (alkaloid).	Nausea, vomiting, mechanical injury.	*
Nutmeg (*Myristica fragrans*)	Seeds (myristicin).	Hallucinations, delirium, convulsions.	*
Physic nut (*Jatropha* species)	Seed.	Nausea, vomiting, bloody diarrhea, unconsciousness.	*
Poinsettia (*Euphorbia pulcherrima*)	Leaves, stems, sap.	Irritation, vesication, gastroenteritis.	* Wash sap from skin with soap and water.
Primrose (*Primula* species)	Stems and leaves (primin).	Skin reddening and irritation, itching, swelling, and blistering on contact with the plant.	Wash skin with rubbing alcohol after handling the plant.
Privet (*Ligustrum vulgare*)	Berries and leaves.	Gastrointestinal irritation and renal damage, fall of blood pressure.	* . Treat as for veratrum (see p 509).
Rayless goldenrod (*Aplopappus heterophyllus*), snakeroot (*Eupatorium rugosum*)	All parts (tremetol).	Drinking milk from animals that have been fed on white snakeroot or rayless goldenrod causes nausea, loss of appetite, weakness, severe vomiting, jaundice from liver damage, constipation, and convulsions. There may be oliguria or anuria from kidney damage.	Treat liver damage (see p 77); treat anuria (see p 72).
Rhododendron	All parts (andromedotoxin).	Salivation, increased tear formation, nasal discharge, vomiting, convulsions, slowing of the pulse, lowering of blood pressure, paralysis.	* . Treat as for veratrum (see p 509).
Sweet pea (*Lathyrus* species)	All parts but especially seeds.	Paralysis, weak pulse, depressed breathing, convulsions.	* . Give artificial respiration; treat convulsions (see p 52).
Tung nut (*Aleurites fordii*)	Seed (a sapotoxin).	Nausea, vomiting, abdominal pain, weakness, fall of blood pressure, shallow respiration.	*
Wisteria	All parts.	Gastric upset, vomiting.	*
Yellow oleander (*Thevetia* species)	All parts (digitalislike).	See Digitalis, p 377.	See p 378.

*Remove ingested poison by activated charcoal, gastric lavage, or emesis (see pp 21–28). Treat symptoms.

cular paralysis similar to that from curare. Nicotinelike ganglionic blockade also occurs.

The pathologic findings in *Cicuta* poisoning are similar to those from picrotoxin (see p 420). The pathologic findings in *Conium* poisoning are inflammation of the gastrointestinal tract with congestion of the abdominal organs.

Clinical Findings

The principal manifestations of hemlock poisoning are convulsions and respiratory failure.

A. Symptoms and Signs: (From ingestion.)

1. *Cicuta* species (eg, water hemlock) cause abdominal pain, nausea and vomiting, sweating, hematemesis, diarrhea, convulsions, cyanosis, and respiratory failure or cardiac arrest.

2. *Conium* (poison hemlock) and *Aethusa* (dog parsley) cause nausea and vomiting, salivation, fever, and gradually increasing muscular weakness followed by paralysis with respiratory failure.

B. Laboratory Findings: The urine may reveal temporary proteinuria.

Prevention

Children and adults should never eat unidentified wild plants.

Treatment

A. Emergency Measures: Remove poison by gastric lavage or emesis with activated charcoal (see p 21–28). Treat respiratory failure by artificial respiration with O_2. Prepare to treat cardiac arrest.

B. General Measures: Control convulsions (see p 52). Diazepam may be useful.

Prognosis

With early and adequate therapy, the death rate should be less than 10%.

MUSHROOMS

Poisonous mushrooms may grow wherever nonpoisonous mushrooms grow. The most dangerous species are *Amanita phalloides*, *Amanita verna*, *Amanita virosa*, *Gyromitra esculenta*, and the *Galerina* species.

Ingestion of part of one mushroom of a dangerous species may be sufficient to cause death. Over 100 fatalities occur each year from eating poisonous mushrooms.

Amanita muscaria contains, in variable amounts, an atropinelike alkaloid and a substance that causes narcosis, convulsions, and hallucinations. Some mushrooms contain the alkaloid muscarine, which produces the same effect as parasympathetic stimulation on smooth muscles and glands. Chronic poisoning does not occur.

Amanita phalloides contains the heat-stable polypeptides amanitin and phalloidin, which damage cells throughout the body. Liver, kidneys, brain, and heart are especially affected. Other mushrooms of the *Amanita* genus as well as of the genus *Galerina* may cause similar poisoning. The toxic principle is rapidly bound to tissues.

The pathologic finding in fatalities from mushroom poisoning is fatty degeneration in the liver, kidneys, heart, and skeletal muscles.

Clinical Findings

The principal manifestations of acute mushroom poisoning are vomiting, respiratory difficulty, and jaundice.

A. Symptoms and Signs: (From ingestion.)

1. Amanitin (amatoxin) type cyclopeptides *(Amanita phalloides, Amanita verna, Amanita virosa; Galerina autumnalis, Galerina marginata, Galerina venenata)*–After a latent interval of 6–24 hours, severe nausea and vomiting begin and progress variably to diarrhea, bloody vomitus and stools, painful tenderness and enlargement of the liver, oliguria or anuria, jaundice, pulmonary edema, headache, mental confusion and depression, hypoglycemia, and signs of cerebral injury with coma or convulsions. The fatality rate is about 50%.

2. Gyromitrin type (monomethylhydrazine) (*Gyromitra* and *Helvella* species)–Vomiting, diarrhea, convulsions, coma, hemolysis. The fatality rate is 15–40%.

3. Muscarine type (*Inocybe* and *Clitocybe* species)–Vomiting, diarrhea, bradycardia, hypotension, salivation, miosis, bronchospasm, lacrimation. Cardiac arrhythmias may occur. The fatality rate is 5%.

4. Anticholinergic type *(Amanita muscaria, Amanita pantherina, Amanita cokeri, Amanita crenulata, Amanita solitaria)*–This type causes a variety of symptoms that may be atropinelike, including excitement, delirium, salivation, wheezing, vomiting, diarrhea, slow pulse, dilated or constricted pupils, and muscular tremors, beginning 1–2 hours after ingestion. Fatalities are rare.

5. Gastrointestinal irritant type (*Boletus, Cantharellus, Clitocybe, Clorophyllum, Hebeloma, Lactarius, Lepiota, Naematoloma, Rhodophyllus, Russula,* and *Tricholoma* species)–Nausea, vomiting, diarrhea, cardiac arrhythmias, and malaise may last up to 1 week. Fatalities are rare.

6. Disulfiram type (*Coprinus* species)–Vomiting, diarrhea, cardiac arrhythmias, and disulfiramlike sensitivity to alcohol that may persist for several days. Fatalities are rare.

7. Hallucinogenic type (*Psilocybe* and *Panaeolus* spe-

cies)–Mydriasis, ataxia, weakness, disorientation, abdominal pain, fever, and convulsions. Fatalities are rare.

B. Laboratory Findings: Increase in creatinine and blood urea nitrogen. Effects on the liver are revealed by SGOT, SGPT, lactate dehydrogenase (LDH), and bilirubin levels. The blood sugar level should be monitored daily or oftener. After gyromitrin, the methemoglobin level may be increased.

Prevention

The frequent occurrence of mushroom poisoning indicates that any ingestion of wild mushrooms is hazardous and should probably be avoided.

Treatment

A. Emergency Measures: Remove ingested mushrooms by ipecac emesis unless the patient has already vomited. After emesis, give activated charcoal in 70% sorbitol to aid in the removal of any unabsorbed poison.

B. Antidote:

1. In amanitin type poisoning, thioctic acid has been suggested, but its use is controversial and not approved in the USA.

2. For mushrooms producing predominantly muscarinic-cholinergic symptoms, give atropine, 1 mg orally or subcutaneously.

3. For gyromitrin poisoning, give pyridoxine, 25 mg/kg intravenously.

4. For cardiac arrhythmias resulting from *Coprinus* or *Clitocybe* ingestion, propranolol may be useful. Avoid alcoholic beverages.

C. General Measures:

1. Careful control of fluid and electrolyte balance, with avoidance of hypoglycemia, must be continued for 5–10 days. In severely poisoned patients, liver function has been known to begin to return 6–8 days after exposure, followed by eventual complete recovery.

2. Repeated hemodialysis or charcoal hemoperfusion has been successful in bringing about complete recovery in cases of *Amanita phalloides* poisoning.

3. Large quantities of carbohydrate appear to help protect the liver from further damage. Give 5–10% dextrose, 4–5 L intravenously every 24 hours, if the urine output is adequate. Give vitamin K for bleeding.

4. As soon as fluids can be given by mouth, give fruit juices fortified by glucose, 120 g/L, up to 4–5 orally daily.

D. Special Problems:

1. Treat anuria (see p 72).

2. Control convulsions (see p 52).

3. Reduce fever by active cooling. Dialysis can be used as a rapid means of reducing body temperature.

4. Maintain respiration but avoid intubation unless necessary.

5. Forced diuresis to 3–6 mL/kg/h with furosemide, 0.25–1 mg/kg/h, is useful.

Prognosis

Approximately 50% of individuals poisoned by *Amanita phalloides* or other mushrooms that damage the liver and other internal organs will die. However, in the absence of injury to internal organs and with adequate atropinization, mushroom poisoning is not likely to be fatal.

Hanrahan JP, Gordon MA: Mushroom poisoning. *JAMA* 1984;**251**:1057.

Olson KR et al: *Amanita phalloides* type mushroom poisoning. *West J Med* 1982;**137**:282.

Vesconi S et al: Therapy of cytotoxic mushroom intoxication. *Crit Care Med* 1985;**13**:402.

Woodle ES et al: Orthotopic liver transplantation in a patient with *Amanita* poisoning. *JAMA* 1985;**253**:69.

POISON IVY (POISON OAK) & POISON SUMAC

Poison ivy *(Rhus radicans)*, poison oak *(Rhus toxicodendron, Rhus diversiloba)*, and poison sumac *(Rhus vernix)* are all related plants that grow widely in the USA.

Fatalities are rare, but at least 50% of those who handle *Rhus* species will have a severe dermatitis, and up to 10% will have temporarily disabling generalized effects.

Rhus toxicodendron and related species contain urushiol, which is a mixture of catechols that may be potent sensitizers, since repeated contact appears to increase the severity of the reaction. Renal irritation occurs after severe exposure. In deaths from poison ivy and related plants, the pathologic findings include renal and myocardial damage.

Clinical Findings

The principal manifestations of poisoning with these plants are vesiculation and generalized edema.

A. Acute Poisoning: (From contact, ingestion, or inhalation of smoke of burning plants.)

1. Local effects–These begin 12 hours to 7 days after contact and include itching, swelling, papulation, vesiculation, oozing, and crusting.

2. General effects–These include generalized edema, pharyngeal or laryngeal edema, oliguria, weakness, malaise, and fever.

B. Chronic Poisoning: Repeated exposure increases the severity of symptoms. Attempts to produce immunity by repeated exposure may lead to severe poisoning.

C. Laboratory Findings: The urine may contain protein, red blood cells, and casts. Blood examination may reveal a high nonprotein nitrogen level.

Prevention

Teach children to recognize and avoid the plants.

Wear heavy clothing and leather gloves if contact with *Rhus* species is unavoidable. The use of silicone base cream appears to give some protection. Avoid touching animals that have been in contact with *Rhus* species. Clean the skin thoroughly with strong soap and water immediately after contact.

Desensitization of hypersensitive individuals may be attempted with commercially available antigens. The use of alum-precipitated antigen is apparently completely ineffective. Do not ingest the plant in an attempt to achieve immunity.

Treatment

A. Emergency Measures: (Must be done within minutes to be effective.) Remove skin contamination by thorough washing with strong laundry soap and water. Remove ingested poison by gastric lavage or emesis followed by saline catharsis (see pp 21–28).

B. General Measures:

1. Treat the exudative stage by exposure to air or, if the irritation is severe, with mild wet dressings such as aluminum acetate, 1%, or potassium permanganate, 1:10,000.

2. In severe generalized reactions to poison ivy, systemic administration of cortisone or related steroids will relieve symptoms but will not shorten the course of the disease. The dosage of cortisone is 25–100 mg orally every 6 hours.

3. Give phenobarbital, 100 mg 3 times daily, to relieve anxiety.

4. Give starch or oatmeal baths to allay itching.

5. Give 2–4 L of fluids daily if urinary output is normal.

6. Launder or expose clothing to air and sunlight for 48 hours.

C. Special Problems: Treat anuria (see p 72).

Prognosis

Recovery is usually complete in 2–3 weeks.

VERATRUM & ZYGADENUS

False hellebore *(Veratrum alba, Veratrum viride,* or *Veratrum californicum)* is widely distributed in the northern temperate zone; the death camas *(Zygadenus venenosus)* grows in the northwest USA. Both are members of the lily family.

A number of cases of poisoning have been reported recently, but fatalities are rare. The fatal dose of the fresh plant may be as small as 1 g.

Veratrum and *Zygadenus* species contain nitrogenous compounds which slow the heart rate and lower blood pressure by a vagus reflex that originates in receptors in the heart and lungs. Larger doses raise the blood pressure by a direct effect on the vasomotor center in the brain.

Clinical Findings

The principal manifestations of poisoning with these plants are vomiting and fall of blood pressure.

A. Acute Poisoning: (From ingestion.) Nausea, severe vomiting, diarrhea, muscular weakness, visual disturbances, slow pulse (down to 30 or below), and low blood pressure (50 mm Hg systolic or less). With excessive amounts, the blood pressure may rise to 200 mm Hg or higher accompanied by a rapid, thready pulse. Use of veratrum alkaloids in high doses medicinally has caused myotonia, muscular spasms, and neuropathy.

B. Chronic Poisoning: Repeated ingestion of small doses may produce tolerance to the blood pressure lowering effect but apparently not to the blood pressure raising effect.

Prevention

Children should be warned to avoid eating strange plants.

Treatment

A. Acute Poisoning:

1. Emergency measures–Remove ingested poison by gastric lavage or emesis (see pp 21–28).

2. General measures–Atropine will block the reflex fall of blood pressure and the bradycardia. Give 0.5–2 mg intravenously; repeat every hour until symptoms are controlled. If hypertension is present, give sympathetic blocking agents, eg, phentolamine hydrochloride (Regitine), 5–10 mg intravenously, or hydralazine, 10–20 mg intramuscularly.

B. Chronic Poisoning: Discontinue the use of veratrum drugs.

Prognosis

If atropine can be given, recovery is likely.

References

Datura poisoning from hamburger—Canada. *MMWR* 1984;**33**:282.

Falconer IR, Beresford AM, Runnegar MT: Evidence of liver damage by toxin from a bloom of the blue-green alga, *Microcystis aeruginosa. Med J Aust* 1983;**1**:511.

Knutsen OH, Paszkowski P: New aspects in the treatment of water hemlock poisoning. *J Toxicol Clin Toxicol* 1984;**22**:157.

Ngindu A et al: Outbreak of acute hepatitis caused by aflatoxin poisoning in Kenya. *Lancet* 1982;**1**:1346.

Ueno Y: The toxicology of mycotoxins. *CRC Crit Rev Toxicol* 1985;**14**:99.

Index*

*Cross-references in the Index are sometimes to synonymous or chemically similar substances that cause the same toxic manifestations. Treat poisoning as for poisoning due to the substance referred to. For mixtures, the approximate concentration of active ingredient is given in square brackets.